KEEPING LIVESTOCK HEALTHY

FOURTH EDITION

N. BRUCE HAYNES, D.V.M.

Foreword by Robert F. Kahrs, D.V.M., Ph.D.

STOREY BOOKS

North Adams, Massachusetts

The mission of Storey Publishing
is to serve our customers by publishing practical information
that encourages personal independence in harmony with the environment.

Edited by Marie Salter
Art direction and cover design by Cindy McFarland
Text design and production by Susan Bernier
Illustrations on pages 68–69 by Elayne Sears
Indexed by Susan Olason/Indexes & Knowledge Maps

Printed in the United States by Versa Press

636.089
HAYN

10 9 8 7 6 5 4 3 2 1

3 2530 60562 3220

Library of Congress Cataloging-in-Publication Data

Haynes, N. Bruce, 1926–
    Keeping livestock healthy / by N. Bruce Haynes.— 4th ed.
        p.   cm.
    Includes index.
    ISBN 1-58017-421-3 (alk. paper) — ISBN 1-58017-435-3 (pbk. : alk. paper)
    1. Livestock—Diseases.   2. Livestock—Diseases—Prevention.   I. Title.
    SF751 .H39 2001
    636.089'—dc21
2001042889

Contents

Foreword

KEEPING LIVESTOCK HEALTHY, while easier said than done, is an essential prerequisite to effective animal husbandry. Although prompt, expert emergency diagnosis and treatment is often essential, health maintenance measures are far more cost effective than treating sick animals.

In the past century, veterinary medicine has been blessed with advanced diagnostic procedures, therapeutic measures, and preventive vaccines. At the same time, livestock rearing methods have become intensively automated, imposing confinement housing and other conditions that are conducive to disease and that create food-safety concerns. Consequently, veterinary medicine has evolved from emphasis on individual animal treatment to preventive medicine and herd-health programming. The latest movement is toward production animal medicine that addresses large integrated operations in which individual animals have minimal value.

Small family farms, often raising several species of animals, still survive as a way of life that emphasizes responsibility, respect for animal life, and preservation of rural ecosystems. Livestock farming promotes a work ethic essential for competitiveness in a global free-market economy and invaluable in all walks of life.

This book is an excellent source of understandable information for livestock owners and farmworkers, be they at home or in the employ of large corporate operations. It offers both concepts and specifics on how to keep cattle, horses, sheep, swine, and goats healthy, and how to take appropriate action, often seeking professional assistance, when they are not.

Readers are urged to peruse the first six chapters to appreciate the concepts of animal health and disease and to refer to later chapters for disease-specific information.

ROBERT F. KAHRS, D.V.M., PH.D.
Dean Emeritus, College of Veterinary Medicine
University of Missouri, Columbia

Preface

As I REFLECT ON MORE THAN HALF A CENTURY of association with the livestock industry and the veterinary profession, I am amazed at the changes and the progress that have occurred. Because of improvements in nutrition, housing, breeding, and disease prevention, an ever-dwindling number of livestock producers are able to provide high-quality food for an increasing domestic population and have enough left over to share with the world.

My colleagues in the veterinary profession can be justly proud of their contributions. In a relatively short span of time, they have helped bring about the advent of many antibiotics, eradication of hog cholera, almost total eradication of bovine tuberculosis and brucellosis, and development of vaccines for protection of livestock from a variety of potentially devastating diseases. We should also note the success of veterinarians in protecting U.S. livestock from serious foreign animal diseases, such as rinderpest, foot-and-mouth disease, African horse sickness, and African swine fever. No less important are the advances made in anesthesia and surgical techniques for the comfort and health of individual animals.

Clearly, great strides have been made in veterinary medicine, but changes in the profession are now occurring that have important implications for the livestock owner. Historically, veterinary medicine has been a combination of art and science. Because our patients cannot verbally communicate with us, we must have a thorough knowledge of their normal behavior and attitudes in order to recognize any departure from normal that might be induced by disease. We must also be aware of their nutritional and housing needs because these have a major effect on health. This knowledge is part of the art of veterinary medicine. The most successful veterinarians are those skilled in both art and science.

It wasn't many years ago that experience with farm animals was a prerequisite for graduation from veterinary college. This is no longer the case, and it is now possible, indeed probable, that some veterinarians graduate without ever having laid a hand on one of the so-called minor species — sheep and goats — not to mention exotic species such as llamas. For many reasons, the art of veterinary medicine is giving way to the science. This is not meant to imply that new veterinarians are incompetent. On the contrary, their technical training is superb, and they are familiar with techniques and equipment that students of my generation could only dream about. They have the ability to step into any laboratory or clinic setting and do a commendable job. And, although some may lack the animal experience required of their predecessors, they certainly have been taught the pathogenesis of animal diseases and methods of prevention or control.

It is this training and the employment opportunities it provides that contributes in part to what may prove to be a looming problem for the small livestock enterprise. For many reasons — among them working conditions, physical ability, technical challenge, and personal preference — the percentage of new veterinary graduates who enter livestock practice is declining steadily. If this trend continues it's quite possible that, except in geographic areas where livestock concentrations are adequate to support practitioners specializing in large-animal practice, it will be difficult to find veterinarians equipped to handle livestock problems.

With this eventuality in mind, it behooves the livestock owner to learn as much as possible about animal health from books such as this. Working cooperatively, a knowledgeable owner and a veterinarian can apply both the art and the science of veterinary medicine for the benefit of animals everywhere.

About This Book

Keeping Livestock Healthy, Fourth Edition, is based on my conviction — after almost fifty years' experience in private practice, as extension veterinarian at Cornell University, and as a veterinary consultant — that the great majority of farm animal disease problems are preventable. On economic grounds alone, any sick animal — no matter how effective the treatment or how speedy the recovery — represents a loss. A less tangible but certainly genuine argument for disease prevention concerns the pain and suffering disease causes.

Farm animals provide us with food, fiber, financial income, and pleasure. In return, we owe them comfortable quarters, adequate feed, compassion, *and* good health. Because the objective is to keep animals healthy, the reader will find that this is not a book on how to treat sick animals. Rather, it attempts to explain the nature of the disease process and outlines, in an understandable way, methods for preventing illnesses of the major farm animals. It by no means covers all the ailments our animals may encounter, focusing instead on those most likely to be seen in the average small herd or flock. If, by applying the information this book contains, the reader is empowered to keep his animals healthier, it will have served its intended purpose.

I would be remiss if I didn't apologize to my female colleagues in large-animal practice for my use of the pronoun *he* when referring to veterinarians in general. I hasten to assure them that it is not a reflection of male chauvinism but, rather, results from a personal aversion to the politically correct phrase *he or she.*

Last, this book is dedicated to my colleagues in the veterinary profession, past and present, whose collective talent and skill made it possible.

PART ONE

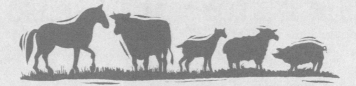

PREVENTING DISEASE

This first part of the book is devoted primarily to a discussion of the various factors that influence the health of farm animals. A good understanding of the disease process, from whatever cause, is essential for the implementation of measures to control or prevent it.

It's important to bear in mind that animals are complex, dynamic, biological individuals and that many factors influence their good health or lack thereof. Comprehension of these factors and their interactions, as described in the chapters that follow, will help the reader understand the logic behind some of the specific disease prevention recommendations in the book's second part, Animal Diseases. With a bit of extrapolation, the reader will also find that many discussions in this part apply to the health of the human animal as well.

The Nature of Disease

ALTHOUGH MOST PEOPLE tend to think of disease as the result of infection, this accounts for only part of the ills that come to humans and animals. Looked at in the broadest sense, *disease* is any condition that results in a departure from normal function. Certainly the infectious agents such as viruses and bacteria produce the most dramatic and contagious diseases resulting in epidemics in humans and epizootics in animals. But there are other important factors as well. Among these are heredity, nutrition, parasitism, accident and injury, and environmental stress. To this list, humans must be added as an indirect and occasionally direct cause of animal disease problems.

Microorganisms

The term *microorganisms* is applied to those living organisms that are microscopic in size. These may be unicellular, such as bacteria, yeasts, and protozoa; multicellular, such as molds; or without cellular structure, such as viruses. All have the capacity to reproduce at astonishing rates under favorable conditions, and some have a remarkable capacity for surviving adverse conditions. For example, the virus causing foot-and-mouth disease will survive boiling, and in the frozen state most viruses will last for years. Some bacteria, such as those causing anthrax, under adverse conditions enter a dormant phase called *sporulation.* Spores will exist in the soil for years, reverting to virulence when the opportunity arises. It has been reported that viable anthrax spores have been found in the tombs of the Egyptian pharaohs! Knowledge of the characteristics of potentially harmful microorganisms is important to the control of infectious diseases and will be discussed in later chapters with the specific animal disease they cause.

There are thousands of species of microorganisms in the world, and they are arbitrarily divided into two broad groups: the good guys, called *saprophytes,* and the bad guys, called *pathogens.* A few, depending on circumstances, will fit either category. We could do without the pathogens, but our survival depends on the saprophytes. All of the higher forms of life depend on the action of saprophytic organisms in the digestive tract for the utilization of conventional diets. Herbivorous animals, such as cows, are especially dependent on microorganisms for the conversion of cellulose in plants to usable forms of energy. Other organisms help to reduce complex protein molecules to their component parts, and themselves, as they die off, provide some nutritional value to the animals. The ability of ruminants such as the cow to utilize economical nonprotein nitrogen sources such as urea and biuret to meet part of their dietary protein need is dependent entirely on the action of microorganisms in the rumen.

Because saprophytic organisms in the digestive tract are essential to digestion, it's important in terms of animal health to maintain an environment conducive to their well-being. Radical changes in the cow's diet such as an abrupt shift to large amounts of grain will increase rumen acidity, unfavorable to some bacteria, resulting in indigestion. Oral administration of large amounts of antibiotics or smaller doses over a longer period will destroy many of the useful organisms in the digestive tract, causing diarrhea and other digestive upsets.

Clearly the saprophytes are important to our health, but they are important in other ways, too. For example, while we rarely think of it, without these beneficial organisms we wouldn't have sauerkraut, cheese, vinegar — or beer. Even worse, without them biodegradable waste would not disappear and our planet would be buried under a layer of refuse, sewage, and even leaves. So the next time someone mentions bacteria, don't throw up your hands in horror! Remember that in every society, even the one-celled variety, there are both good guys and bad guys, and we can't get along without the good ones. But we do have to contend with the bad guys, so let's look now at how the animal body copes with pathogens.

Disease Resistance

Most pathogens are parasitic in that they survive at the expense of their host. Many tend to have an affinity for certain tissues. For example, the viruses of rabies and equine encephalomyelitis prefer to attack the cells of the nervous system, as does the bacterium *Listeria monocytogenes,* which causes circling disease. *Streptococcus agalactiae* is rarely found outside the udder, whereas some species of staphylococci will invade tissues anywhere when circumstances are favorable. Some members of the mold family, such as *Trichophyton* species, prefer the skin, where they cause ringworm. Others, such as *Aspergillus* species, prefer the internal body surfaces, including as the lungs and reproductive tract. The list goes on and on.

Aside from tissue preference, pathogens also vary in their mode of action. Some will invade and destroy body cells. Others, such as *Clostridium tetani,* produce metabolic poisons, called *toxins,* that are harmful. Some molds never invade the body at all but produce toxins in feedstuffs, called *mycotoxins,* that are equally harmful when consumed by the animal. Last, pathogens vary in their affinity for some animal species. While this host specificity is not absolute, it is sometimes helpful in arriving at a diagnosis. For example, rabies can affect any animal, while eastern equine encephalomyelitis virus will be found only in horses, humans, and some birds. Therefore, that disease can be ruled out in a cow with evidence of central nervous system disease.

The first line of body defense against the invasion of pathogens is the skin and mucous membranes. Mucous membrane is the highly specialized epithelial tissue that lines body cavities that are exposed to the environment, such as the digestive and respiratory tracts. This tissue acts partly as a mechanical barrier to the invasion of bacteria, yeasts, viruses, and molds. But in addition, the mucous membranes contain cells that produce fluids that tend to wash away invaders. The respiratory tract epithelium, lining the trachea and bronchi, also is lined with cells that have hairlike projections called *cilia.* These move with rhythmic undulating regularity to help wash out bacteria and particulate matter. Because of the extremely small size of virus particles, this protective screen is much less effective in preventing viral infections. In fact, some viruses readily invade between the cells of the mucous membranes to produce disease.

If the integrity of this first line of defense is breached by cuts, abrasions, burns, and so on, infection may result. Note that *infection* and *disease* are not synonymous. *Infection* means only that the organism is in the body. Depending on a number of factors, infection may or may not produce disease, and, in fact, each of us and our animals carry a number of potential pathogens at any given time without any evidence of disease. This accounts for the epizootics that frequently occur when animals from a variety of sources are brought together, such as at fairs and shows. Unaffected carriers of a contagious infection will transmit the infection to all the others; disease may result if they are susceptible. Bringing your animals into contact with others, therefore, carries an element of risk that must be weighed against the potential benefits.

Let's use a cut in the skin as an example of how the primary bacterial defense mechanism works. At the moment skin integrity is destroyed, a chain of events is set in motion that determines whether or not disease will result. First, bleeding tends to wash out any bacteria that may have been carried into the wound. Concurrently, large numbers of specialized white blood cells called *phagocytes,* which have the capacity to engulf and destroy bacteria, appear at the site. If the invading force of bacteria is small, that's the end of it and healing occurs. If, however, the invading force is large, inflammation occurs with heat and swelling produced and some discharge of pus. *Pus* is an accumulation of dead bacteria and tissue cells. When pus accumulates in a closed wound, it is called an *abscess.* As a part of the defense mechanism, abscesses become walled off with connective tissue to prevent extension of the infection, and in some cases abscesses may persist for weeks or months after active infection has subsided. These are sometimes referred to as *sterile abscesses.*

In response to the need at the wound site, the healthy body rapidly will produce additional white blood cells, called *leukocytes,* and if the invaders get beyond the point of introduction, leukocytes will attack wherever needed. Thus, with active bacterial infection, there is almost always an increase in the white blood cell count, called *leukocytosis.* The opposite, *leukopenia,* is commonly seen with viral diseases. A white cell count is useful, therefore, in determining the presence of a bacterial infection and in distinguishing between a bacterial and a viral infection.

Under normal circumstances, this first line of defense is adequate to cope with most common infections. If it weren't, every cut and scratch would be the beginning of disaster. But failures do occasionally occur with serious results. The capacity of the body to produce leukocytes in response to need is reduced in the presence of malnutrition, during long-term disease, as a result of stress, when corticosteroid drugs have been recently used, in patients undergoing cancer chemotherapy, and as a result of a few specific diseases in humans such as acquired immunodeficiency syndrome (AIDS). Under these circumstances, invading bacteria are carried via the bloodstream to all parts of the body, a condition called *bacteremia* or *septicemia.* These migrating bacteria multiply rapidly, creating microabscesses wherever they may lodge. The kidney, liver, and brain are frequent sites of secondary infection, the serious implications of which are obvious. In this era of antibiotics, septicemic infection is not the catastrophe it once was, but it remains a serious concern that requires prompt and correct specific and supportive therapy.

Viral Infections

While the foregoing discussion is true of defense mechanisms against infection with bacteria, yeasts, and molds, it does not hold true for viral infections. Viruses are so small that they can slip through tissues with minimal disruption and tissue response. Viruses generally don't result in pus formation, and phagocytosis is not an important factor in defense against viral infections. In fact, an engulfed virus will often continue replicating in the phagocyte and actually be carried therein via the bloodstream to its preferred tissue site. Once at that site, it will begin destroying tissue cells or, in the case of tumor-inducing viruses, causing cell alteration. When viruses are circulating in the bloodstream, the condition is called *viremia.* It is during this phase, early in the disease, that an infected animal poses the greatest risk to others. The first evidence that viral infection has taken place may be fever, which in itself has some protective effect as far as defense is concerned. A body temperature rise of only a few degrees will make the body a less desirable place from the point of view of the virus. A prolonged fever, however, has detrimental effects on the body, such as dehydration, so it becomes a fine line in therapeutic judgment how long to let a fever continue and when to reduce it with the aid of drugs such as aspirin.

Immunity

Defense against viral infections relies heavily on a complex mechanism called *humoral immunity.* While humoral immunity may be considered a secondary, though important, defense against the larger pathogens such as bacteria, it is the primary defense against viral infections. It is highly selective in that immunity against one virus will not protect against another. There are a few minor exceptions to this rule that will be mentioned under specific diseases.

The science of immunology is developing rapidly, and new frontiers are being explored daily. It's not surprising, then, that new concepts are coming to light that help to explain the successes and failures of the immune system. In its simplest terms, immunity results when the body produces a protein *(antibody)* in response to stimulation by a foreign protein *(antigen). Pathogens* are foreign proteins. Antibody found in the globulin fraction of the blood *(humoral antibody)* combines physically or chemically with the antigen to inactivate it. In the normal animal, some immunity begins to develop whenever infection occurs. If the invading organism is low in virulence or present in small numbers, immunity develops fast enough that clinical disease doesn't occur or, if it does, recovery results. If all the defense mechanisms including immunity are overwhelmed, death usually results. Drugs, in part, are used to buy time for the animal to develop immunity by holding the infection in check and preventing secondary infections. Unfortunately, with few exceptions, drugs have virtually *no* effect against viruses. The exceptions include acyclovir and related compounds, drugs moderately effective against the herpes simplex virus responsible for cold sores and genital herpes in humans.

The primary sites of humoral antibody development are the liver, bone marrow, and, in the young animal, the thymus gland. Lymphoid tissue, such as tonsils and lymph nodes, plays a role that is less clear. Certain cells in other tissues respond to antigens by producing a general antiviral compound called *interferon,* which appears to block the entry of viruses into target cells. Interferon production is more rapid than humoral antibody, and it exerts its effect locally at the site of infection. Vaccines such as the intranasal vaccine for infectious bovine rhinotracheitis take advantage of this phenomenon. In general, however, it takes about two weeks for a protective level of antibody to be produced, in response to either infection or vaccination. For this reason, vaccination after a disease appears in a herd is usually of little value.

Types of Immunity

With this brief background of immunology we can take a look at immunization and immunizing agents. Basically there are two types of immunity: passive and active.

Passive Immunity

Passive immunity occurs without the active participation of the antibody production system of the immunized animal. For example, blood serum from an immune animal contains antibody that, when injected into another compatible animal, will make the latter immune. This is mechanical transfer of immunity in which the recipient plays no part; therefore, it is passive immunity. Because only antibody, not antigen, is transferred, however, the recipient's immune system is not stimulated and the recipient will be immune only as long as the transferred antibody lasts, which may be as short as 2 weeks or as long as 6 months. Passive immunity, although of short duration, has the advantage of being immediate. Unfortunately, antiserum or its antibody-containing fraction, gamma globulin, is not without risk and is expensive, precluding routine use in veterinary medicine.

In nature, passive immunity results from transfer of maternal antibody to the offspring via colostrum. *Colostrum,* or first milk, contains about twice the total solids of normal milk. Much of this excess is globulin, containing the same antibodies as found in the dam's blood. The developing fetus has a very limited capacity for antibody production, and, therefore, most animals are born with little or no immunity. If we stop to think how vulnerable the newborn is to infection and about the stress to which it is subjected at birth, it's not hard to imagine how important it is that newborns acquire some immunity as rapidly as possible. Nature has provided for this by equipping colostrum with high concentrations of antibody and at the same time providing a mechanism for the newborn to absorb antibody molecules intact.

Antibody is a complex protein that, when ingested by an adult, is broken down into its amino acid components prior to absorption. This digestive process destroys the usefulness of antibody as an immunizing agent. The newborn, however, has an undeveloped intestinal epithelium that permits absorption of intact antibody. But this capacity diminishes rapidly, being almost gone 24 hours after birth. It is vitally important, therefore, that the newborn animal receive colostrum as soon as possible after birth — even by hand-feeding if necessary. Once this specialized absorptive capacity disappears, colostrum has value primarily as a nutrient, although it continues to provide some local protection against diseases affecting the digestive tract. Surplus colostrum is valuable and should not be discarded. It can be stored in clean covered containers at room temperature for 7 to 10 days or frozen and stored for months while still retaining antibody content sufficient to protect other newborns if the need arises.

Active Immunity

Active immunity occurs when the animal itself produces antibody in response to antigen. It may be the result of infection and recovery or may result from deliberate exposure to antigen, as through vaccination. The duration of active immunity may range from several months to a lifetime depending on the stimulative effect *(antigenicity)* of the organism involved. Some organisms, notably those having limited local effect on the animal, are not strong antigens and attempts to produce vaccines to protect against them have not been very successful. Examples of these are the several species of bacteria causing mastitis in cattle. Conversely, some, such as the virus causing virus diarrhea in cattle, produce a strong immunity.

Passive/Active Immunity

We have talked about passive and active immunity. There is a situation in which both mechanisms come into play, complementing each other. When the dam develops active immunity in response to infection, she will pass that immunity on to her offspring via colostral antibody to produce a temporary passive immunity in the newborn. However, since her infection resulted from natural exposure, in many cases the pathogen will still be on the premises and will infect the newborn. While this infection usually will not result in disease due to the passive immunity the newborn animal has acquired, the constant exposure to the infectious agent will stimulate active antibody production to reinforce the colostral antibody, providing protection long after the passive immunity has disappeared.

From this one might conclude that the best time to vaccinate an animal for maximum protection would be during the period of passive immunity. Such is not the case, and frequency of exposure makes the difference. Vaccines (antigens) given once or even twice would be rapidly inactivated by the maternal antibody. On the other hand, natural exposure in our hypothetical illustration takes place daily. Thus, while the maternal antibody is gradually dissipating, repeated exposure to infection is stimulating active antibody production. It is possible in the laboratory to measure circulating antibody, the measurement being called *antibody titer*. Ideally, one should determine maternal antibody titer periodically in the young animal and vaccinate when it declines. Unfortunately, this is not an economical practice. In most cases, therefore, attempts to immunize permanently by vaccination should be postponed until most of the maternal antibody is gone, generally at about 6 months. An exception to this rule of thumb is the situation where the disease does not exist. For example, calves are vaccinated against brucellosis even though the herd may be free of infection, solely because many states require it as a prerequisite to interstate shipment. In this case, they should be vaccinated at the minimum legal age.

Immunization

Medical research has been able to capitalize on this immunity phenomenon by producing a variety of immunizing agents for protection against infectious diseases, and we are now able to protect humans and animals against the great majority of serious illnesses. Although all immunizing agents are commonly called *vaccines,* there are three basic types, each with important differences.

The first and simplest is *antiserum.* This is the serum component of whole blood that contains antibody. It is produced by hyperimmunizing animals, through either vaccination or actual infection, so that they produce a high level of antibody. Blood is then taken from them and refined, so that the finished product contains a high percentage of *globulin,* the protein fraction containing antibody. The resulting product has the advantage of producing immediate immunity when injected, but its duration is very short. It does not stimulate immunity in the animal to which it is given but merely passively transfers antibody to that animal. Antiserum is quite perishable, relatively expensive, and must be refrigerated until used. It is typically used in the specific species from which it was prepared. For example, bovine antiserum should not be given to a horse because it may produce a severe allergic response. There are times, however, when immediate protection is necessary, and antiserum is the best way to provide it.

Bacterins by definition are killed bacterial cultures. These are produced by growing bacteria in artificial media in the laboratory and then killing the bacteria with chemicals, ultraviolet light, irradiation, or gene modification. They represent a method of getting a specific bacterial protein (antigen) into the animal without risk of clinical disease. After the bacteria are destroyed, the culture is refined and then packaged for marketing as a single organism antigen, such as *Leptospira pomona* bacterin, or mixed bacterins prepared from cultures of more than one organism. The effectiveness of bacterins as immunizing agents is determined by the antigenicity of the organism, the number of killed organisms present in the product, the quality of its manufacture, and the addition of special adjuvants to delay absorption following injection. Bacterins are widely used to protect against leptospirosis, blackleg, malignant edema, swine erysipelas, and a variety of other diseases. Bacterin-induced immunity is usually of medium duration and rarely lasts more than 1 year. Two or more doses may have to be given to yield satisfactory protection.

Vaccines

Immunizing agents are commonly lumped together as *vaccines,* but the term technically is reserved for those products containing living antigen, although new technological advances have made this definition less accurate. One of the vaccines in veterinary medicine is the *Brucella abortus* strain 19 vaccine (and its current replacement, RB51), designed to protect cows against brucellosis. This vaccine is a living culture of a variant of *B. abortus*. The variant retains the antigenic identity of the naturally occurring organism but generally doesn't cause clinical disease, although there have been exceptions where it caused both systemic and local infection. Such exceptions are always a risk when living immunizing agents are used.

The most common vaccines used today are for protection against viral diseases in animals and humans. Viruses generally will not survive long except in living tissue. Therefore, the production procedures for viral vaccines differ significantly from those used for bacterins or bacterial vaccines. The virus must first be adapted to an unusual host cell and propagated through serial passage until it ultimately loses its virulence and capacity to produce disease, a process called *attenuation*.

The early viral vaccine work utilized living chick embryos as the unusual host. Since then, however, virologists have developed techniques of culturing living tissue cells in the laboratory, which has greatly simplified the production of viral vaccines. Tissues commonly used, for example, are kidney cells taken from swine or sometimes laboratory animals such as hamsters. The end result is safer products, better standardization, and greater antigenicity.

Spectacular advances in molecular biology in recent years have made it possible to incorporate only the immunogenic portion of some organisms in a vaccine. More effective *Escherichia coli* vaccines have been produced this way. In a few cases, where sufficient antigenic material cannot be produced by separating it from the pathogen, antigenic genetic material can be placed in other harmless organisms, a process called *gene cloning*. These organisms are then propagated in quantity to produce vaccine. Undoubtedly, even more exotic techniques will be devised to produce vaccines as time goes on.

Sometimes, because of the nature of the disease or for convenience, it is desirable to use a mixed vaccine. Bovine respiratory disease complex (BRDC) in cattle, for example, is caused by the interaction of viruses and bacteria, and a vaccine is available containing antigenic fractions of several viruses as well as the *Pasteurella* species responsible for the disease. Leptospira bacterin may contain fractions of one or several of the serovars of leptospira known to cause disease.

Although commercial mixed vaccines are available, remember that these have been tested and proved effective. Do not mix vaccines on the farm because, mixed together, they may be incompatible and rendered totally ineffective. If it is desirable to use two or more vaccines concurrently, keep them separate and use different injection sites.

The modified live-virus (MLV) vaccines have an important disadvantage: although they generally produce a long-lasting immunity, they occasionally will cause the illness because most are a compromise between antigenicity and attenuation. The most effective in producing immunity are those having the least attenuation. Thus, when they are given to an animal weakened by malnutrition or stress, or to those without a responsive immune mechanism, clinical disease may result. Their use should be restricted to healthy animals not under stress, and they should be given at a stage in life when economic effects will be minimized if the animal does get sick. Largely because of the risk associated with MLV vaccines, new vaccines utilizing inactivated virus have been developed. They produce immunity of shorter duration but are not as hazardous to use.

Generally the killed virus vaccines need to be given annually to maintain a protective antibody titer, whereas the MLV vaccines such as bovine virus diarrhea vaccine will produce immunity lasting several years.

Planned Infection

Planned infection with the actual or closely related disease organism is another technique for producing immunity. A disease such as infectious bronchitis in chickens, for example, exerts its principal effect economically by lowering egg production. This loss is averted by deliberately exposing young birds to the virus before they begin laying. This technique is almost universally applied by commercial poultry growers. It also has been demonstrated that hog cholera can be prevented by infecting swine with the virus causing bovine virus diarrhea. This virus does not produce apparent disease in swine but does exert a blocking effect against hog cholera virus. This method was never widely used, and with total eradication of hog cholera in the United States, the need for immunization has disappeared.

There is one obvious and important disadvantage in the planned infection approach to disease control that is best exemplified by a former use of rhinopneumonitis virus in horses. This virus causes a mild upper respiratory infection, but it also causes abortion, a matter of serious concern on breeding farms. To minimize abortions from this disease, all horses on the farm were deliberately infected at a time when risk of abortion was minimal, so mares had a good antibody titer during pregnancy. This practice resulted in wide dissemination of virus and precluded any possibility of eradicating the disease. Fortunately, this method of immunization against equine rhinopneumonitis fell out of favor.

Summary

We will talk more about immunization against specific diseases, but there are several important points to remember. The need to vaccinate depends on the prevalence of a disease, the risk of disease transmission, and the degree of risk one is willing to assume. A single animal kept in the backyard and never in contact with others of its species does not share the same risk as an animal in a large commercial herd to which new animals are frequently added. For the former, vaccination against contagious diseases is less important, but for the latter it would be essential.

Once a decision to vaccinate has been made, then you need to keep in mind that as a general rule, killed products do not produce as long an immunity as MLV vaccines, although killed products are safer to use.

In any case, bear in mind that vaccination and immunity are not synonymous. Vaccination is not a simple mechanical procedure that automatically produces immunity. Under the best of circumstances, no vaccine is 100 percent effective. Vaccines must be properly handled from point of manufacture to point of injection. Generally, this means refrigeration, protection from sunlight, and use prior to expiration date. Last, for maximum immune response, vaccines must be given at the proper time to healthy animals. Once a disease appears in a herd, vaccination is of very limited value, and in some cases may actually be harmful.

There are a great variety of vaccines available, and often several types to protect against the same disease. In a matter as important as immunization, the prudent livestock owner would be well advised to seek the advice of a veterinarian on the necessity of vaccination and the best form to use. Don't forget that vaccination should take place before the disease appears.

If by choice or necessity you plan to vaccinate animals yourself, there are several things to keep in mind. Although there are many different vaccines and combinations thereof on the market produced under U.S. Department of Agriculture (USDA) license, some are better than others. Don't let your choice be dependent on the producer's advertising; instead, get advice on which to use from your veterinarian or someone who has used it. Second, follow the directions for use carefully. And last, with animals used for food such as beef and pork, don't inject vaccines or other drugs in the "region of the high-priced cuts" — the hind leg, for example. Intramuscular injection in the neck is preferable because any resulting scars will not depreciate the value of the carcass.

Other Causes of Disease

If animal diseases were limited to those caused by infectious organisms, the diagnostic problem would be greatly simplified. Unfortunately, this is not the case, and other factors must always be considered.

Nutrition

Nutrition is a factor often overlooked. When animals roamed wild, nutritional deficiencies were less of a factor because the animal would eat a variety of grasses and leaves when these were available. Although this diet was inadequate and precluded maximum growth rate and productivity, the variety generally prevented some of the mineral and vitamin deficiencies we see today. The chief nutritional problem of animals in the wild was outright starvation.

While this is a rare and inexcusable condition in domestic animals today, we now see nutritional deficiencies that are more subtle and difficult to diagnose.

Domestic animals are dependent on the feed we offer them, and the science of animal nutrition has become extremely important. Any successful animal husbandry manager must have a good understanding of the nutrient needs of the animals he feeds. Many good textbooks are available for the serious student of animal nutrition. The National Academy of Sciences has a series of booklets on the nutrient requirements of all the major animal species. These booklets (called the Nutrient Requirement series) are concise and current, and they contain everything the husbandry manager needs to know about the nutrition of his or her animals. (See Other Resources on page 330 for ordering information.)

Without some understanding of nutrition, it's not easy to be sure animals are being properly fed. Nutrition will be discussed in more detail later.

Trace Minerals and Vitamins

Animals grazing on land with a high molybdenum content may develop a copper deficiency because molybdenum ties up copper, making it unavailable to the animal. Copper deficiency leads to anemia, causing, among other things, poor reproduction. Zinc deficiency causes a skin disease in swine called *parakeratosis.* Calves and lambs frequently suffer from white muscle disease, an often fatal condition resulting from a deficiency of selenium or vitamin E.

Unfortunately, deficiency diseases are insidious and slow developing, although the final result may be dramatic. White muscle disease may cause sudden death of the healthiest-looking calf, and the comatose cow with milk fever is a real emergency. But the deficiencies leading to these conditions prevail over a long period of time. Once a diagnosis is made, further problems in the herd can usually be prevented by varying the diet and, if necessary, adding mineral supplements. Commercial interests have capitalized on the latter by marketing complicated mineral mixes at exorbitant prices for the unwary buyer. Generally speaking, if herbivorous animals are offered a diet of good-quality mixed hay and grain to which has been added 1 percent dicalcium phosphate and 1 percent trace mineral salt, no additional supplementation is necessary. Exceptions are dairy cattle and animals not fed grain. These should also have free-choice access to a mixture of equal parts of dicalcium phosphate and trace mineral salt.

Parasitism

Parasitism is another common cause of disease in animals that ranges from dramatic to innocuous. Animal parasites vary from single-celled coccidia to more complex organisms such as worms and insects. Some are free-living part of the time; others are totally dependent on the host animal for survival. Many have intricate life cycles that are absolutely fascinating to the biologist.

One of the more interesting parasites is the common horse bot, *Gasterophilus intestinalis*. The adult bot fly deposits its eggs on the hair, particularly on the front legs and shoulders. These eggs have a yellowish color and are about the size of pinheads. There they remain until, stimulated by the animal's licking, they hatch. The larvae then enter the mouth, where they penetrate the tongue and oral mucosa, and eventually migrate to the stomach, where they attach themselves to the wall, sometimes in very large numbers. They not only damage the wall but may also cause indigestion. After a developmental period of 8 to 10 months, they pass out in the feces to the soil, where they pupate. In about a month, an adult fly emerges to repeat the cycle.

Knowledge of parasite life cycles often presents an opportunity for control programs not dependent on drugs. For example, liver flukes, which affect most animal species, must spend a part of their life cycle in the snail. Because snails must have moisture to survive, a simple control procedure is to keep animals out of wet areas.

Parasitologists debate the merit of attempting to maintain internal parasite–free livestock. The relationship of many parasites to their host is *commensalistic* — that is, the parasite derives benefit from the host without harming the host. If it were otherwise, the host would die and the parasite would be homeless. Also, some parasites, such as *Haemonchus* species in sheep and hookworms in the dog, produce a degree of immune response, and modest infestations stimulate enough immunity so that overwhelming infections normally don't occur. However, when the animal has no immunity or is debilitated from other causes, such as malnutrition and stress, overwhelming infection may ultimately be fatal.

Proponents of limited infection argue that it is necessary for immunity. Those of the opposite school argue that with eradication or even control with medication, reinfection will not be a problem and immunity then is inconsequential. The practical course seems to lie somewhere between and is based on control through good sanitation and maintaining animals in a healthy state as well as interrupting parasite life cycles when feasible. Parasite control through medication alone is a continuing expense without lasting benefit that frequently doesn't work and in some cases may not even be necessary. Internal parasitism is generally a problem primarily of the young and the debilitated, especially when coupled with unsanitary housing and feeding conditions or malnutrition.

External Parasitism. Most often found in animals that are debilitated or kept under unsanitary housing conditions, external parasitism presents a different problem. The principal external parasites of farm animals are ticks, lice, and mites. While ticks cause some discomfort and do suck blood from the unlucky animal or human to which they become attached, they are chiefly important as vectors, or carriers of disease-producing organisms. The tick *Boophilus annulatus* was the vector of a serious cattle disease in the Southwest called *piroplasmosis,* or Texas fever, which caused losses running into millions of dollars. Once this vector relationship was recognized, the disease was eradicated by eliminating the specific tick that carried it. Ticks are responsible for transmission of diseases such as Rocky Mountain spotted fever, equine piroplasmosis, tularemia, and Lyme disease.

Lice are divided into two groups: biting and sucking. The biting lice feed on cellular debris on the skin surface and cause intense itching. Sucking lice, on the other hand, suck blood from the host. Severe infestations can cause fatal blood loss. Adult ticks and lice are visible to the naked eye, and frequent grooming of the animal may be sufficient to control them.

Mites are microscopic in size and are the cause of mange, or scabies, found in almost all species. This condition, which can become severe, causes itching and loss of weight. Psoroptic mange in sheep causes the wool to fall out in patches, which is a direct economic loss.

Where external parasites are a problem, one effective control measure is the use of insecticides on the animal as a spray, dip, or powder. Some insecticides may be given orally, by injection, or by the pour-on method for systemic effect. The use of many of the best insecticides is severely restricted by federal and state governments, however, because of associated risks of environmental contamination. Restrictions are even greater if the compound is to be used on food-producing animals, especially lactating dairy cattle, because of possible residue in milk or meat. Fortunately, the avermectin class of drugs, administered as a pour-on injection or orally, has provided alternatives.

Hereditary and Congenital Defects

Sixty-four hereditary defects have been identified in cattle alone. The influence of relatively few bulls on large numbers of offspring through artificial insemination has made hereditary defects in cattle a matter of concern. Two of the most common are umbilical hernia, recognizable at birth, and spastic syndrome, which doesn't appear until the animal approaches maturity.

Congenital defects are those that result either from developmental accident during the embryonic stage or from the influence of a toxic or infectious agent during prenatal development. The former are uncontrollable accidents; the latter have an external cause and are preventable if one knows the contributing factors. For example, consumption of a weed *(Veratrum californicum)* by the ewe at about day 14 of pregnancy results in birth of a high percentage of deformed cyclopian lambs. Knowing this, the shepherd can prevent it by keeping ewes out of pastures where the weed grows during early pregnancy, or he can eliminate the weeds in the pasture with herbicides.

Infection with bovine virus diarrhea during early pregnancy has been shown to cause cerebellar hypoplasia and cataracts in calves as well as abortion in some cases. This can be prevented by vaccination of the dam at least 30 days prior to breeding.

It is vitally important, regardless of species, that developmental defects or diseases that may be hereditary in origin be reported to the appropriate breed associations. Identification of hereditary defects is always retrospective and dependent on large numbers of reports. Just as we keep careful production records on purebred animals and plan matings to improve the breed, so should we keep good records of matings that result in offspring detrimental to the breed. Fortunately, most hereditary defects are lethal or at least render the animal uneconomical to raise to maturity. But not all of them are, and we need to identify those individuals that carry the genes leading to defective offspring so they can be removed from the population or at least neutered. Too many breeders adopt the opposite approach and go to great lengths to conceal the birth of defective offspring. Such conduct is irresponsible, to say the least.

The Human Contribution

Thus far in this chapter, a variety of agents contributing to animal disease have been described. To these, people are often the unwitting accomplices in myriad ways. Accident and injury are not uncommon, and frequently they are our fault. It's easier to clean a smooth barn floor, so we trowel the concrete smooth and wonder why the cows slip and fall, sometimes breaking a leg. The problem of spraddle-legged pigs is directly attributable to slippery floors. We build barbed-wire fences because barbed wire is cheaper than woven wire and then call the animals that get tangled in it "stupid." And when the wire gets chopped up in the hay baler and the resulting pieces pierce the cow's stomach, we call it bad luck.

Barns are expensive, so in the name of efficiency, we crowd in as many animals as possible. This improves the opportunity for disease transmission, and the problem is compounded during cold weather when, because we don't like to work in the cold, we shut the barn up tight. This raises temperatures and particularly humidity, fostering the production of ammonia from manure and urine. The respiratory tract irritation this causes is one of the leading factors predisposing young animals to pneumonia. From a health standpoint, they would be better off outside with an open shed for shelter. All too often we design animal housing with our own comfort and convenience in mind rather than that of the animals.

Every animal harbors pathogens to which it has become immune but that are transmissible to other animals in the herd. It's a rare buyer who insists on a complete physical examination or immunization record of the animal he buys. And it's an even rarer individual who isolates a purchased addition from the herd to be sure it isn't in the incubation period of a contagious disease before putting it with the others. If you have young children, you are familiar with the outbreaks of head colds and other ailments that occur soon after school starts. The situation is the same whether people or animals are brought together in close confinement.

Exhibiting at Fairs

A special word of caution is in order for people who exhibit at fairs and shows. This is an ideal place for transmission of contagious diseases. Not only is a large group of animals (and pathogens) brought together from a variety of areas, but the animals are also under stress from trucking, a strange environment, and often a complete change of diet. This makes them much more susceptible to infection, which in turn spreads to the rest of the herd when they are returned. The prudent exhibitor will minimize stress as much as possible; will immunize his animal against every disease for which safe, reliable vaccines are available; and will isolate the animal from the herd for 2 weeks after the show is over.

Biosecurity

Regardless of the species involved, much can be done at minimal cost to reduce the risk of disease:

■ Have animal born in a clean area uncontaminated by recent previous births or manure from other animals. Ideally, clean and disinfect birthing area between uses.

■ Good health should start at birth. Bear in mind that, in the northern climates especially, the newborn arrival may experience an ambient temperature drop of 100 degrees or more in a matter of minutes and, to make matters worse, is born wet. Be prepared to dry the newborn with clean towels, and provide supplemental heat if necessary. Avoid chilling!

■ Be certain the new arrival gets colostrum within an hour of birth. Calves should get at least a gallon, and other species in proportion to body weight. Have a supply of frozen colostrum on hand to use if needed.

■ Keep the stable area clean, dry, and well ventilated. If the barn smells like a barn, ventilation is probably inadequate. Avoid draft situations such as from broken windows.

■ Eliminate mechanical hazards such as slippery floors, protruding nails, and machinery in the pasture.

■ Avoid feed contamination. Use separate implements for feed and manure handling. Keep dogs and cats out of the feed alleys.

■ Implement a rodent and fly control program.

■ Isolate purchased additions and show animal returnees for at least 2 weeks.

■ Discourage visitors in the barn and have a sanitizing footbath available for those who must enter.

■ Teach employees how to recognize signs of disease and explain what they can do to reduce these hazards.

■ Follow a set routine for feeding, exercise, milking, and so on, and always move slowly and quietly around your animals. Quiet, relaxed animals will produce better and be healthier.

If after reading this far you have gotten the impression that animal health and disease are highly complex, the chapter will have served its purpose. Keep in mind that nothing is absolute in medicine, whether human or veterinary. Each animal is unique in its response to extraneous influences, as are the pathogens that affect its health. The variables are infinite, and the line between health and disease is easily breached. It behooves us, and in fact it's our obligation, to do everything possible to maintain our animals in good health.

Fortunately, medical research has made tremendous gains in techniques for disease control and prevention. What has been lacking generally in veterinary medicine is the application of that knowledge on the farm to prevent animal disease. Your veterinarian and the information in this book can help you correct that deficiency. Remember that animal disease is not always bad luck; it's more often a reflection of bad management. Fully 90 percent of the animal health problems we encounter could have been prevented.

Nutrition and Health

IT GOES WITHOUT SAYING that a well-fed animal is more likely to be a healthy animal. But what is a well-fed animal? What does *well-fed* mean? There is no simple answer because nutrient requirements vary with age, body weight, stage of gestation, and, for the dairy cow, level of milk production. Extensive research has produced guidelines that help, but they are guidelines only. Feeding cattle or other animals is part science and part art because of individual variation. Animals respond much like people to nutrient intake: at a given level some get thin, some stay the same, and some get fat. A good herd manager recognizes the individual variations in the herd and adjusts feed intake accordingly.

Cattle

Good cattle nutrition begins with the newborn calf. There are some differences between the dairy and the beef calf that will be pointed out as we go along. As a rule of thumb, young calves should receive 10 percent of their body weight daily of whole milk equivalent. For example, a 100-pound calf should have 10 pounds of milk, or about 5 quarts, daily.

For the first 12 hours of life, calves should have all of the antibody-rich first milk, or colostrum, they can consume. After that period, the calves' ability to absorb antibody from colostrum diminishes rapidly, and its value then becomes primarily nutritional. Because the dairy cow typically produces colostrum far in excess of the needs of her calf and because colostrum is higher in total solids than is whole milk, overfeeding it can cause digestive upset and diarrhea.

The situation differs somewhat with beef calves, and it's customary to leave them with their dams to nurse. Overfeeding problems generally don't occur because most beef cows don't produce milk significantly in excess of need. In fact, beef breeders usually select for cows with extra milking capacity so they will have enough milk to raise a good calf.

Don't Waste Colostrum

While the dairy cow gives more colostrum than her calf needs, the excess need not be wasted. It can be diluted 50 percent with water and fed to other calves or can be stored. It can be frozen and kept indefinitely or stored at room temperature and fed as sour or "pickled" colostrum. It can be held this way for about 3 weeks. While it doesn't look or smell the greatest to us, calves like it and thrive on it.

Where dairy calves are held in group pens, another health consideration related to feeding arises. Young calves will instinctively suck after they are fed and will suck one another's ears and udders if given the opportunity. They should be tied after each feeding for about an hour or until the sucking urge disappears. While sucking ears is not especially harmful, wet ears will freeze if it is below freezing where the calves are housed. Sucking udders may introduce infection that will flare up as mastitis when the udder begins to develop. Equally important, the sucking habit may become fixed as a lifelong habit, and it's not rare for cows to suck their own udders or that of a willing neighbor. This is a vice carried over from calfhood that makes the animal a liability.

Before leaving the subject of feeding milk to calves, there is one recurring question that should be answered. Dairy farmers often ask if it's all right to feed milk from cows with mastitis to calves. Nutritionally it's probably satisfactory and economically it makes sense, but in my opinion such milk should not be used, for two reasons. First, it is usually teeming with pathogenic organisms that caused the mastitis. From a health standpoint, it doesn't make sense to expose the calf to these organisms and at the same time spread them to other areas of the barn. Second, if the infected quarters have been treated with antibiotics and milk from them is fed to calves, the calves will absorb some of the antibiotics and have tissue residues of these antibiotics for varying periods of time thereafter. In the case of streptomycin, it may be over a month, and it is illegal to market veal containing drug residues.

Milk Replacers

Purely for economic reasons, it's sometimes advantageous to use commercially prepared milk replacer rather than whole milk for calves. These powdered products, when reconstituted with water, make a satisfactory milk substitute. Many companies market milk replacers that vary widely in price — and in quality. All of them indicate on the label the composition analysis in terms of protein and fat. But the quality of the protein, for calves, is as important as the amount. The cheaper ones use vegetable sources such as soybean oil meal as the protein source, whereas the better ones use milk by-products. Very young calves do not utilize vegetable protein well, and calves maintained on this type of diet are often stunted and unthrifty. With milk replacers, as with most things, you get about what you pay for.

Frequency of feeding apparently has little significant effect on overall growth of calves. The nursing calf, of course, will get a little milk whenever he feels like it, which is the way nature intended it and which, perhaps, should be considered the ideal. Hand-feeding is almost a necessity for dairy calves, and this creates a labor problem. Most dairy farmers feed their calves twice daily, but research at Cornell University indicates that calves do about as well when fed only once a day. Similarly, it seems to make little difference whether the milk is fed warm or cold. Feeding the total daily intake in one meal of ice cold milk, however, may cause chilling and stomach cramps.

Sanitation

Whatever method is used — once a day, twice a day, warm or cold — sanitation is important. Whether you use ordinary pails, nipple pails, or automatic feeders, these should be scrubbed and sanitized after each use. Milk is the most nearly complete food, and this attribute, which is desirable for young animals, also makes it suitable for bacterial growth. Any amount of milk left in the pail at room temperature becomes a thriving bacterial culture in a few hours. If these happen to be pathogenic, such as some of the *Salmonella* species, every calf that subsequently drinks from that pail is likely to get sick. Always remember that the calf has virtually no immunity at birth and is vulnerable to every pathogen it encounters. The health of your calves will be proportional to your success in reducing that exposure.

At 1 week of age, calves will begin to eat a little grain and hay. The hay offered should be early cut and of high quality. Consumption will be insignificant at first but will gradually increase to become a major part of the diet at the end of a month. The amount of milk being fed can be reduced commensurately as grain and roughage consumption increases. Calves can usually be weaned from milk at 4 to 6 weeks of age, but it's part of the art of husbandry to tell how fast and how soon. The nutritional problems of the calf, once weaned, become similar to those of the mature cow. The important thing is to keep calves growing and gaining weight steadily. An animal in a weight-gaining condition is more likely to be a healthy animal.

Clean Water

In addition to whatever it eats, whole milk or milk replacer, the growing calf needs clean water. It's ideal to have a supply of fresh water available at all times. However, where physical conditions won't permit this, additional water must be hand-fed by adding it to the milk or separately. A good way to wean calves as they get older is to add increasing amounts of water to a constant amount of milk. Eventually, the solution gets so dilute that when the milk is stopped, the calves hardly miss it. Mature animals should have access to free-choice water at all times.

A complete discussion of the nutrition of the growing and mature cow is beyond the scope of this book. For a concise summary, the reader is referred to Nutrient Requirements of Dairy Cattle and its counterpart for beef cattle, both published by the National Academy of Sciences (see page 330). In it one will find the recommendations for protein, energy, minerals, and vitamins for growing and mature cattle in various weight ranges. For mature cattle, a basic amount is given for maintenance and to this must be added an increment for advanced pregnancy and for milk production.

Balancing the Ration

Also given are examples of how to balance a ration using readily available feedstuffs. Ability to balance a ration is a must for the serious herd manager who wants to feed the animals adequately at minimum cost. Also given is the average nutrient composition of several hundred feed ingredients. These can be used as a guide in formulation of rations, but it's much more reliable to have a forage analysis done on your own hay and silage and, using that as a base, determine how much additional grain is needed to balance the daily ration.

Analysis of forage is a laboratory procedure that, in most states, can be arranged by your Cooperative Extension agent, veterinarian, feed dealer, or a commercial laboratory. Analyses are usually reported in terms of percentage of total digestible nutrients (TDN) and total or crude protein (CP). Mineral and some vitamin analyses can be obtained as well, but usually at added cost.

To illustrate how this information is used, let's assume we have a 700 kg dairy cow giving 20 kg of 3.5 percent butterfat milk daily and due to calve in 2 months. Her daily intake, according to the National Research Council (NRC) standards, should meet the amounts outlined in Table 2-1.

Let's further assume that we have available good-quality mixed alfalfa-brome grass hay to feed this cow. How much will she need to eat to meet her nutritional needs? Looking first at TDN in the feedstuff composition tables, we find that this mixed hay will average 55 percent TDN on a dry-matter basis but that it is only 82.5 percent dry matter with the balance moisture. Our cow needs 6.9 kg of TDN daily. By simple arithmetic, we find that 15 kg of hay daily will meet her energy needs, but will it supply enough protein? The same hay is composed of 16.2 percent total protein on a dry-matter basis. By multi-

TABLE 2-1	**DAILY INTAKE FOR DAIRY COW**			
	TOTAL PROTEIN (KG)	TDN (KG)	CALCIUM (G)	PHOSPHORUS (G)
For maintenance and pregnancy	1.00	6.30	39.00	30.00
For milk production	1.48	0.60	52.00	38.00
TOTAL	2.48	6.90	91.00	68.00

plying, we find that 15 kg contains 2.4 kg of protein. But since the hay is only 82.5 percent dry matter, the actual total protein is only 2 kg, or 0.4 kg less than recommended. While the cow would undoubtedly survive with this modest protein deficiency, her milk production would suffer.

Mineral Components

Let's look at the important mineral components in this all-hay diet. This hay averages 1.03 percent calcium (Ca) and 0.3 percent phosphorus (P), both on a dry-matter basis. Fifteen kilograms of this hay calculates out to 127 grams of calcium and 37 grams of phosphorus daily. This is more calcium than the cow needs and considerably less phosphorus than she requires. Further, the Ca:P ratio is wide, being 3.4:1.0. With a phosphorus-deficient ration and a wide Ca:P ratio, the cow on this diet would likely have parturient paresis (milk fever, hypocalcemia) when she calves. Nutrition influences health.

Well, we have all this good alfalfa-brome hay on hand, which, incidentally, is higher in protein and energy than most hay. What can we do so it can be used and still give the cow an adequate diet? Depending on available feeds, several things can be done. Corn silage can be substituted for part of the hay. This will narrow the Ca:P ratio but also reduce the protein. To balance the diet using this hay, some mixed-grain dairy ration containing 1 percent dicalcium phosphate or liquid protein supplement will have to be used.

A word or two should be said about grain used to balance rations for livestock. The science of genetic engineering has produced grains, especially corn, that not only produce better yields but also are resistant to some plant diseases. There is no evidence at this writing that the nutrient content of genetically engineered grain is any different from that of the parent stock or that it is harmful to animals or people who consume it.

The same procedure can be used to determine adequacy of other essential minerals and vitamins. If all the mathematics scares you or you don't feel confident trying to balance a ration yourself, your local Cooperative Extension agent or feed dealer will be glad to help.

Using a total mixed ration (TMR) composed of chopped hay and/or silage and grain lends itself well to mechanical handling and thus lower labor costs. It creates a problem, however, in meeting the needs of the cow for energy intake in proportion to milk production. In large herds, it is less of a problem because cows can be grouped according to production level and fed accordingly. In smaller herds, any energy deficit can be made up by feeding additional grain in the milking parlor. And, of course, in the traditional stanchion barn where cows are fed individually, adjustments can be easily made.

The purpose of this discussion is to demonstrate that feeding the dairy cow adequately is not a hit-or-miss proposition and that nutrition does have an important bearing on health. Just how important can be seen in Table 2-2.

TABLE 2-2	NUTRIENTS AND THEIR FUNCTIONS	
NUTRIENT	FUNCTION	REQUIREMENT
Energy (glucose, fats, fatty acids)	Muscle and nerve activity; growth; fattening; milk secretion	Variable with size, rate of growth, milk production, and milk-fat percentage
Fiber	Stimulates rumination and secretion of saliva; helps maintain rumen pH near neutral ±6.8	Minimum 15% of ration dry matter for lactating cows; higher with finely chopped feeds
Protein	Cell formation; muscle, hair, blood proteins, enzymes; milk protein secretion	11–15% of ration dry matter depending on age and rate of production; proportional to energy intake
Salt: sodium (Na) and chloride (Cl)	Acid-base balance; nerve and muscle action; water retention; hydrochloric acid	2–3 g/cwt/day; estimated 0.18% sodium or 0.45% salt (NaCl) in dry ration
Calcium (Ca)	Skeletal growth and milk production; muscle quiescence	Maintenance 10–15 g/day plus 1 g/lb milk; 0.3–0.4% in dry ration for lactation
Phosphorus (P)	Energy metabolism, skeletal growth, milk production	Maintenance 10–15 g + 0.75 g/lb milk; 0.25–0.3% in dry ration
Vitamin D	Absorption of Ca and P; reduced excretion of P; mobilization of Ca and P from skeleton	300–400 IU/cwt/day; D2 or D3, 5000–15,000 IU/head/day
Magnesium (Mg)	Muscle irritability; electrolyte balance; enzymes	Calves: 0.4–0.6 g/cwt/day; or 0.15–0.20% in the dry ration of milking cows
Potassium (K)	Acid-base balance in intracellular fluid; osmotic pressure; activates enzymes; heart, muscle tone	0.5% of dry ration for growth of lambs; 0.7% suggested for cattle, more for high-producing cows
Iron (Fe)	Formation of hemoglobin	Growth, 150 mg/cwt/day for growth, 100 ppm; in adult ration 2 g/day
Iodine (I)	Thyroxine synthesis; metabolic rate	0.1 ppm in dry ration (for nonlactation, 2 mg/head daily); 0.8 ppm for pregnancy or 8–12 mg; more may be required when soybean meal or other goitrogenic feeds are fed heavily
Fluorine (F)	Small amount appears to prevent dental caries	Toxic above 10 ppm
Manganese (Mn)	Growth, enzymes	Cows: 20 ppm in dry ration for normal reproduction and offspring; normal growth at lower levels

DEFICIENCY SYMPTOMS

Low milk production; slow growth rate; poor body condition; silent estrus (heat). Lowered protein content of milk. Energy in excess of requirement; fattening, high blood fat levels; fatty liver; tendency for depressed appetite and ketosis post-calving. Unsaturated fats in tissue and fat deposits; tendency toward low resistence to infectious diseases, retained placentas, and metritis; sudden increase causes lactic acidosis, death.

Rumenitis, founder, rumen stasis; tendency toward displaced abomasum post-calving. Low milk-fat test; higher unsaturated fats in tissue fats; may contribute to poor muscle contractility.

Emaciation (poor body condition), retarded growth, low milk production. Reduced digestion of feed, poor conversion of feed to growth, fat, or milk; lower blood protein and possibly antibody fractions. Underdeveloped reproductive organs possibly due to retarded growth.

Lack of appetite; unthrifty; low production; craving for salt, appetite for soil, clothing, licking objects, drinking of urine from other cows.

Bones and teeth easily broken. Low Ca content in bones.

Lack of appetite, irregular estrus; depraved appetite for bones, wood, bark, etc.

Rickets, enlarged joints, wobbly gait, lack of appetite, stiff legs, arched back, swelling of pasterns, lameness; calves deficient in Ca, P, or vitamin D.

Grass tetany (or grass staggers), twitching of the skin, staggering or unsteady on feet, down and unable to rise. Common with cattle grazing rapidly growing, succulent pasture or similar green chop and occasionally stored feeds. May be aggravated by high nitrogen (N) and K levels in feeds.

Overall muscle weakness, loss of appetite; poor intestinal tone with intestinal distension; cardiac and respiratory muscle weakness and failure.

Anemia — particularly in calves maintained on milk. Seldom in adult cattle.

Goiterous (big neck) calves frequently born dead or hairless. Failure to show estrus, high incidence of retained placentas in mature cows.

Deformed teeth and bones.

Newborn: deformed bones, enlarged joints, stiffness, twisted legs, shorter humeri (forelegs), general physical weakness. Deficiency could occur in cattle fed high-grain, low-roughage rations, where symptom could be ataxia (uncoordinated movements).

TABLE 2-2   NUTRIENTS AND THEIR FUNCTIONS *(continued)*

NUTRIENT	FUNCTION	REQUIREMENT
Copper (Cu)	Respiratory pigments of blood; some enzymes	5 ppm dry ration, 6–8 ppm suggested; increases with high molybdenum intake
Cobalt (Co)	Microbial synthesis of vitamin B_{12} in rumen	0.1 ppm in dry ration (2 mg/day)
Vitamin B_{12} (cobalamin)	Energy metabolism; maturation of red blood cells	Calves 1.5 mg/cwt/day
Selenium (Se)	Muscle integrity	Uncertain: believed 0.05 ppm minimum
Sulfur (S)	Synthesis of S-amino acids, coenzyme A	0.2% in dry ration; 1 S to 10 parts N in high NPN rations
Zinc	Enzyme systems	Calves: 9 ppm in ration was adequate for normal growth and appearance; about 20 ppm may be desirable for lactation
Vitamin A	Growth, differentiation, and health of epithelial tissue, especially of eyes, alimentary tract, and respiratory mucosa	3000 IU/cwt/day or 6 mg carotene/cwt/day; no lactation requirement except for health of animal
B Vitamins	Synthesized by organisms in normal-functioning rumen to meet requirement	Calves to weaning; contained in milk
Niacin, nicotin, or nicotinamide		Energy metabolism enzymes
Thiamin B_1		Prevented by 0.65 mg thiamin-HCl per kg of liquid diet or 0.065 mg per kg live weight
Riboflavin B_2		Calves <0.075 mg/kg live weight or 0.65 ppm in liquid diet
Biotin		0.01 mg/kg liquid diet; 1.0 µg/kg body weight
Pantothenic acid		<1.3 mg/kg liquid diet
Folic acid		0.39 mg/kg liquid prevented in lamb
Vitamin B_{12}		0.34–0.68 (µg) per kg live weight
Pyridoxine		<0.065 mg/kg body weight
Choline		260 mg/kg liquid promoted recovery

DEFICIENCY SYMPTOMS

"Coast disease" or "salt sick" in Florida. Anemia, stillbirth of young, loss of wool in sheep, incoordination of hind legs, sudden death in cows due to heart degeneration. Baby pig "thumps" due to Cu and Fe deficiency.

Loss of appetite, anemia, emaciation, low appetite for grain. Calves unthrifty, poor appetite, first to exhibit symptoms because low vitamin B_{12} content of milk.

See above.

Nutritional muscular dystrophy; high calf and lamb mortality; retained placentas increased; liver necrosis (degeneration) in pigs. Toxic above 3 ppm.

Lowered production, poor N utilization. Cellulose digestion and conversion of lactate to propionate.

Itch, hair slicking, stiff gait, swelling of hocks and knees, soft swelling above rear feet, rough and thickened skin, dermatitis between rear legs and behind elbows. Undersize testicles in bull calves and low fertility in cows have been attributed to zinc (Zn) deficiency.

Night blindness, bulging and watery eyes, muscle incoordination. Bronchitis and coughing may progress to pneumonia. Chronic symptoms: roughened haircoat, emaciation; hairless or blind calves if dam deficient; edema or swelling of the brisket and forelegs (anasarca); abortion. Young calves: weakness at birth, susceptible to pneumonia and digestive infections, watering of the eyes, cloudiness of the cornea, protrusion or "bulging" of eye followed by permanent blindness and death.

Deficiency symptoms produced only with abnormal restricted diets. May occur in calves with prolonged severe scours or fed artificial milk diets.

Dermatitis and necrotic lesions in mouth.

Polioencephalomalacia; necrosis in the gray matter of the brain. Muscular incoordination, tremor, grinding of teeth, convulsions. High blood and urine lactate and pyruvate.

Lesions around the corner of the mouth, eyes, and nose; damp haircoat; loss of hair; copious salivation; lacrimation.

Paralysis of hindquarters.

Lack of growth and emaciation. Scaly dermatitis around eyes and muzzle; susceptible to respiratory infection.

Lack of growth and emaciation, leukopenia (low WBC).

Lack of growth and emaciation (see Cobalt).

Lack of appetite, epileptiform fits, demyelination of peripheral nerves.

Extreme weakenss, labored breathing within 6–8 days.

TABLE 2-2	NUTRIENTS AND THEIR FUNCTIONS *(continued)*	
NUTRIENT	FUNCTION	REQUIREMENT
Vitamin C (ascorbic acid)	Synthesized in tissue of calves and adult bovines	
Vitamin E (alpha-tocopherol)	Antioxidant, muscle integrity	Calves: <40 mg/day; adults: not established

NPN = nonprotein nitrogen source.
Data compiled by Hillman and Newman, Michigan State University.

Water

Last, water is the most important constituent of the cow's diet, although it is seldom thought of as such. The cow can go several days without feed but one day without water will cause a precipitous drop in milk production; two days without will make a very sick animal; and three days without will likely kill the animal. Adult cattle consume water in proportion to the amount and moisture content of feed consumed, level of milk production, and environmental temperatures. An average cow eating 20 kg of dry matter daily and producing 20 kg of milk will consume about 120 liters or approximately 30 gallons of water daily. Milk production will be higher if water is available free choice.

Digestion in Cows

From a health standpoint, there are some other important factors about cattle nutrition to keep in mind. The first is the nature of the beast. Cattle are ruminants, as are sheep and goats, with a digestive system that differs markedly from simple-stomached animals such as the horse, the pig, and humans. The cow's stomach is divided into four distinct compartments, designated in order of progression as rumen, reticulum, omasum, and abomasum. The rumen is basically a large fermentation vat where the action of bacteria and other microorganisms begins the digestive process by converting fiber into usable energy forms. It's this capacity to utilize fiber that makes the ruminant unique.

We hear a lot these days about how cattle compete with humans for available grain, thereby contributing to the world food shortages. Nothing could be further from the truth. Even under our system of finishing beef cattle in feedlots, less than 20 percent of the animal's lifetime feed intake is grain. Most of it comes from grass, which humans couldn't digest even if they could swallow it. In terms of food resource utilization alone, beef is a real bargain.

DEFICIENCY SYMPTOMS

Other species — scurvy, loosening of teeth, subepithelial hemorrhage and other problems related to faulty collagen formation.

Nutritional muscular dystrophy; white muscle disease in calves; stiff lamb disease; stiff legs; sudden death from heart muscle degeneration. Heart, diaphragm, and intercostal muscles show light streaking.

The cow doesn't have upper incisor teeth and eats grass more by pulling it off than by biting it off, as a horse does. Similarly, a cow will take a mouthful of hay and chew it very little before swallowing it. Most of her jaw motions when eating are directed toward mixing the hay with saliva, wadding it into a bolus, and swallowing it. It's this failure to chew that contributes to the cow's propensity for swallowing foreign objects, especially pieces of wire that are tangled in hay. These eventually gravitate to the lowest part of the digestive tract, the reticulum, where they sometimes perforate the wall, causing peritonitis and/or pericarditis.

Ingested feed in the rumen is churned by rhythmic contractions that normally occur two to four times a minute. The fermentation and digestion process, aided by rumen microorganisms, is going on constantly. When the cow is at rest, she voluntarily regurgitates part of the rumen contents, chews it a while, and swallows it again. The process is called *rumination,* and the regurgitated ingesta is called a *cud.* Most of the cud, when swallowed, passes into the reticulum.

Occasionally a cow will drop a cud out of her mouth, and a favorite wives' tale professed that losing a cud would make a cow go off feed. There is no truth in this. It is good therapy, however, to give a cud from a healthy cow to one that has been or is off feed. When you see a cow chewing, simply

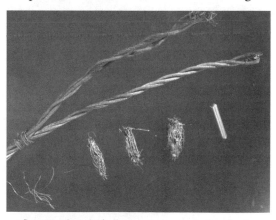

Because they don't chew, cows have a propensity for ingesting foreign obejcts. These pieces of metal were found in a cow's rumen.

open her mouth and remove the cud she is chewing. Then put it in the mouth of the cow that has been off feed. This has the effect of inoculating the rumen of the cow that has been off feed with normal rumen microorganisms, which will frequently restore digestive function and improve appetite.

Rumination and Health

Normal rumination is a good indicator of the animal's health. Rumination is absent in such diseases as traumatic gastritis, milk fever, and most digestive disorders. Rumen activity may be greater than normal in some diseases causing diarrhea. Because digestion in the cow is first a fermentation process, she is subject to some problems rarely seen in nonruminants. Radical changes in diet, such as excessive amounts of grain, change the rumen pH from slightly alkaline to acidic, which is not desirable for rumen microorganisms, causing them to die. This leads to incomplete digestion and rumen stasis, the results of which can be fatal. Fermentation with evolution of gas is a normal digestive function. However, if the cow eats large amounts of lush green pasture, especially clover or alfalfa, excess gas will be trapped in a froth causing bloat, which can be rapidly fatal.

If the cow is sick and not eating, important alterations in rumen digestive activity take place that have a bearing on her recovery. Without a daily addition of nutrients to the rumen, protozoa decrease almost to zero, bacteria decrease to 10 to 25 percent of normal, and the balance between bacterial species is altered. All of these changes reduce fermentation activity, which

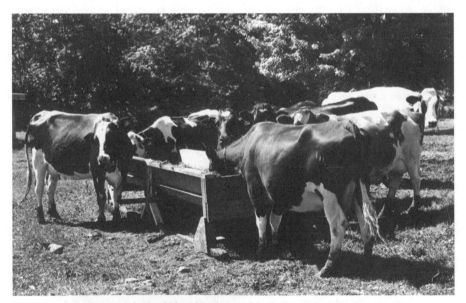

Feed for animals should be placed in raised troughs and not on the ground. Fecal contamination leads to internal parasitism.

reduces the animal's energy supply in both quantity and quality, cuts off the supply of water-soluble vitamins, and increases susceptibility to acidosis and other digestive disturbances.

Restoration of normal rumen activity is an important consideration in restoring the sick animal to health. Poor-quality hay high in fiber and poor-quality silage should be avoided. Instead, the best-quality hay available should be selected and grain intake should be increased gradually as appetite improves.

Although some absorption of nutrients takes place in the rumen, most occurs farther along in the digestive tract. From the reticulum, ingesta passes to the omasum and then to the abomasum. From the abomasum down through the intestinal tract, the digestive process is comparable to that of simple-stomached animals. The difference is primarily one of size. The gut is subject to the same ailments seen in other animals.

Two Systems of Ruminant Nutrition

Ruminant nutrition really concerns two biological systems: (1) the microorganisms in the rumen and (2) the animal itself. The feed offered must be conducive to proper microbiological metabolism and the end product must meet the nutrient needs of the animal. Because digestion is dependent on rumen microorganisms, it follows that their activity must be the first concern. Abrupt changes in diet are often detrimental. The most common example is what happens every spring when cows are put on pasture for the first time after a winter diet of perhaps dry hay, corn silage, and grain. If they are turned out directly on pasture without being fed some hay first, a few cows will bloat in a matter of several hours, but almost all will have diarrhea within 12 hours. This is not so much because fresh grass has a laxative effect, which it does to some degree. Rather, it occurs primarily because the rumen organisms are not adapted to it. After a week or so at pasture, the cows' manure will return to a normal consistency.

The matter of rumen microorganism adaptation is especially important when alternate protein sources are used. Protein is usually the most expensive ingredient in the cow's diet, and it is frequently advantageous to use a substitute.

Urea is the chemical usually used, and the cow can derive up to 30 percent of her protein needs from it. It may be added to the grain or to the silage as long as it is thoroughly mixed. Urea itself has no nutritional value whatsoever. But in the rumen, it breaks down to its component elements, and the rumen microorganisms utilize the nitrogen ion to synthesize amino acids, which are protein precursors used by the cow.

This conditioning, or adaptation of rumen flora, is rapidly lost if the cow goes off feed for a day or two for any reason. Feed containing urea must then be reintroduced gradually to the diet to avoid toxicity. If too much urea is accidentally fed or if it is fed at too high a level for cows not conditioned to it, death may result. This happens because the nitrogen is not utilized fast enough by the rumen organisms, and an excess of ammonia, fatal to the cow, is produced. Urea, not exceeding 3 percent of the grain ration, can safely provide 30 percent of the cow's protein needs once the rumen flora have been adapted to it. The majority of formula dairy feeds contain some urea, and it is commonly used in liquid protein supplements.

Vitamins and Minerals

Although the chief concern in cattle nutrition is with energy, protein, and the minerals calcium and phosphorus, attention must be given as well to vitamins, trace minerals, and salt. The B vitamins are largely synthesized by rumen microorganisms, so supplementation for the healthy cow is generally not required. The fat-soluble vitamins, A, D, and E, are more of a concern. Vitamin A is the most important of the three. It and its precursor, carotene, are found in green feeds and grain, so supplementation is not required when cows are on pasture. It oxidizes rather rapidly in storage, however, so hay that was high in vitamin A when cut will have very little after 6 months in storage. If stored hay or silage is a major part of the diet, vitamin A supplementation, in the feed or by injection, is usually necessary. Vitamin A is routinely added to most commercial grain mixes.

Vitamin D plays an important role in calcium metabolism and is sometimes used prophylactically in high doses prior to calving for the prevention of milk fever. It is synthesized by specialized cells in the skin, under the action of sunlight. Deficiencies are unlikely to occur in adult cattle except where cattle are constantly housed indoors. Deficiency in calves causes rickets; thus vitamin D is usually added to milk replacers to prevent this possibility.

Vitamin E plays a role, with selenium, in muscle metabolism. A deficiency of either leads to a sometimes-fatal condition in calves and lambs called *white muscle disease*. This is more likely to occur on an all-milk diet, which is a reason for getting some grain and hay into the diet as early as possible.

The need for the essential trace elements and salt can be met by giving cattle free access to trace mineralized salt (sometimes called *blue salt*). The addition of an equal part of dicalcium phosphate will help to maintain an adequate calcium and phosphorus intake. The mixture should be put in a container protected from rain and placed in an area where the cattle have daily access.

Horses

With the advent of the tractor and automobile, horse numbers declined precipitously during the 1930s and 1940s to a point where, immediately after World War II, many people believed the future of the horse was seriously limited. As a consequence, most colleges and experiment stations discontinued equine research and husbandry programs. However, with the unpredictable resurgence of interest in the light horse, it is obvious that this was a mistake.

One result of the temporary decline of interest in the horse is a lack of good research data on equine nutrition. Only within recent years has this important area begun to get the attention it deserves, and there is still much to learn. Until this time, equine diets have been largely a matter of trial and error, unfounded opinion, and even superstition. There are horse owners today who believe the only safe and satisfactory diet for horses is timothy hay and oats. This opinion has been thoroughly discredited, but there are factors about the horse and diet that have a profound influence on health.

Although the horse is an herbivore like the cow, its digestive system is entirely different. The horse has only a simple stomach, comparable to the fourth compartment of the cow's stomach; it has limited capacity. The horse, although it needs some roughage, cannot handle the volume the cow does to meet its energy requirements, especially when heavy work is required. If fed enough, the horse can survive on hay alone, but the volume required frequently results in chronic abdominal distention referred to as *hay belly,* which is undesirable, particularly for a show animal. The horse doing heavy work must get most of its energy needs from concentrates.

The energy requirements of the horse are comparable in some ways to those of the gasoline engine. The greater the power output required, the greater the fuel consumption. As a rule of thumb, the horse needs 1½ to 1¾ pounds of good-quality hay per 100 pounds of body weight to maintain his condition. In addition, if he is doing light work, he needs ¾ to 1½ pounds of grain per hour of work, and for heavy work, this need goes up to 8 pounds of grain per hour of work. Like the cow, the mare during advanced pregnancy or during lactation has an additional requirement for energy ranging from 1½ to 1¾ pounds of grain per 100 pounds of body weight. While these figures are good guides, they are not absolute, and the horse owner must feed according to the needs of the individual animal. The most common error in feeding light horses is overfeeding. The resulting obesity contributes to lack of stamina, liver disease, and leg problems, as well as foaling complications for the mare.

Which Grain?

A variety of grains can be used to meet the energy needs of the horse. Oats are traditional and good. They are higher in fiber and lower in energy than corn and wheat, and therefore overfeeding is less likely to have health repercussions. Many horse owners feel that corn is "too hot" for the horse and will cause indigestion and even laminitis. This is not true if the corn is fed on an energy-equivalent basis. It's common practice to feed grain to horses on a volume rather than a weight basis, as is done with other species.

If, for example, you are feeding 6 quarts of oats twice a day to a working horse and decide to use shelled corn instead, the same measure will provide almost twice the energy needs because an equal volume of corn weighs 1.7 times as much as oats. Cut the volume in half and you will have no difficulty, but make any feed change gradually over a period of several days because the horse is particularly sensitive to radical changes in diet. Abrupt change frequently causes indigestion and colic.

The protein requirement of the mature horse is much less critical than that of the dairy cow or dairy goat. The horse needs protein at the level of about 8 to 10 percent of the total ration, and this is readily met by a combination of hay and grain. The requirement increases during pregnancy and lactation and can be met by switching to mixed hay with a higher percentage of legumes or to a grain-mix formula that includes a higher percentage of protein. The weanling needs considerably more high-quality protein than the mature horse. To provide the 14 to 18 percent of protein needed in the weanling's diet, creep feeding is usually necessary.

Quality of Feed

A word of caution should be given about hay. Any grass or legume hay of good quality is satisfactory from a nutritional standpoint, but *never* feed moldy or "smoky" hay to horses. Mold spores and dust are largely responsible for *pulmonary emphysema,* a chronic lung disease, or "heaves" in the horse. Moldy grain is equally hazardous from the standpoint of mycotoxicosis. The

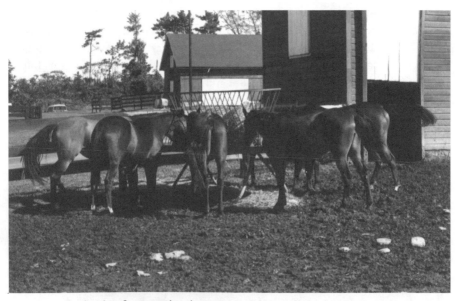

Feeding hay from a rack reduces waste and prevents fecal contamination.

horse, the pig, and the chicken seem to be particularly susceptible to poisoning by the toxins that some molds produce. Both of these problems can be avoided largely by paying attention to feed quality.

Grain for the horse (and in fact for all livestock) should be coarsely ground or pelleted. Finely ground grain is less palatable and dusty, and, more important, when swallowed it may lodge in the esophagus, causing the animal to choke. This is a serious condition requiring prompt professional attention.

Although the specific nutrient requirements of the horse have not been investigated as thoroughly as those for the cow and pig, enough information is available to make some valid recommendations. If you know the composition of your own hay from forage analysis or use the average composition from feed analysis tables, the recommendations in Table 2-3 will be useful.

Note that the calcium and phosphorus requirements for the weanling as a percent of daily intake are much higher than those for the mature horse. This is to meet the need for rapid skeletal growth. Calcium and phosphorus are the two most important minerals for the horse. Grains are rich sources of phosphorus, and if the horse is being fed relatively large amounts of grain, phosphorus is likely to be consumed in excess in proportion to calcium, unless legume hay is also being fed. Over a period of time, this imbalance will cause a demineralization of bone and a disease called *nutritional secondary hyperparathyroidism,* or "big head." To avoid this condition, more calcium must usually be added to the diet.

The horse also has a relatively high requirement for salt, especially when sweating from hot weather or strenuous exercise. The mature horse needs 50 to 60 grams of salt daily, and considerably more when sweating. The need for salt and extra calcium can be met by free-choice feeding of dicalcium phosphate and trace mineralized salt as recommended for cattle. When salt is first fed free choice, be sure an ample amount of fresh water is available in case the horse eats too much. Once his initial craving for salt is satisfied, he will consume only enough to meet his needs.

TABLE 2-3   **REQUIREMENTS EXPRESSED AS PERCENTAGE OF DIET**

CATEGORY	PROTEIN	CALCIUM	PHOSPHORUS
Weanling	14–16	0.70	0.40
Mature	8–10	0.35	0.25
Late Pregnancy	11–12	0.40	0.30
Lactating	13–15	0.60	0.35

Swine

Of all the farm animals, the dietary needs of swine most nearly parallel those of humans. Pigs are omnivores — that is, they can utilize energy and protein from both vegetable and animal sources to meet their requirements. This ability, coupled with economics, for years made garbage feeding a part of many swine enterprises. From a disease-control standpoint, however, feeding garbage is hazardous because pathogenic organisms that will infect pigs may be present in the meat scraps. The last outbreak of foot-and-mouth disease in the United States occurred this way in 1929, and many outbreaks of hog cholera have occurred since then. Because of the disease transmission hazard, feeding raw garbage to pigs has been made illegal, and some states have banned the feeding of cooked garbage as well. Undoubtedly, many people who keep one or two pigs for their own use continue to feed their own household garbage because it reduces the feed costs and helps to solve a disposal problem. There is nothing wrong with the practice provided raw meat scraps are not included. But for all practical purposes, garbage feeding in a commercial enterprise is no longer a consideration in swine nutrition.

The question, then, is what to feed for maximum economical rate of gain and for a minimum of nutrition-related disease problems. Perhaps because of its rapid growth rate and small stomach capacity compared with the ruminant, the pig seems more susceptible to disease conditions resulting from vitamin, mineral, or amino acid deficiencies. There is a wealth of information available as a result of intensive research on these conditions that, with a few exceptions, is beyond the scope of this book. Such information is important to the professional swine nutritionist responsible for formulating commercial rations. Most of the land-grant universities have good bulletins available on swine nutrition for those needing more detail, and there are a number of good texts on the subject. *Nutrient Requirements of Swine,* published by the NRC, is the most authoritative.

Formula Feed

If you are raising just a few pigs as a hobby or for your own use, probably the easiest way to avoid nutritional problems is to use a formula feed prepared by a reputable milling company for the class of pig you are feeding. Most companies have rations available as prestarters for pigs 1 to 4 weeks old, starters for pigs 1 to 4 months of age, finishers for pigs 4 months to market weight, and maintenance rations for sows and boars. Although perhaps not the least expensive approach, in the long run this may be the simplest course to follow.

If you have some homegrown feed available, however, it certainly can be used if a few basic nutritional needs of the pig are kept in mind. Pigs have a very limited capacity for roughage, and total fiber in the diet for young pigs

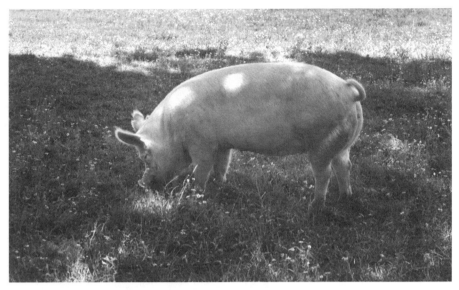

Pigs can make good use of pasture, but formula feeding is also an excellent option.

probably should not exceed 7 percent. For sows, there is some advantage to increasing this to 15 percent, to keep them from getting too fat and to reduce the problem of constipation so common when sows are put in crates at far-rowing time. Good-quality alfalfa or other legume hay can provide up to 20 percent of swine diets. This can be in the form of pasture or as alfalfa meal in the ration, with the balance being grain.

The general need of swine for diets containing 75 to 80 percent energy and 16 percent protein (higher for young growing pigs) dictates that most of the diet must be grain when both composition and economy are consid-ered. To avoid deficiency disease problems, ideally a combination of grains should be used.

Corn is an excellent source of energy for pigs. It is usually the cheapest and is commonly equated with fattening. Whenever we think of high-quality meat we usually think of "corn-fed" pork or "corn-fed" beef. During the short finishing period, a high percentage of corn *can* be used without difficulty. But if corn makes up most of the diet for the pig's lifetime, disease problems will occur because corn is deficient in the amino acids lysine and tryptophan, as well as in calcium and total protein. Without supplementa-tion, pigs maintained on a corn diet will suffer stunting and skeletal disease problems such as osteodystrophy. Using a mixture of grains will reduce this possibility.

Of course, the various amino acids, fatty acids, vitamins, or minerals that may be deficient in a diet can be supplemented. How much and what to add is a job for a professional nutritionist. Compared with the herbivores, such as cattle and horses, the pig is much more sensitive to dietary deficiencies because much less of the digestive process is done by microorganisms, which in the cow, for instance, synthesize the B vitamins the cow needs.

Health Problems

A few nutrition-related health problems, in addition to deficiencies, should be mentioned. Moldy feed should *never* be fed to pigs because pigs are extremely sensitive to the toxins that some molds produce. *Gibberella zeae,* a common grain mold, produces a toxin that has the same effect on the pig as female hormones. Sows and gilts fed diets contaminated with this mold have lowered conception rates and sometimes reddening and swelling of the vulva as well as enlargement of the mammary glands. The condition is reversible when the contaminated feed is removed, but it may take several months for normal fertility to be restored.

Baby pigs frequently suffer from iron-deficiency anemia because they are born with little iron reserve and sow's milk is very low in iron. Symptoms generally appear 1 to 3 weeks after birth and include listlessness and failure to grow. Perhaps the most dramatic symptom, aside from sudden death, is the oxygen deficiency that results in spasmodic contraction of the diaphragm and simultaneous expansion of the rib cage. Feeding additional iron to the sow has no value because it is not passed through in the milk.

Fortunately, the condition is readily preventable by several methods. One of the early and still widely used practices is to put a few chunks of sod in the pen where the baby pigs can root around in it and even lick or eat some of it. A second method is to swab the udder of the sow with a ferrous sulfate solution (1 pound in 3 quarts of water), so that when the piglets nurse, they also get some iron. Perhaps the most certain way to be sure they get adequate iron supplementation is by intramuscular injection of iron dextran when they are 2 or 3 days old. A number of preparations are commercially available for this purpose. Once piglets begin to eat some starter ration, their iron intake usually will be adequate to prevent further problems.

Use of Dairy Rations

Some people raising just a few pigs for their own use will feed them dairy ration or even horse feed. The pigs will usually do all right on it, but a note of caution should be injected regarding the use of dairy ration. Many formula dairy feeds contain urea, which, we have explained, the cow's rumen bacteria can convert into protein components. Pigs don't have this capacity, and if dairy ration is their only feed, protein deficiency may result, which will cause poor growth rates. If, for example, the tag on a 16 percent protein dairy ration feed bag says something like "contains 3 percent protein equivalent from nonprotein nitrogen sources (NPN)," it means that the feed actually contains only 13 percent natural protein. This would be too low for optimum long-term maintenance of swine. Urea by itself has no nutritional value, and it is also a highly toxic chemical when consumed in excess. It could easily kill a pig.

Salt and Water

Last, in addition to the usual nutrients, pigs need salt and a good supply of clean water at all times. On a comparative weight basis, pigs will consume twice as much water as dry feed; in hot weather, their consumption will double. Young growing pigs may drink water equivalent to 20 percent of their body weight daily, but as they get older, this amount declines to about 7 percent. In any case, the water should be fresh, preferably from fountains or drinking cups. If you must water them by hand, don't just add to what is left in the trough or pan. Empty it out and give them a clean supply daily, because any feed rinsed off their mouths when they drink will settle to the bottom, where it not only sours but also provides a good place for pathogenic bacteria such as *Salmonella* species to grow. For the same reasons, a mud hole is not a healthful water supply for pigs.

If you are using some homegrown grains to build your own swine ration, I'd strongly advise you to get some professional help in making up its formulation. Your local Cooperative Extension agent may be able to help, or will at least steer you in the right direction to get some help. Because you will need some supplements, your feed dealer can help, too. Making up a swine ration on a "by-guess-or-by-gosh" basis will sooner or later lead to deficiency disease problems, especially if your pigs are raised in total confinement where they must depend solely on you for a balanced diet.

Sheep and Goats

Some goat enthusiasts will no doubt take offense at having their favorite species lumped together with sheep in this brief discussion of nutrition. Let me assure them now that this is purely for pragmatic reasons. Very little work has been done on the specific nutrient needs of the goat. Anatomically and physiologically, as far as diet goes their needs are essentially the same as that of the cow and the sheep for proportional body weight.

Goats are unique in only one respect. Goats are browsers, and for its size the goat can consume substantially more foliage than the cow or the sheep. Goats will consume leaves and fresh twigs in preference to lush grass. Their ability to consume twice the volume makes it possible for goats to survive and produce milk on marginal pastures where a cow would starve. It is this capacity that makes goats the predominant food animal in many parts of the world. It does not, however, confer on them the ability to recycle tin cans, as some people seem to think. For a dairy goat to be productive, it must have adequate good pasture or hay to meet at least half its needs, with the balance coming from concentrates such as dairy ration. As a rule of thumb, the milking doe should get about ½ pound of dairy ration daily for each quart of milk produced, in addition to as much pasture or hay as she wants. Between lactations, pasture or hay alone will usually suffice. When fed in this manner, with a clean water supply available, a goat generally will have a minimum of nutrition-related health problems.

It is important, however, to keep in mind that goats tend to be finicky eaters and will often leave 10 to 15 percent of the forage offered. If you interpret this as an indication of overfeeding and then reduce the amount fed, a decline in milk production and body weight is likely to ensue. It's better to waste a little hay than to feed too little. Also, goats tend to develop a well-defined social order, and the dominant doe or buck may keep the others from getting their fair share.

The nutrient needs of sheep have been extensively studied. In fact, because of its size and economy, the sheep has served as the experimental model for most of the basic nutrition research that has subsequently been extrapolated to the cow. From this, you can correctly infer that the needs of the sheep are the same as those of the cow in proportion to its body weight. An important difference, however, is that cattle have about twice the copper requirement of sheep. Therefore, feeding cattle grain (rather than sheep grain) to sheep may result in copper toxicity.

For the person who keeps a few sheep as a hobby, with costs secondary to the pleasures of ownership, this knowledge simplifies the feeding problem. Good pasture or hay, supplemented with some grain during advanced pregnancy, will usually free the animals of nutritional problems. Commercially, however, the situation may be quite different. Sheep not only have a relatively low unit value but also the margin of profit is small. Because feed costs make up about 75 percent of the cost of production, this is where the greatest savings can be made. Unfortunately some growers try to save too much, and the end result is poor fertility, small lamb crops, reduced rate of gain, and a variety of disease problems — not the least of which is sometimes starvation.

The Right Combination

Sheep get along well on combinations of pasture, hay, silage, and grain. The possible combinations are almost infinite, and the choice will depend on available feeds and their cost. No single combination can be said to be the best, but the serious sheep grower can find guidance in the NRC recommendations referred to earlier or in the *Sheepman's Production Handbook*. (See page 330 for ordering information.)

While it's important to maintain sheep on an adequate diet, it's also important from a health standpoint to recognize that individual animals respond differently to the same nutrient intake and that nutritional needs vary depending on the status of the animal. With most species, the owner's eyeball is usually the best diagnostic tool to determine whether the animal is getting enough to eat. If your animals look thin, feed them more; if they look too fat, feed less. Except in the head of the experienced shepherd, however, the eyeball is not nearly as useful to determine the status of sheep, because of their wool covering. I have seen sheep that were actually emaciated and yet the owner was unaware of it. To determine body condition on a sheep, one has to feel down over the shoulder and loin with the fingertips. If all you feel is bone, you'd better feed them more. Conversely, if you have trouble feeling bone through the fat, feed them less.

Always remember that while we may have good data on the protein and energy needs of animals, the numbers given are only averages, not absolutes. Judgment must be used. Economically, it's important to feed sheep the minimum needed, recognizing that minimum needs change. For example a 140-pound dry ewe early in gestation will get along on about 3½ pounds of alfalfa hay daily without supplementation. The same ewe during the first months of lactation will need 5 pounds of alfalfa and ¾ pounds of corn daily and even then will probably lose some body weight. Like cows, most sheep cannot consume enough feed to replace the energy lost through high milk production. Especially in ewes with twins or triplets, this negative energy balance is largely responsible for *ketosis,* or "pregnancy disease." This common metabolic disease is largely preventable by keeping ewes on a minimum maintenance diet early in gestation to prevent obesity and then raising energy intake during the last 4 to 6 weeks of pregnancy and during early lactation.

Loose Salt

Like other livestock, sheep and goats need salt in addition to the usual nutrients. This should be fed loose rather than in salt blocks. Sheep are more inclined to bite a block rather than lick it like a cow or horse, and in so doing may break their teeth. Depending on diet, they usually need additional calcium and phosphorus. The best way to provide all three is to feed a mixture of equal parts of dicalcium phosphate and trace mineralized salt. This may be fed free choice. However, as a management technique for sheep at pasture, it's a good idea to hand-feed the mixture in a feed trough about once weekly. This not only gives you a chance to observe the flock at close quarters, but it also keeps the sheep accustomed to people in the pasture, making them easier to handle when the need arises. Especially for the novice, anything that makes sheep easier to handle is desirable.

Feeding Orphan Lambs

Orphan lambs, unfortunately, are a common part of the sheep business, and keeping them alive presents a problem. Sometimes a ewe with adequate milk and only a single offspring can be persuaded to adopt orphan lambs. But more often it's a bottle-feeding proposition best delegated to one of the children in the family. Cow's milk or milk replacer can be used with the lamb bottles and nipples commercially available or with a baby bottle. The orphans always should have colostrum early in life from their dam or another ewe. If calf milk replacer must be used, select one formulated for veal calf production that has a fat content of 25 percent or more. Older (3- to 4-week-old) lambs usually can be taught to drink from a nipple or from a conventional pail.

An ample supply of clean fresh water is important for all livestock. But it has added importance in preventing the common problem of urolithiasis, seen in wethers and rams. Because of anatomical differences, urolithiasis rarely happens in the female. This condition results when stones composed of precipitated mineral salts form in the urinary bladder and are flushed down the urethra, where they may lodge in the urethral process of the male. Especially in wethers on full feed, these calculi may plug several centimeters of the urethra. This makes urination difficult or impossible, and a ruptured bladder is the usual fatal sequel. Increased water intake to reduce the concentration of dissolved salts in the urine effectively reduces the prevalence of this condition. In the lamb feedlots where this condition is seen most frequently, it is common practice to encourage water consumption by adding additional salt up to 10 percent of the daily ration.

Summary

A great variety of nutrients is available to feed livestock. The ruminants — cattle, sheep, and goats — have similar needs as far as dietary components are concerned, and, generally speaking, the amounts needed vary only according to body weight and stage of lactation. The horse is closely related, although its energy needs are higher when working and its stomach capacity is less. The pig is quite different in its needs.

Remember that good nutrition is fundamental to good health. Deficiency diseases are usually insidious and slow in onset, and the response to correction of a deficiency in most cases is not dramatic. Diagnosis is often difficult. Help, if you need it, is available from your veterinarian, your Cooperative Extension agent, the animal science departments of the land-grant universities, and most of the larger feed companies. If you suspect a problem, don't hesitate to seek advice.

To prevent problems, use only good-quality nutrients undamaged by weather or spoilage, in recommended amounts, and keep a supply of fresh clean water available at all times.

Proper feeding of livestock has become a much more scientific process than it was formerly. There is a wealth of good research information available from the animal science departments of the land-grant universities pertaining to nutrient requirements and composition of feedstuffs. It remains for the herd manager to utilize this information to best advantage.

Even the process of ration formulation has been simplified. It is possible to buy computer programs that, when your data are entered, will do all of the calculations for you. The same type of service is available from most feed companies and animal science departments, and, in the major livestock production areas, from private nutrition consulting firms.

Remember, though, that nutrition recommendations are averages, not absolutes. No two animals respond alike, and the best scientific information available will not totally replace the judgment of the good herd manager.

Housing 3 and Health

HOUSING FOR ANIMALS may vary from nothing to palatial, depending on the species to be housed, the climate, and the resources of the owner. Whether facilities are dictated by the use to which the animals are put or are merely intended to provide protection from inclement weather, housing can have a significant effect on health.

This chapter offers a few suggestions, from a veterinarian's perspective, that will make animal housing facilities more satisfactory.

Cattle

The environment in which the cow is kept plays an important role in health. If survival is the only consideration, shelter requirements of cattle — regardless of temperature — are minimal. If cattle have enough to eat, they get along very nicely with nothing more than an open shed to provide shade in summer and protection from wind, snow, and freezing rain in winter. In fact, this is the way most beef cattle are kept. Range cattle manage to get along with nothing except perhaps a grove of trees as a windbreak. It's when humans intervene that health problems related to housing are likely to arise. Keep in mind, however, that when cattle are outside in cold weather, they utilize more energy to maintain body heat and must be fed accordingly.

Without exception, dairy cattle housing is designed to facilitate materials handling, to make milking more convenient, to comply with sanitary codes, and always to provide the owner with a way to handle cattle with minimum effort and maximum comfort. There is nothing wrong with these objectives, provided the health of the cow is considered, too. But when people build facilities for their cows, they often overlook or subordinate the cows' needs to their own personal comfort.

The Traditional Barn

The traditional dairy barn in northern climates has a concrete floor, with the cows confined to stanchions or tied in stalls. The barn is tightly enclosed in winter and body heat keeps it warm. High density of cows per square foot not only keeps construction costs to a minimum but also keeps the barn warmer. This sounds logical and efficient, but what does it imply for the cow?

The sanitary codes governing commercial milk production require that barn floors be constructed of impervious material and kept clean: concrete is really the only choice. Troweling the concrete smooth when installed facilitates cleaning but makes the floor so slippery it's a hazard for cows that must walk on it. Even if it isn't smooth when installed, it soon becomes smooth from constant cleaning and scraping.

To avoid falls, provide better footing for cows. Some dairy farmers scatter superphosphate on the barn floor to improve traction. In theory, this is good because it is also a valuable fertilizer when later spread on the land with the manure. In practice, it's poor because many of the superphosphate prills are round, making it somewhat like walking on marbles. Calcite, which is finely crushed limestone, provides excellent traction but the particles are sharp and get ground into the feet and cause lameness. Ground limestone is better than crushed limestone but tends to be slippery when wet. For good traction, nothing is better than sand or gravel spread lightly where the cows walk. A few wood shavings or sawdust add to the appearance and help keep the floor dry. Mechanical grooving of the floor is helpful, and some contractors provide this service.

Another health detriment inherent in the stanchion barn is lack of exercise. This contributes to rapid hoof growth, the need for more frequent hoof trimming, and, equally important, loss of muscle tone. When total body weight is considered, the dairy cow is not heavily muscled. In fact, the description of "a big bag of guts supported by four posts" is not inappropriate. When there is loss of muscle tone due to physical inactivity, the stage is set for difficulties at calving time. Some of the so-called downer cows following calving are that way because they don't have the strength to get up unassisted and often injure themselves trying. Entirely too many cows are unnecessarily lost this way.

The Stall Bed

The stall bed must be considered, too, because that's where the cow must stand or lie, day and night. Particularly in stanchion barns, the size of the stall is critical for the cleanliness, comfort, and health of the cow. Short stalls force the cow to stand with hind legs in the gutter; long stalls mean manure in the stall and on the udder; and narrow stalls increase teat injuries. Concrete stalls must be padded or bedded in some manner to protect the cow from the constant bruising and irritation that concrete causes. This becomes especially apparent on the hocks and knees. Adequate amounts of straw, dry shavings, sawdust, or shredded paper are satisfactory bedding, but because they are a recurring expense, many dairy farmers use heavy rubber mats designed for the purpose or even indoor-outdoor carpet. Either is a help, but the cows will stay cleaner if some additional bedding is used. Green hardwood sawdust or shavings and especially bark chips are *not* recommended for bedding because they may be contaminated with *Klebsiella* species, a bacterium that can cause mastitis.

Ventilation

Ventilation is another problem directly influencing health. Most barns have a combination of windows and forced ventilation to provide air circulation, and frequently the combination is inadequate. Inadequate ventilation leads to high humidity, condensation on ceiling and walls, and accumulation of stale air — an ideal environment for pneumonia to start in the herd. With an outside temperature of 50°F, for example, a ventilation rate of 174 cubic feet per minute is required per 1000 pounds of animal housed to maintain the inside temperature at 60°F. From a health standpoint, an inside temperature of 50°F in winter is preferable. The agricultural engineering departments at most of the land-grant universities have excellent technical bulletins on barn construction and ventilation available. Anyone contemplating barn construction should take advantage of their advice.

Avoiding Drafts

Another point should be emphasized with respect to ventilation and health. Cold is not harmful to the cow, but drafts can be deadly. In winter the cow stanchioned next to a broken or open window with cold air pouring in is almost certain to get pneumonia. If allowed to move, cows will always avoid these situations.

I was called some years ago as a consultant to investigate what was reported to be an unusual outbreak of calf pneumonia. It was midwinter and on this farm calves 3 months and older were consistently getting pneumonia. The mortality rate was very high. It didn't take long to confirm that the calves were dying from pneumonia; several had obvious signs of pneumonia when I was there. Nor did it take long to figure out the underlying cause.

This dairy farmer made it a practice to move calves to a separate barn after they were weaned. His "calf barn" was an old, former dairy barn oriented north and south on a hillside. One side of the barn was below grade and on the other, westerly, side he had built five box stalls, each large enough to hold five calves. Windows extended the whole length of the west side. Doors were located at the north and south ends and the south door was open. So far, so good. But windows adjacent to three pens were broken and the prevailing westerly wind at 10°F was whistling through those openings, with a velocity that must have approached 30 mph, directly on the calves in those pens. Even with a heavy coat on, I was uncomfortable examining the calves in the pens.

The answer to the problem was simple: Replace the broken glass in the windows to stop the draft. This was done and the mysterious pneumonia outbreak came to a rapid close. Ironically, this man's veterinarian had given him the same advice a month previously but he couldn't believe the answer was that simple. As he told me, "I thought fresh air was good for calves." It is, but not in a wind tunnel.

The Free-Stall Barn

One of the reasons for the rapidly increasing popularity of free-stall barns, aside from construction economy, is improved herd health. In free-stall barns cows are free to move about at will, the stall beds are elevated, bedded usually with deep sand or mattresses and sawdust, and the cows lie in them as they choose. The slippery-floor problem remains and, in fact, is worse than in the traditional barn, but because the cows move about at their leisure, falls are less frequent. They get some exercise, and drafts are not a problem because the cow can move. In fact, in the "cold" system of free-stall housing (open and uninsulated), only natural ventilation is required, if the design is right, to get an adequate change of air. Most dairy farmers with free-stall barns report improved reproductive performance because more pronounced signs of estrus make it easier to detect.

Even in northern climates we are now beginning to see free-stall barns built without rigid sides but with movable sidewall curtains that can be raised or lowered as wind conditions dictate. Greenhouse-type barns are receiving considerable attention as housing alternatives for calves and cows. They offer the advantages of economy, flexibility, and sunshine, which may keep animals healthier.

Teat Injuries

Another housing-related health problem is the matter of teat injury. This occurs with both traditional and free-stall housing systems but is more prevalent in stanchion barns, particularly when the stall beds are narrow or when the cows are fidgety because they have lice. Cows are not especially bright, are certainly clumsy, and seem to have a great propensity for stepping on one another's teats. Sometimes they even step on their own when they get up. A teat caught between concrete and the foot of an animal weighing over half a ton suffers a variety of injuries, ranging from, at the least, a severe bruise to amputation. In any case, it makes milking difficult and frequently leads to mastitis. This type of accident is more common when cows are spaced too close together. For the larger breeds such as the Holstein, stall beds should be at least 4 feet wide, and a partition between cows is helpful. A curb of concrete in stanchion barns or plank in free stalls at the bottom of the partition helps to keep the cow's feet away from her neighbor.

A word of caution about partitions, especially in free-stall barns: These should be designed so that cows can't get caught underneath them. Cows may suffer fractured legs or backs when they are caught under a partition and struggle to get up.

Teat injuries are much less frequent in free-stall barns because cows have more room to get up and down, and the bedding — whether it be sand, sawdust, or mattresses — is generally deeper and softer than in stanchion barns.

Without belaboring the point, it should be obvious by now that with a little forethought, many potential health problems can be eliminated by proper building design. If you are building a new barn or remodeling an old one, visit some newly constructed barns in your area to get some good ideas. And talk with your veterinarian. In practice, all of us see accidents to animals that could have been avoided, and we pick up ideas in the many barns that we visit in the course of our daily work.

Shelters and Sheds

If you are concerned only about the family cow or live in the South, discussion of construction and housing is moot. The family cow usually survives in whatever shelter is provided, although the same consideration should be given to ventilation, drafts, and floors. In warm climates, the shelter requirement is reversed and the prime necessity is shade. Similarly, the housing requirements for beef cattle are minimal. All they need is a dry place to lie down and protection from driving rain or snow. An open shed facing south in a well-drained area is adequate. A few translucent fiberglass panels in the shed roof let some sunlight in, making it more comfortable for the cattle.

Calf Housing

Housing probably has a greater influence on the health of dairy calves than on any other class of cattle. Because of their vulnerability to infectious diseases, calves ideally should be kept isolated from one another and from other animals. Unfortunately, this adds to housing costs and labor requirements, but some practical compromises have been developed.

The system of having a pen in the barn, in which calves are kept loose and to which new ones are added as they are born, is most likely to lead to disease problems and so has fallen out of favor. Most commercial dairy farmers are moving away from this housing method as rapidly as possible. The typical history of calf pens is that for the first year or so, health problems are minimal. But in the second and ensuing years, they increase to a point where every calf

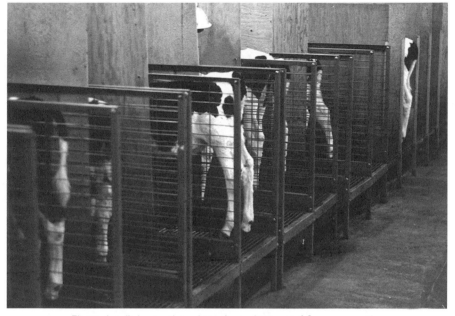

Elevated stalls keep calves clean, dry, and separated from one another.

put in the pen will develop diarrhea, septicemia, or pneumonia and die. Calf pens are difficult to keep clean and dry, and they are often located in a section of the barn that is difficult to ventilate. These problems are compounded if sunlight is not available. Together, these factors create an ideal environment for pathogens to survive, and when new susceptible calves are constantly added to the group, the level of pathogens such as *Escherichia coli* and *Salmonella* species increases rapidly, infecting every calf. Any factor that then lowers resistance results in disease.

Use Pens in Rotation

It's well established that, to use this housing system successfully over a period of years, more than one pen must be available and pens must be used in rotation. If a pen can be vacated, thoroughly cleaned and disinfected (preferably with steam), and left vacant for 6 to 8 weeks, pathogens in it will die and it can be used again.

Elevated Calf Stall

A modification of this system that works well is the elevated calf stall, in which calves are kept tied until weaned. These are often built on skids in units of four so that the whole assembly can be moved outside for cleaning and left out in the sunlight to kill any pathogenic organisms. This system has the advantage of preventing direct contact among calves. It makes it easier to observe individuals for signs of illness and gives calves a dry place to lie down; cleaning the floor underneath is also easier. This system is widely used in commercial veal production.

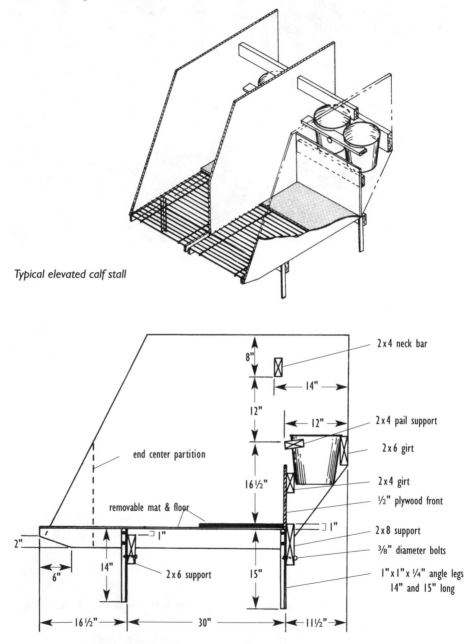

Typical elevated calf stall

Cross-section layout plan for elevated calf stall

Calf Hutch

From a disease-control standpoint, probably the best innovation is the calf hutch. This is a small open shed, usually made with three and one-half sheets of 4×8 exterior plywood, and has a small exercise area attached that is designed to accommodate one calf. Commercially available translucent fiberglass hutches are even better.

Hutches provide isolation, ventilation, and sunlight, all of which are important. Furthermore, they can be moved easily to clean ground before the next calf is brought in, so pathogen buildup is not a problem. Of course, it is cold in the winter, but this is only a problem for the person feeding the calves. With ample bedding, calves in hutches tolerate below-zero temperatures very well and, in fact, will be far healthier than in a warm barn. It should be noted, however, that the feed (energy) requirement of calves increases up to two to three times normal during extended

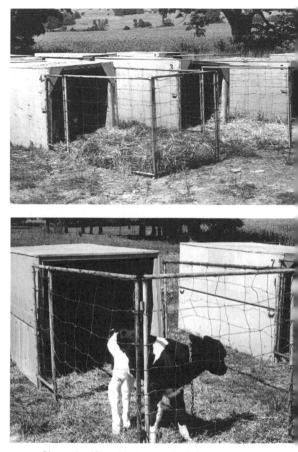

Plywood calf hutches provide isolation, ventilation, and sunlight.

below-zero temperature periods, and they should be fed accordingly.

Choice of the optimum housing system for dairy calves is a trade-off between disease risk for the calf and labor-saving convenience for the operator. No system rates highest in both categories except perhaps the old method of putting three or four calves with a good motherly nurse cow and turning them loose at pasture. Economically, even that has disadvantages.

Maternity Pens

A word should also be said here about the use of maternity stalls or pens. For a variety of reasons, not the least of which is comfort of the cow, it's common practice to put cows into box stalls just prior to calving so they have ample room to move at will when parturition is imminent. A dimension of roughly 10 feet by 10 feet is adequate, and it's a good idea to have a strong ring fastened to the ceiling to which a sling can be attached to help the cow to her feet after calving, if necessary. Ideally, for reasons that will become apparent, the walls and floors of the maternity pens should be constructed of impervious material that is easily cleaned and disinfected.

There is little doubt that, on many dairy farms, problems with metritis and mastitis in the cow, as well as navel infection, septicemia, and diarrhea in newborn calves, can be traced directly to contaminated maternity pens. When the same pens are in constant use, a buildup of pathogens occurs that makes infection inevitable. The pens must be cleaned and disinfected thoroughly after each use. Construction with smooth impervious material makes the job easier, especially when the floor slopes toward a drain so that ample water can be used.

Electrical System

Last, be sure your electrical system is in good repair and properly grounded. There is nothing more disconcerting than seeing a whole row of cows drop to their knees because of electric shock when the milking machine pump or the water pump is turned on. While that is an extreme that doesn't happen often, a low-voltage tingle, called *stray voltage,* which makes cows very uneasy, is fairly common. It can originate anywhere on the line, and it may require the help of a master electrician and the power company to find the source. If the cow associates the tingle with the milking machine, a precipitous drop in milk production is likely to occur.

Electrically heated water troughs or buckets in the cold free-stall barn are also a potential source of electric shock. Be sure the wiring is properly done and is in good repair. Use of metallic water pipe instead of plastic helps ensure that grounding is adequate.

Horses

Housing for horses generally is more dependent on the desires of the owner than on the needs of the horse. In terms of need, horses are akin to beef cattle, and an open shed or other windbreak is adequate. In fact, it is not unusual to see horses, if they have a choice, out in a pasture on the most inclement winter day pawing through the snow to reach a bit of grass, even though there is hay in the shed under cover where they could be. We are talking, of course, about the minimum needs of the horse that has grown a winter hair coat and is being left to his own devices. The horse that is kept groomed and ready for the show circuit all year is a different matter. This horse requires warmer housing and, in very cold weather, blanketing as well.

The show horse usually is kept in a box stall and perhaps put in an exercise yard during the day. The type of barn in which the stall is located is limited only by the imagination and financial resources of the owner. Nevertheless, the same need for fresh air in a draft-free environment prevails for the same reasons given in the section on cattle housing.

Flooring

There are some peculiarities of the horse that influence the choice and design of housing for health. Fortunately, the sanitary codes that require impervious flooring for dairy cattle do not apply to horses, because concrete is perhaps the least desirable flooring material for the horse. Clay or a mixture of clay and sand covered with a bedding material of some sort is very good. Clean, bright straw makes a good absorbent bedding, but some horses will eat it. This provides the opportunity for worm infestation when the bedding is contaminated with manure, but, more important, it takes the place of the nutritious hay that the horse needs. The horse that makes a habit of filling up on straw will gradually lose weight because the straw is high in fiber and low in both protein and digestible energy. For horses that eat straw bedding, something less palatable such as wood shavings can be used. Keep an eye on your horses bedded with shavings, though. Some of them, out of curiosity, will eat enough shavings to cause indigestion.

Accidents related to housing conditions are probably more common with horses than with any other species. Horses tend to be quick in their movements and are more inclined, with a quick toss of the head, to break unprotected lightbulbs or windows. This may cause serious lacerations. For the same reason, the stalls and areas where horses walk should be free from projecting nails or sharp protrusions of any kind. This also applies to the fencing around the exercise yard. The horse has a thin skin that cuts very easily. At best, a laceration will probably leave a scar; at worst, it may lead to tetanus and death. With a little care on the owner's part, this type of accident is easily preventable.

Cribbing

Some horses, out of boredom, develop a habit called *cribbing*, in which they will bite and chew on the edge of a board, and at the same time arch the neck and swallow air. This leads to indigestion, colic, an unthrifty horse, and an unsightly stall. To reduce this possibility, build or alter the stall so that insofar as possible there will be no edges for the horse to grab. Where an edge can't be prevented, such as the top edge of the gate or door, sheathing the top 4 to 6 inches with sheet metal will help.

Last, be sure the stall is strong enough that the horse can't kick a hole in it. This is more likely to happen when horses are kept in adjoining stalls. The average horse easily can kick a hole in a 1-inch board and, in fact, can knock down a whole wall constructed of such light material. In so doing, the horse is very likely to injure his legs. To avoid such injuries, the lower 4 feet of the stall should be plank, preferably oak, 2 inches thick.

Hauling Horses

One more thing, although not directly related to housing, has bearing on it, and that is the trailers and trucks used to haul horses. One of the factors contributing to the popularity of the horse is the ease of mobility using modern trailers. It's not at all unusual to put a horse in a trailer behind the family car and travel 100 miles to take part in a show and return the same day. Before you load your horse in a vehicle, be sure that the vehicle is strong enough to carry the load. I think the most pitiful sight I ever saw was a horse who had one foot fall through the rotted floor of a trailer. The foot was caught and dragged there until it was worn off up to the coronet by the pavement. All I could do was put the suffering horse to sleep, and I was sorely tempted to do the same to the owner. Such accidents are not bad luck. They are the result of carelessness and stupidity.

With regard to health and housing for the horse, perhaps the best rule of thumb to keep in mind is that what can go wrong probably will. Granted, horses shouldn't kick holes in the wall, get tangled in the wire, or step in the hole, but sooner or later they do, and injury results. Perhaps because of the closeness that develops between horse and owner, we tend to attribute a measure of intelligence to them that is undeserved. When it comes to accidents, the behavior of the horse is perhaps the least predictable of the large domestic animals. It's up to us to foresee the potential hazards and eliminate them before accidents occur.

Swine

The nature of the beast and the business tends to make several aspects of swine housing unique from a health standpoint. Separation or isolation of susceptible individuals is a valid fundamental of disease control that must be compromised in the swine operation, first because pigs come in litters rather than singly, and second because profitable swine production is a high-volume business. To the hobbyist with only one or two pigs, this is less of a concern, but even then the need for good sanitation and management prevails.

The housing needs of different age groups of pigs vary, with the farrowing house being most critical. Because of the need for good sanitation, ventilation, and environmental temperature control, the commercial farrowing house is usually a specialized building used for that purpose only. In fact, it is possible to buy prefabricated farrowing houses that outwardly resemble mobile homes. When moved to the site and when utilities are connected, the farrowing houses are ready for operation. With liquid manure handling, forced ventilation, automatic feeders, electric heat, and other conveniences installed, these farrowing houses are a delight to behold, but baby pigs will die in them just as fast as anywhere else if you forget the basics of disease control.

Preventing Infection

Preventing spread of infection by separation of susceptible individuals is one of the basics of disease control. But how do you separate newborn pigs that come a dozen or more at a time and that all have to nurse the same sow? Obviously, modifications have to be made.

Two things are important. One is to prevent the introduction of contagious disease. As part of this effort related to housing, place a conspicuous sign on the door of the farrowing house asking visitors to stay out. Some swine diseases can be carried from farm to farm on clothing and equipment. The other thing that helps to cut down disease spread is scrupulous cleanliness in the farrowing house, paying particular attention to feeding equipment, floors, and farrowing crates. The risk of spreading disease will be reduced further if separate cleaning equipment, shovels, brooms, and buckets are kept in the farrowing house and not used anywhere else.

I recall some years ago being asked to investigate a long-standing problem of high baby pig mortality. For several years, half or more of every litter born would be dead within a week, despite the use of all kinds of medications. Diarrhea, lack of appetite, weakness, and death were commonplace, and a major contributing factor was obvious. The farrowing area was incredibly filthy, with sour feed in the troughs and manure not only built up on the floor but also spattered to the ceiling. Ironically, this was on a state prison farm, where, considering the cost and availability of labor, the place should have been spotless. The manager simply didn't recognize the importance of sanitation and was an advocate of the popular fallacy that pigs are inherently dirty animals. Nothing could be further from the truth. Given the opportunity, pigs will be as clean or cleaner than most other species.

Protecting Baby Pigs

Apart from the need for good sanitation, there are some other specialized requirements in the farrowing house. One of these is heat in the colder climates. Baby pigs are born with virtually no hair and little if any body fat to insulate them from the cold. Chilling is a common cause of death. To prevent it, supplemental heat to provide a temperature of about 85 to 90°F at floor level is necessary for the first two or three days, after which it can be reduced gradually. Heat lamps are used for this purpose, but a word of caution is in order, especially if you use heat lamps on a temporary, makeshift basis. Be sure the wiring is adequate to carry the load, and be sure, too, that the lamps are far enough away from combustible bedding, such as straw, so you don't end up with barbecued pigs instead of warm pigs. The ideal way to warm the floor is with hot-water pipes or hot-air ducts buried in the concrete.

Another consideration in the farrowing house is a means of protecting the baby pigs from their mother. A clumsy 300-pound sow lying down can flatten a

2-pound piglet. This kind of accident happens too often, especially when the sow and piglets are in a pen or box stall. One way of reducing the risk when a pen is the only farrowing place available is to fasten a strong rail around the inside of the pen 6 inches out from the wall and about 8 inches above the floor. This provides an avenue of escape for a piglet that might otherwise be crushed against the wall. A better device used almost universally by commercial hog producers is the farrowing crate. This is a steel framework that gives the sow freedom to eat, drink, stand, or lie down but keeps her in one place, reducing the opportunity for her to lie on the pigs. Except when nursing, the piglets will stay alongside the crate under the heat lamp or brooder, whichever is provided.

Every precaution must be taken to avoid introducing infectious diseases into the farrowing house. This begins with preparation of the sow. Sows should be immunized against the common diseases such as erysipelas and leptospirosis, of course. But beyond that they should be scrubbed thoroughly with soap and warm water before being put into the farrowing house. This removes dirt and manure that usually is teeming with bacteria and frequently with worm eggs as well. A preparation room adjacent to the farrowing house where washing can be done with a reasonable degree of convenience and comfort for both sow and operator, regardless of the weather, is a necessity for a farrowing operation of any size.

The Farrowing House Floor

Some attention should be given to the farrowing house floor. Concrete is most satisfactory for ease of cleaning, but very smooth, slippery floors are a major contributing factor to the condition known as *spraddle-legged pigs*. New concrete should not be troweled smooth, nor should it be brushed to leave it rough because the roughness causes abrasions on the piglets' knees and legs. Once over with a wooden float is about right. If you are stuck with an existing facility that has a glass-smooth floor, it can be mechanically roughened or you can use bedding on the floor. Some people use wooden floors successfully in the farrowing house, but they are difficult to clean and sanitize. However, they are warmer and more comfortable for the pigs.

Once the piglets are weaned, usually at 4 weeks of age, they can be separated from the sow and grouped together in another building. What happens to them thereafter depends on the type of swine operation. In some instances, they will be sold as feeder pigs at about 40 pounds body weight. In other cases, they will be fed to market weight (200–220 pounds) on the original farm.

Ventilation and Sanitation

In any event, housing for the older pigs is much less critical from a health standpoint as long as ventilation and sanitation are adequate. Inside temperatures should be above freezing, preferably about 50°F in winter and no warmer than outside air temperature in summer. The latter can be a major problem on a hot day. The body heat of a large number of pigs in a building dependent on forced ventilation can quickly increase the inside temperature to well over 100°F on a summer day if the electric power goes off. Pigs have a dismal cooling system and are extremely vulnerable to heatstroke. Therefore, if you are operating a confinement-raising system, a standby generator is a worthwhile investment.

One innovation that has made total confinement finishing systems practical is the use of slotted floors and liquid manure handling systems. In these the pigs trample manure down through slots in the floor to a pit underneath. This eliminates the need for manure removal in the pens, greatly reducing the labor requirements. However, a means of ventilating the manure pit should be provided. As manure decomposes, methane gas is produced. It is highly explosive. In Iowa some years ago, a spark ignited methane in a manure pit and the resulting explosion blew the finishing house and pigs sky-high.

Sheep and Goats

One of the factors leading to the current popularity of the goat and one making sheep raising economically feasible is that housing requirements are minimal. Except for the very young, a good windbreak or shed to provide protection from severely inclement weather is all that is required. However, the dairy goats will produce a little more and it's certainly easier for the milker if dairy goats are housed in a stable in winter, but the health-related housing requirements are not unique. A word of advice to those selling goat milk: The product sometimes gets a bad name because of objectionable odors and flavor. Have the milking room separate from the stable and keep it, the milking stand, and the milking utensils scrupulously clean. By doing so you will have a tasteful, nutritious product.

Sheep require extra attention at lambing time, and a lambing shed is a necessity in the North not only for the comfort of the ewe but for the survival of the lambs as well. Sheep tend to be seasonal breeders, and lambs are usually born in early spring when weather is likely to be the worst. The lambs are wet and often weak when born, so supplemental heat for a short period is usually a necessity. For the small flock, heat lamps are probably the most practical heat source. Check the adequacy of wiring and the proximity of combustible bedding. Don't set the shed on fire with them.

Washroom and Hot Water

It's not unusual for ewes and sometimes does to require assistance when giving birth. This means that you will need clean warm water available to thoroughly scrub the vulva and surrounding area before putting a hand in to straighten out a twisted lamb or kid. And you will need water to clean yourself up after you get through. Cleanliness is absolutely essential to prevent uterine infection following lambing, and the cleanup job will be more thorough if the materials to do it are readily at hand. Therefore, a washroom with ample hot water available should be part of the lambing shed. I might add that you may find your veterinarian more responsive to a call for help with parturition problems if he knows you have a decent place where he can clean up before he goes on to the next call.

Summary

A few suggestions have been presented in this chapter that will help to prevent some of the housing-related health problems that veterinarians and livestock owners see. Keep in mind, however, that there is no one best system and that livestock housing frequently must be governed by circumstances unrelated to animal welfare.

But regardless of the constraints imposed by finances and other matters, keep the comfort and safety of your animals uppermost in mind. Be safety conscious! Pick up the loose wire, junk, machinery, and other obstacles in the pasture. Pull out the projecting nails and other sharp objects in the barn where animals move. The injuries these cause are easily avoided if you look ahead and anticipate what might happen.

Animal housing facilities need not be warm, but they must be dry, well-ventilated, and free from drafts. Above all, keep the animal quarters clean. All it takes is a little ambition and energy, and if you don't have that, you shouldn't have animals. It's heartbreaking to see the conditions under which some people keep their livestock and the needless health problems that arise. If you have any doubt about the adequacy of your facilities, ask yourself this simple question: "Even if I had a fur coat, would I be comfortable living in there?" If the answer is no, some changes are in order.

Animal Reproduction

WHILE IT MAY SEEM STRANGE to include reproduction in a book on animal health, veterinarians get more questions about reproduction and infertility than about any other condition, and nothing else is more vital to a profitable livestock enterprise. While we could survive without meat and milk, most of us would find vegetables and grain a rather dull diet. Furthermore, cattle, sheep, and goats can convert otherwise useless roughage into high-quality protein and energy to supplement the world's food supply, so it's important that we keep them producing and reproducing.

Reproduction is truly a remarkable process that, for many people, is also mysterious. In the next few pages I try to remove some of the mystery by describing the reproductive functions common to all species and then pointing out differences that make the various livestock species unique, starting with the male, the most important individual in livestock breeding and often the most neglected. Why the most important? First, because the traits of the herd sire will appear in all the offspring in the herd, whereas the dam will influence only her own progeny. Second, if the herd sire is sterile, there will be no herd offspring. If the dam is infertile, she is the only one affected.

Male Anatomy

The primary sex glands of the male are the two testicles. During embryonic and fetal development, the testicles are formed within the abdominal cavity. Just prior to or soon after birth they descend through the inguinal canal into an external pouch called the *scrotum*. Each testicle has its own nerve and blood supply and a duct called the *vas deferens* connecting to the urethra. Sperm cells, or *spermatozoa,* are transported through the vas deferens, and a section of it is removed in the sterilizing operation called a *vasectomy.* Occasionally one or both testicles fail to descend, leading to conditions called *monorchidism* and *cryptorchidism,* respectively. A cryptorchid animal will have the external sex characteristics of a male but will be sterile if the testicles remain within the abdomen. If the testicles are near the external inguinal ring, the animal may or may not be fertile. If only one testicle is undescended, the animal will be fertile.

Cryptorchidism sometimes presents a dilemma when castration to control aggressive behavior or to render an animal sterile is a consideration. Removal of only the descended testicle will not change behavior and may or may not make the animal sterile. But it greatly complicates the surgical procedure if a decision is made later to go in and find the undescended testicle, because there is usually no way to tell which side it is on. Castration of the monorchid should be done completely the first time to avoid confusion later. Castration of the cryptorchid is a major surgical procedure requiring general anesthesia and aseptic technique.

Testicular Functions

The testicles serve two primary functions. They are the source of the male hormone, *testosterone,* which gives the male his secondary sex characteristics, larger size, heavy shoulders, and deeper voice. It also influences aggressive behavior and *libido,* or sex drive. The testicles also produce spermatozoa in a gradual developmental process called *spermatogenesis.* As the animal reaches sexual maturity, or puberty, mature sperm cells are produced constantly by the millions. Fertility of the male is governed primarily by the numbers of live sperm cells produced and libido. Sperm count is influenced by general health and frequency of ejaculation. It declines during prolonged illness, periods of fevers, and strangely enough periods of high environmental temperature.

Nature has provided a way to maintain the testicles at a temperature slightly below body temperature for maximum fertility. On a hot day, involuntary muscles relax, allowing the testicles to drop farther from the body in the scrotum. Conversely, on a cold day they will be drawn close to the body wall. The "short scrotum" method of castrating bull calves destined for the feedlot capitalizes on this phenomenon. With this technique, the testicles are left intact but the lower half of the scrotum is removed so that the testicles are held tightly against the body wall, where the higher temperature inhibits spermatogenesis. The advantage claimed is that testosterone production continues, resulting in a larger animal with improved rate of gain, but I advise against this technique if the goal is to guarantee infertility.

The secondary sex organ of the male is the penis. It has a rich blood supply that becomes important in erection. The penis must be fully erect before copulation can occur. The mechanisms by which this occurs comprise a simple lesson in hydraulics. Blood comes in under arterial pressure and returns, in part, through spongy cavernous tissue, sometimes called *erectile tissue.* When the animal is sexually aroused, the return blood flow is restricted by smooth muscle contraction. Pressure then builds in the cavernous tissue. The penis becomes extended, enlarges some in diameter, especially in the horse, and becomes rigid. This change is completely involuntary and cannot be controlled by the animal. It is the result of external sex stimuli, such as sight and smell, coupled with libido. Libido is most marked in young animals and sometimes leads to aberrant behavior, such as mounting other males or masturbation. With young healthy animals, except boars, libido is rarely absent. Some young boars, especially if exposed to an aggressive, domineering sow, must be taught what their function is.

Female Anatomy

While the anatomy and physiology of the male reproductive system is quite uncomplicated, that of the female is considerably more complex. This complexity probably accounts for infertility problems, which are more frequent in the female. The primary sex glands of the female are the two ovaries, located, roughly, behind the kidneys and supported by the broad ligament attached to the uterus. Like the testicles, the ovaries serve a dual role, production of germ cells, called *ova,* and hormones. Unlike the male, in whom new sperm cells are constantly developing, the female is born with all the ova that she will ever have. They are released in a precisely orchestrated sequence of events controlled by several interacting hormones. This sequence is called the *estrous cycle,* and although its length varies in different species, the events are the same.

The Estrous Cycle

The estrous cycle is initiated by a portion of the brain called the *hypothalamus,* which acts through the pituitary gland located at the base of the brain. The pituitary gland produces follicle-stimulating hormone (FSH). This hormone brings about the development of follicle on the ovary. Follicles normally occur singly in the mare and the cow but are multiple in the sow and are frequently in pairs in the ewe and doe. In the cow, the follicle resembles a large blister on the surface of the ovary and when mature will be about half the size of the ovary. The follicle contains an ovum and is lined with specialized cells that produce the estrogenic hormones, estrone and estradiol. These hormones have a twofold effect. In animals they bring about the period of sexual desire called *estrus,* or heat, and they initiate changes in the cellular lining of the uterus to prepare it for attachment of a fertilized ovum.

Through a feedback mechanism, as estrogen levels peak and the follicle reaches maturity, further production of FSH is inhibited and, in its place, luteinizing hormone (LH) is produced by the pituitary gland. Luteinizing hormone brings about rupture of the follicle and release of the ovum, and counteracts estrogen to terminate signs of heat. It also initiates development of a *corpus luteum,* or yellow body, at the site of the ruptured follicle. The corpus luteum, through its production of progesterone, plays an essential role in the attachment and maintenance of the fertilized ovum. It also temporarily overrides or counteracts further FSH production. If the animal becomes pregnant, the placenta produces additional progesterone, which prevents resumption of the estrous cycle for the duration of the pregnancy. If pregnancy does not occur, FSH levels again increase and the entire cycle is repeated.

A Multistep Process

Numerous physiological changes that we haven't yet mentioned take place during the estrous cycle. To provide a sense of the complexity of the reproductive process, some of these changes are mentioned below in the sequence in which they occur.

■ **Proestrum:** The period during which the follicle is enlarging. Concurrently, there is an increase in the growth of cells and cilia lining the oviduct, in the blood supply to the endometrium (uterine lining), and in the amount of mucus produced in the vagina. In the sow, the vulva swells slightly, and in all species there is increased muscular activity of the oviduct and uterus. Estrogen levels are increasing and the corpus luteum from the previous cycle is rapidly getting smaller.

■ **Estrum:** The period during which the female is receptive to the male and will stand to be mounted. The uterus is contracted, the cervix is dilated, and mucus in the vagina is copious. *Ovulation,* or release of the ovum, occurs soon after the period of estrum.

■ **Diestrum:** A period of several days during which the corpus luteum is developing and producing progesterone, which brings about what might best be described as a return to the status quo. The estrogen level drops rapidly and the uterus becomes soft and relaxed. In the cow, there may be some capillary bleeding from the endometrium, with blood visible at the vulva or on the tail about 48 to 72 hours after signs of estrum have passed. This can be a very useful indicator of the stage of estrus. Some cows, especially high-producing ones, do not show strong signs of heat and it's difficult to know when to breed them. If you see blood on the tail, you know a heat period has just passed. About half of cows will conceive if you breed them artificially 18 days later, whether or not they show signs of heat.

■ **Anestrum:** Best described as a resting period during which little uterine or ovarian activity takes place. Anestrum is prolonged in the mare during late fall and early winter and in the ewe and doe during late spring and summer. These species are called *seasonally polyestrous* because they cycle seasonally. The cow and the sow, on the other hand, cycle year-round and are called *polyestrous.* The mare is polyestrous, except in late fall and early winter.

While the foregoing discussion has outlined the principal hormonal activity and its effects in the female, the thyroid and adrenal glands play a role as well. Other factors are important, too. An animal that is well fed will reach sexual maturity earlier and will cycle regularly. Those whose energy intake is low often fail to cycle. Generally, fertility will be best when the animal is in a weight-gaining condition. But, of course, this can be carried to an extreme; obesity is also a cause of infertility.

Sight, sound, and smell play a less well-defined role, but it is well known that putting a boar near a pen of gilts or a stallion near a mare will often initiate signs of heat. Hours of daylight influence the onset of the estrous cycle in the mare, and the use of artificial light will often advance the time of first estrus in the spring. Extremes of temperature, especially heat, induce a stress that interferes with reproduction and is a major problem for dairy farmers in southern climates. With so many factors involved in the estrous cycle alone, it's remarkable that reproductive failures are not more frequent.

Conception

Assuming that all systems are functioning normally, the follicle ruptures, marking the end of estrus or standing heat, and the ovum is released. It is trapped in the open, funnel-shaped, fimbriated end of the oviduct and is worked down in the oviduct toward the horns of the uterus. The oviduct is a tubelike structure (about the diameter of a pencil lead in the cow) that leads from the ovary to the tip of the uterine horn. It is lined with ciliated cells and mucus-producing cells whose action and secretions help move the ovum to its final destination in the uterus. The trip requires about 3 days in the sow and 5 days in the other domestic species.

A Y-shaped organ in domestic animals, the uterus consists of two horns and a body. It has a capacity for tremendous distention during advanced pregnancy and a very rapid return to normal size following birth of the fetus. The normal nonpregnant uterus in the cow and mare can easily be held in both hands and is proportionately smaller in other species. It has a rich blood supply and a cellular lining, the *endometrium,* that responds to hormonal influence. The fertilized ovum develops to maturity in the uterus. The uterus is separated from the vagina by the *cervix,* a firm muscular band that during pregnancy remains tightly closed. It relaxes slightly during estrus, and during parturition dilates to a point where it is almost imperceptible. Incomplete dilation makes parturition difficult, if not impossible, and may lead to tears or lacerations that occasionally cause complications, such as scar tissue or incomplete closure, which impairs subsequent fertility. The cervix opens into the vagina, which in turn is open to the outside world at the vulva.

Copulation

During copulation, the male mounts the female and thrusts the erect penis into the vagina, a process called *intromission.* Intromission, or copulation, terminates with ejaculation of semen at the cervical opening. The female seeks out, and in fact will tolerate, this procedure only during the period of standing heat. Depending on the libido of the male, copulation will take place several times during the heat period. Frequency, duration of coitus, and volume of ejaculate vary with different species. Keep in mind that simply because the male goes through the right motions doesn't mean he is fertile. He can look and act normal and be sterile. For that reason, test matings, or fertility examination of the male prior to the breeding season, are a good investment.

Sperm cells have the capacity of independent movement with the aid of the *flagellum*, or long tail, that swishes back and forth to propel them through the copious mucus that is always present during estrus. This, coupled with capillary action and muscular contractions in the uterus and oviducts, transports spermatozoa through the genital tract quite rapidly. Bovine spermatozoa have been found at the ovarian end of the oviduct 2 to 4 minutes after deposition at the cervix. Despite this rapid transport, attrition of spermatozoa en route is high. Although millions of spermatazoa are deposited during ejaculation, only a few hundred get into the oviduct where fertilization takes place, and they rarely remain viable more than 24 hours. Similarly, the fertile life of the ova is short — only about 12 hours. Timing of the mating, therefore, becomes extremely critical except, of course, when the animals are left to their own devices and nature takes its course. Then repeated copulation removes the element of timing chance.

Fertilization

Only one active sperm cell is necessary for fertilization to take place, but the sperm cell must be at the right place at the right time. With frequent natural breeding during the heat period, spermatozoa will be in the oviduct at the time of ovulation. With artificial insemination, however, the timing may not be as precise, leading to conception failures. Fertilization takes place in the oviduct, at which time a single sperm cell will penetrate the ovum and all others will be blocked out.

Each germ cell, sperm and ovum, contains half the normal complement of chromosomes for the species. The cow, for example, has sixty pairs of chromosomes. Each chromosome contains the genes that determine the physical characteristics of the offspring. At fertilization, these combine in a random manner so that no two offspring of the same mating will be identical, but each will have some of the characteristics of both parents. Cell division commences immediately following fertilization and about 3 to 5 days later the aggregation of cells, at this time called a *zygote*, arrives in the uterus. At this point the corpus luteum has formed, and progesterone from it has brought about the changes in the uterine lining necessary for attachment and further development of the embryo.

In animals such as the pig, a dozen or more ova are fertilized at the same time, but otherwise the process is the same. As a matter of interest, if the sow is bred to more than one boar during the heat period, as is commonly done, spermatozoa from different boars will fertilize different ova, so the piglets, although born at the same time, will be half brothers or half sisters, genetically related to each other only on the sow's side.

Twinning

In animals such as the mare and cow that normally have single births, twinning, if it is going to occur, is determined at this time. Twins can form in two different ways. The more common is when two ova are released from the ovary and fertilized. In this case the twins will not be identical, since there is a different combination of genes in each zygote. Identical twins result when a fertilized ovum divides into two independent cells that then continue to develop in the normal manner. While identical twins may be considered a developmental accident, there is some hereditary predisposition to multiple ovulation in some individuals and families.

In *uniparous* animals (animals having a single offspring), the embryo usually develops in the uterine horn on the same side where ovulation occurred, whereas in multiparous species such as the pig, the zygotes will be spaced throughout both uterine horns. Development of the zygote to an embryo is by cell division and differentiation. Without going into all the details of embryology, suffice to say that different cell types form that develop into muscle, bone, nerve, tissue, and so on, in a coherent manner that ultimately terminates in a functional animal at the time of birth. Occasionally, cellular differentiation and organization gets disorganized, resulting in a fetal monster. This can be caused by exposure to chemicals and poisonous plants during gestation.

Some of these cells become the *placenta,* a membranous three-layered sac within which the fetus develops. It is attached to the uterine wall and is filled with fluid. On the fetal side, it is, for descriptive purposes, an outgrowth of the umbilical cord. The umbilical blood vessels branch out through it to the point of uterine attachment. The type of attachment varies in different species from sixty to seventy isolated structures called *cotyledons* in ruminants, to complete attachment, called *diffuse placentation,* in the pig. Function is the same in any case, and it is through the placenta that the fetus gets nutrients from the dam and eliminates the waste products of cell metabolism. There is no direct interchange of blood between the dam and the fetus, the only exception being when as a result of rare injury there is some bleeding from the uterine lining. The placenta is a very important structure for the well-being of the fetus, and anything that disrupts it may result in abortion. It is a common site of infection by bacteria, viruses, and fungi. Diseases causing abortion, such as brucellosis, affect the placenta primarily.

Rate of Growth

Because fetal development takes place by cell division in geometric progression, rate of growth accelerates throughout gestation, with the greatest increase in size coming during the last third of pregnancy. Allowance must be made for this in the feeding program or the dam will lose weight during late pregnancy. It's a marvel of nature that with an inadequate diet the pregnant animal will utilize all her stored reserves of energy, protein, vitamins, and minerals for fetal nourishment at her own expense and can be at the verge of death from starvation before any adverse changes in the fetus occur. This is not as true in humans, where protein deficiency in the maternal diet has been linked to some types of mental retardation in the newborn.

When all goes according to plan, pregnancy terminates in parturition, or birth of the young. This is often a time of anxiety for the novice animal owner, but it need not be if you know what to expect and are prepared. The most elementary thing is to note the date of breeding so you know when to expect parturition. Although the length of the gestation period is not always precise, it does fall within a narrow range of days, so you shouldn't be taken by surprise.

In all species, there will be some premonitory signs of impending parturition. A few days before, the udder begins to get distended with milk. The ligaments around the tail head will relax to give a sunken appearance, although this may not be noticeable in swine. Concurrently, the vulva may become distended and relaxed and some sticky tenacious mucus may appear. Just before labor begins, the animal may be restless, may seek out an isolated area, and may refuse feed. Of course, with animals such as sheep that are pasture bred and kept in flocks, these signs usually will not be observed even though they occur. That's why it's advisable to pen them up in a lambing shed about 140 days after the ram is put into the flock.

Most, but not all, animals will lie down when giving birth. In fact, as the onset of labor begins, they may act very restless, getting up and down several times before getting on with the business at hand.

TABLE 4-1	GESTATION PERIODS
SPECIES	AVERAGE GESTATION PERIOD
Cow	280 days
Mare	340 days
Sow	114 days
Ewe	145 days
Doe	150 days

The Birth Process

Normally, the young are born front feet first, followed by the head and shoulders. The placenta usually appears first, and because it is filled with fluid, it exerts a cushioning effect as it is forced against the cervix by uterine contractions. This helps to dilate the cervix, and as the feet and nose follow along, the cervix is dilated even further to permit birth of the animal. As the feet enter the vagina, strong abdominal contractions begin that hasten the whole process. As the intensity of contractions increases, the placenta frequently ruptures, releasing its fluid contents. This is not a cause for concern when everything else is normal; in fact, it helps to lubricate the birth canal. The duration of labor is generally longer in animals giving birth for the first time and varies considerably in different species, ranging from as little as 15 minutes in the mare to 6 to 8 hours in the sow until the last piglet is born.

Is Assistance Needed?

People frequently ask if it's necessary to assist an animal giving birth by pulling on the fetus. Generally speaking, assuming the dam is healthy and the presentation is normal, the answer is no. Millions of animals have been born without help, and forced extraction of the fetus may actually precipitate the complication of retained placenta. But the decision when to intervene is a matter of judgment that improves with experience. The cow that labors over an hour with the front feet and nose of the calf showing and no signs of further progress would certainly appreciate a little help. The cow that labors over an hour with nothing showing obviously needs help.

With the front feet showing and the head started, it's a simple matter to apply traction by pulling on the front legs of the calf. That traction should be gentle, however, and should coincide with abdominal contractions. This is not a time for brute strength and determination. I have seen dairy farmers go at the job as if it had to be done right now at all costs, even to the point, one time, of hooking a tractor to the calf and trying to pull it out. Such brutality is uncalled for and frequently results in a dead calf and a paralyzed cow.

Assuming the presentation is normal and the feet are out where you can reach them, there is no reason why you cannot give the animal some help if necessary. But remember that presentations are not always normal, and that's when your veterinarian should be called. If labor continues more than an hour, it's quite possible that the presentation is something other than normal; the possibilities are numerous and often quite difficult to handle. For that reason, these are best left to a person with training, experience, and the equipment to handle the situation. Figures 4-1 through 4-12 illustrate some of the unusual presentations of the fetus. In all species the *anterior presentation,* or front feet first (Figure 4-3), is normal and most common.

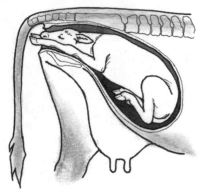

Figure 4-1. Anterior presentation, forelegs flexed. For delivery, the head must be pushed back and the legs pulled to an extended position.

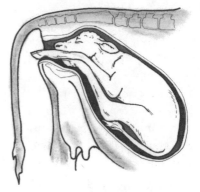

Figure 4-2. Anterior position, hind legs in the pelvic canal. Hind legs must be pushed back out of the pelvic canal while maintaining traction on the forelegs.

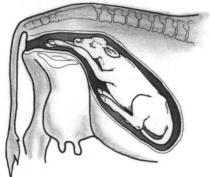

Figure 4-3. Normal anterior position

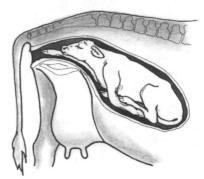

Figure 4-4. Anterior position, one foreleg retained. Head and foreleg must be pushed back while the retained leg is flexed and brought into position.

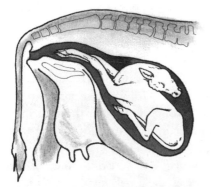

Figure 4-5. Head deviated to the side. Push forelegs back to get room and bring the head into position.

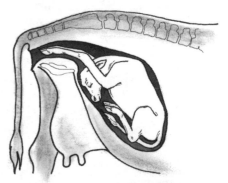

Figure 4-6. Head deviated ventrally. Push head and shoulders back and bring head up into position.

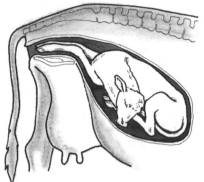

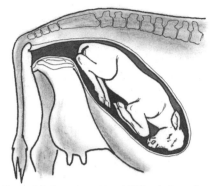

Figure 4-7. Anterior position, head and neck deviated to the side. Head must be brought into the pelvic canal. Difficult to handle. Sometimes requires fetotomy or cesarean section.

Figure 4-8. Breech position. While applying forward pressure to the rump, bring the hind legs into the pelvic canal.

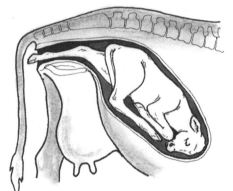

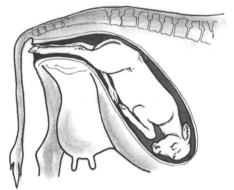

Figure 4-9. Posterior position, one leg retained. Push forward on the leg presented and bring the retained leg into position.

Figure 4-10. Normal posterior position. Frequently requires traction for delivery.

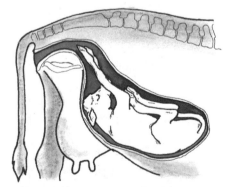

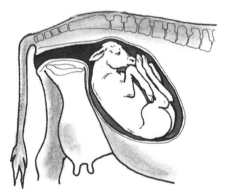

Figure 4-11. Anterior position, fetus upside down. Rotate 180 degrees and the normal delivery follows.

Figure 4-12. Anterior position, head and legs flexed. Rotate 180 degrees, and bring head and front legs into pelvic canal for normal delivery.

The next most common is the *posterior presentation,* or hind feet first, and it's easy to tell the two apart, even if the head isn't visible. If the soles of the feet are on the down side toward the dam's feet, the presentation is anterior; if they are up toward the dam's tail, the presentation is posterior. While this rule of thumb is not infallible, it is true at least 99 percent of the time and it's helpful early in the game to know what kind of problem you may be getting into so you can decide early on whether to call your veterinarian. He can do you more good at the early stages than after you have struggled with the situation for a couple of hours, exhausting yourself and the dam. Those of us in practice encounter this circumstance all too often, and the end result is usually a dead fetus, sometimes a dead dam, and always short tempers all the way around, especially when the owner gets the bill for what has unnecessarily become a salvage operation.

How to Help

If it's a normal anterior presentation with only a little added traction necessary, you can handle it. You will find the legs slippery to handle and, in the larger species, attaching a clean rope or, better yet, an obstetrical chain makes the job easier. Be sure that this is placed above the fetlock joint. If it's attached lower, it may slide off when you pull, tearing the hoof wall. The direction of pull should be outward and downward, coinciding with the dam's abdominal straining. Having an assistant rotate the fetus slightly back and forth each way on its longitudinal axis at the same time will often facilitate matters. The dam's pelvic canal is longer in the vertical axis than in the horizontal; therefore, the fetus must be in the vertical position with its backbone next to the dam's.

There may be times when, for whatever reason, you can't get a veterinarian to help with a complicated delivery. For those in this unenviable circumstance, the following will provide a little guidance. But I hasten to add, whenever possible get a veterinarian to help with the complicated cases, because the outcome is likely to be far better.

Cleanliness is extremely important when assisting with a delivery. The uterus is exceedingly susceptible to infection, especially following the trauma of birth. The first step is to get the dam on her feet and thoroughly scrub the vulva area with soap and water; scrub your hands and arms with soap and water as well. Next, lubricate one hand thoroughly using soap solution, or, if available, a neutral lubricant such as K-Y jelly or even mineral oil.

Gently put your hand in the vagina and try to ascertain what is wrong. If the cervix is not dilated, just wait awhile longer and try again. But any number of other malpresentations may be encountered. Before delivery can be accomplished, the fetus must be in the anterior or posterior position.

In attempting to correct malposition, it might be useful to list what can't be done so you don't waste time trying.

■ You can't change a posterior to an anterior presentation or vice versa — there isn't room.

■ You can't deliver an anterior presentation unless both legs and the head are started through the cervix. Sometimes only the legs come through and the head turns to the side. The head must be straightened around before the fetus can be delivered.

■ You can't make a delivery when three or more legs are through the cervix. They may all be from the same fetus or from two. In any event, the proper two legs have to be sorted out and the other pushed back out of the way.

■ Only rarely can you deliver a fetus when just the head is through the cervix. It must be pushed back and the forelegs brought through first. If the head is swollen, and it usually is in this case, it frequently must first be amputated to make room to get the legs through.

■ Another impossible situation seen more commonly in the sow is when the fetus lies across the cervix and extends into both uterine horns. It must first be slid one way or the other to place it in an anterior or posterior position before it can be delivered. With limited space available, this is easier said than done.

In fact, none of these procedures is easy. In all animals, space is limited and in the mare and cow you may be working at the limit of your reach. Also, your arm in the vagina stimulates the animal's straining reflex, and working conditions are not the best, to say the least. Add to this the fact that with an animal that can't get up, you may have to lie on your belly to reach as far as necessary. I think you can visualize how difficult this may be.

Torsion of the Uterus

The last impossible situation, encountered most frequently in the cow, ewe, and doe, is torsion of the uterus. This condition is simply an accident in which the uterus becomes twisted on its long axis. The end result is analogous to a bag, the opening of which has been twisted until it is partially or completely closed. A 180-degree rotation is most common, and it is enough to constrict the cervical opening so that birth cannot occur until the twist is reversed. The diagnosis is not difficult, but correction sometimes is. Generally, with a uterine torsion, the early signs of parturition — restlessness, perineal relaxation, and leaking milk — will appear but the state of true labor will not. In fact, in a few hours the animal may act entirely normal again, but this is transitory. A uterine torsion, if uncorrected, will ultimately lead to death. When the hand is placed in the vagina, spiral folds reflecting the direction of the twist can usually be felt.

Two methods are commonly used to correct a torsion. If it's only a partial torsion and one or two feet can be reached, it is often possible to rotate the fetus longitudinally in a direction opposite from the twist. The uterus will rotate along with the fetus to relieve the condition. The other method is to roll the entire animal sideways in the direction of the twist. If the animal is rolled fast enough, inertia will hold the uterus in place long enough for the twist to unwind.

A modification makes this somewhat more successful in the cow. If, for example, the cow needs to be rolled on her right, lay her on her right side (see chapter 5) and place one end of an 8-foot plank on her belly with the other end on the ground to her left. Have an assistant stand on the plank. This helps to hold the uterus in place. Then roll the cow over quickly. It may be necessary to repeat this several times, but reexamine the cow each time first or you may overdo it. If neither technique succeeds, a cesarean section is the only recourse. In the ewe and doe, with less weight to move, torsions can usually be corrected manually.

While there is much satisfaction to be derived from successful correction of *dystocia*, or difficult birth, in the large animals it is physically hard work that can be exhausting. Occasionally, a dystocia may be such that the fetus cannot be manipulated to accomplish a normal delivery. When this is the case, there are only two alternatives. One is a *fetotomy*, in which the fetus is cut up and removed piece by piece; the other is a *cesarean section*. Either technique is a job for the veterinary surgeon.

Except for the impossible situations described, correction of a malpresentation is mainly a matter of mechanics, common sense, and hard work. Remember to be clean and be gentle. Not only is the fetus delicate, but also the uterine wall is thin in advanced pregnancy and lacerates easily. Small tears may cause enough hemorrhage to be fatal, but even without that complication peritonitis and death may result. So be careful in straightening out a fetus and in the application of traction when necessary. And if at all possible, get veterinary help for the complicated cases, especially for the mare. Mares are in a class by themselves when it comes to complications, but fortunately they have complications less frequently than do other species.

The Offspring

Immediately following parturition there is a second animal to contend with, and what you do in the few minutes after birth may determine whether the offspring lives or dies. Remember that up until the moment of birth the young animal was in a completely protected aquatic environment at a constant temperature, well protected from infection, and totally dependent on its mother for survival. Consider the stress to which the newborn is subjected! It is pushed and squeezed through a very narrow opening and at the moment it reaches the outside world, depending on where and when it is born, the environmental temperature may be 100 degrees lower. At the same time, it is cut loose from oxygen via the umbilical blood supply and immediately must begin to breathe.

Care of the Newborn

Normally, the dam will lick the newborn vigorously after birth to help dry it and stimulate respiration. This is instinctive in animals with good "mothering" ability, but sometimes they are either physically unable or simply will ignore their offspring. I have seen young heifers and ewes that actually seem to be afraid of their first-born. In any event, what they can't or won't do you may have to do if the newborn animal is to survive.

First, be sure all the mucus and fluid is out of the nostrils so the airway is clear. If a lot of mucus is present, suspending the animal by the rear legs for a few minutes may help drain it out. Tickling the nostrils with a straw initiates sneezing, which also helps. Once the air passages are clear, the animal will usually breathe on its own, but rubbing the chest vigorously with a cloth will help the process and at the same time dry the animal so it can better withstand the temperature change.

Once breathing is established, the next step is to dip the navel in tincture of iodine. It should be literally dipped rather than just swabbing some on the outside. This has two purposes. It kills any bacteria present, which could travel up the umbilical vessels to establish a septicemic infection, and the astringent action of the alcohol in tincture of iodine helps to close the ends of the umbilical vessels so bacteria can't enter. Frequently with horses and less frequently with others species, the umbilical vessels don't rupture at birth. When this happens, wait a few minutes to let the foal recover as much blood as possible from the placenta, then tie the cord with string about 2 to 3 inches from the abdominal wall, and cut the cord on the placental side of the ligature.

Colostrum

By the time all this has been done, the animal is usually strong enough to stand and be introduced to the dairy bar for its first meal of colostrum, important in establishing disease immunity as well as for nutrition, as explained in chapter 1. If for any reason the animal doesn't nurse during the first hour, colostrum should be milked from the dam by hand and fed to the newborn. This will do much to ensure that the newborn animal survives the rigors of the outside world.

The importance of animal reproduction has fostered intensive research throughout the world. This has been highly successful and new knowledge is still being gained, much of it applicable to human reproduction as well.

Artificial Insemination

Perhaps the single most important development in animal reproduction has been the technique of artificial insemination (AI). While used to some degree in all species, it has thus far found greatest application in dairy cattle. Probably more than 90 percent of the dairy cattle in the United States are now bred by bulls they never see. Improved reliability of estrus synchronization has made artificial insemination more useful for the beef industry as well. With this technique, semen from a single ejaculate is collected and extended with a diluent, usually about a hundred times. Thus, instead of siring a single calf per ejaculation, the bull can sire a hundred calves. The genetic advantages are obvious. Bulls with superior milk-production-transmitting capability or conformation can now sire thousands more calves than they could by natural service. In fact, the average sire in AI service produces 40,000 breeding units annually, and some go as high as 60,000 breeding units. Economically, it means that the individual farmer can have the use of superior sires that he otherwise could never afford. For the person with a small herd, it is now cheaper to breed cows artificially than it is to keep a bull. The technique has proved so successful that there are many companies and cooperatives whose sole business is the production of high-quality semen from superior sires. The semen is then used on the farm by the company's own technicians on a fee basis and is available for direct sale to the farmer who wants to do his own insemination.

Although genetic improvement and economics are important advantages for AI, disease control is equally important. Bulls that are AI studs are not put into service until they have had extensive examinations to be sure they are free of contagious diseases, especially venereal diseases such as trichomoniasis. Similarly, every batch of semen is carefully evaluated and then standardized for the number of spermatozoa. And their genetic potential is proved by test matings *before* their semen is offered for sale. The advantages of AI are substantial.

Although the technique is feasible in other species, it has not been as widely accepted in other species as it has in dairy cattle. It is being done more frequently in swine and beef cattle, but the need for individual handling increases the labor requirement, thus reducing the economic advantage. Conception rates in mares bred artificially are somewhat less than in cattle and the extended semen is not as stable. But it's probable that additional research could overcome this deficiency if there were sufficient demand. The concept has not been accepted enthusiastically by the industry, however. When top stallions can command stud fees of $10,000 or more, it isn't hard to see why.

Initially, extended bovine semen was stored and used in a liquid state and its life was limited. Further research led to techniques for freezing it, and semen stored in liquid nitrogen remains viable for years. In fact, calves are being born today from sires long since dead. Frozen semen is regularly being shipped to all parts of the world.

International shipment of frozen semen is a matter of some concern because it creates an opportunity for transmission of foreign animal diseases, particularly those caused by viruses. In the United States, importation of semen as well as animals is regulated by the U.S. Department of Agriculture.

Learning the Technique

The technique of inseminating cows is not difficult, although proficiency certainly improves with practice. Most of the AI organizations conduct periodic training schools for farmers who want to do their own insemination. Although AI has advantages, it does place an added burden on management. Because the cows are usually inseminated only once, timing becomes critical as sperm and ovum must meet at precisely the right time. In the absence of a bull, heat detection is a major problem for the dairy farmer and more time must be devoted to watching the herd for signs of heat.

Planned Matings

Research has led to another significant development that is a useful management tool. Sometimes it is desirable to plan matings within a short time period. By feeding synthetic progesterone to a group of females, it is possible to synchronize their estrous cycles so that all of them will come in heat about 48 hours after the drug is withdrawn. I had the opportunity years ago as a practitioner to participate in some of the early clinical trials of this technique, and I'll never forget the sight of about four hundred beef cows in heat at the same time. It was like a three-ring circus.

The same technique is applicable to other species and, as a matter of interest, forms the basis for the oral contraceptives used by women. Heat synchronization is most applicable in special situations where it is desirable either to shorten the breeding season, such as breeding range cattle by AI, or to have all offspring born within a short span of time. Needless to say, where large numbers of females are in heat at the same time, AI is a must.

More recent endocrine research has centered on the effect of a unique class of compounds called *prostaglandins*. A series of prostaglandin $F_2\alpha$ injections will reliably induce estrus 2 to 5 days after administration to animals that are cycling normally. Its use is most applicable when a precisely timed mating is desirable. Neither technique will correct major infertility problems.

Embryo Transfer

The success of AI, particularly with the advent of frozen semen, has had a major impact not only on the economics of animal husbandry but also on genetic improvement of livestock. But the rate of improvement was limited by the length of the gestation period because, even though bred to a superior sire, a cow still could have only one calf per year.

Improvement in the technique and reliability of embryo transfer during the 1980s brought about change that would have been considered science fiction not many years before. Transferable embryos are obtained by inducing the donor animal, through the use of hormones, to superovulate. The many ova that are released are then fertilized by AI. At the same time, recipient or surrogate animals are given hormones to synchronize their estrous cycles with that of the donor.

Fertilized ova (embryos), generally five or six in each cow, are collected by flushing them from the uterus of the donor cow. They are then examined microscopically for viability and, if satisfactory, are transferred to the surrogate or frozen in liquid nitrogen for transfer at a later time. This technique is being used in all livestock species, although swine embryos do not withstand freezing well. The technique is not widely used in horses because the major breed associations don't favor it, just as they oppose AI. With the technique of embryo transfer, genetic improvement of the breed can proceed more rapidly than before. A single cow, for example, could theoretically produce twenty-five to thirty calves per year. Obviously, the technique requires specialized skills and is not inexpensive, but costs are coming down and the procedure is being more widely used.

With the ability to examine living embryos *in vitro* well established, related procedures are on the horizon that present some potentially frightening prospects. For example, using microsurgery it is now possible to split a single embryo into two, producing identical twins. It's conceivable then that one of these embryos could be stored frozen and later transferred to its twin, so that a cow could give birth to her genetically identical sister. And if one embryo can be divided into two, it won't be long before two will become four, four eight, and so on. In the twenty-first century, we may see entire herds of genetically identical animals. Cloned calves and lambs have already been produced.

A bit farther down the road, but not far, is the application of gene-splicing techniques to determine the sex of the embryo and, by modifying its genetic makeup, to "engineer" an animal more suited for a particular purpose. Perhaps we can remove genetic weaknesses and genetically add disease resistance to create a more healthy and productive animal. There is limited availability now of bovine semen that has been sorted by X and Y chromosomes so that the sex of the calf can be predetermined with 90 percent accuracy. These achievements are all possible, but they must be produced by responsible scientists with due regard for the welfare of the species as a whole.

To this point, we have been discussing embryo transfer in animals, but the same techniques are applicable to the human species. It was reported in 1993, for example, that a group of British scientists propagated cloned human embryos *in vitro* to the sixty-cell stage before allowing them to die. Think what a moral and ethical dilemma this type of research presents!

Let's look now at some of the reproduction characteristics that make the various species unique.

Cattle

Cows are polyestrous, normally coming into heat or estrus every 21 days from the onset of puberty. Some individuals will have estrous cycles a couple of days shorter or a few days longer, but as long as the cycle is consistent, it doesn't matter. Onset of puberty in the heifer is governed more by physical size than chronological age. Well-fed, rapidly growing animals may show signs of heat as early as 4 months of age. Conversely, those grown on a marginal diet may not come into heat until they are almost 2 years old. Young bulls will show signs of sexual activity at 4 months and are usually fertile at 6 months. They should be separated from the females by that time.

When to Breed

Because calving difficulties are inversely proportional to size, heifers should not be bred until they are big enough, but they should be bred when they reach optimal weight. Proper breeding weight varies with the breed, but 800 pounds is considered the optimum for Holsteins, with others in proportion. Holstein heifers should reach 800 pounds at about 15 months of age and, given an adequate diet, will continue to grow during pregnancy until they reach their definitive weight. The gestation period of the cow is 280 days, so heifers bred at 15 months will calve at 2 years old.

There is great controversy over the merit of breeding heifers to bulls of smaller breeds to yield a small calf the first time so that there are fewer calving complications. Geneticists argue that this causes a wasteful loss of genetic potential because the resulting crossbred offspring have limited value for milk production. Many veterinarians, myself included, who have seen too many good heifers injured by oversized calves will argue that the loss of any genetic potential is more than offset by the reduced injury and death loss at calving time and the increased milk production during the first lactation as a result of less calving stress. Fortunately, better selection of sires for calving ease, combined with better heifer nutrition, has greatly improved this problem in recent years.

Changes in Behavior

Signs of impending estrus in the bovine are generally marked by well-defined behavioral change. The lactating cow may have a transitory decline in production lasting about a day. Concurrently, there will be restlessness, occasionally bawling, and usually some clear mucus discharge from the vulva. The most definitive sign is standing to be mounted by other cows, the period of standing heat. When a bull is placed with a cow in standing heat, there is very little foreplay involved. The bull will usually sniff the vulva once or twice, curling his upper lip in a characteristic manner. Smell seems to increase libido, and the bull quickly gets an erection and mounts the cow. The whole procedure is accomplished speedily, with the interval between intromission and ejaculation averaging 7 seconds. Depending on the vigor of the bull, ejaculation occurs at the moment of a violent thrust, during which the bull's hind feet actually leave the ground. It's important, therefore, that the bull and cow have good footing during copulation. Heavy bulls can knock down a small cow or heifer during breeding. Similarly, if they slip, injury may result, making them useless for further service. To avoid injury, mating should not take place on a slippery floor.

Intromission terminates in ejaculation of 3 to 10 mL of semen, containing up to a billion spermatozoa. Volume and concentration decline somewhat with frequency of mating. Copulation will usually occur several times during the heat period. For that reason, if a single bull is turned out with a herd at pasture and several cows come into heat the same day, conception rates may be lower than anticipated. Controlled mating, sometimes called *hand breeding,* will conserve bull power and generally yield higher first-service conception rates.

Using a Breeding Rack

When a heavy bull must be used on a small heifer or cow, the use of a breeding rack is advisable. This is basically a stanchion, in which the cow is placed, that on each side has a strong plank extending from the stanchion frame at the level of the cow's shoulders back to the ground at her hind feet. When the bull mounts, his weight is supported by his front legs on the plank rather than by putting all his weight on the cow. The risk of injury can be eliminated entirely, of course, by AI. More will be said about that later.

Keeping Good Records

For good breeding efficiency, it's vitally important that records be kept of dates of heat periods, breeding, and calving. In addition, all cows should be examined by a veterinarian about 30 days after calving to be sure the uterus is normal and that no infection is present; this also should be part of the record. Examination of the ovaries at the same time will indicate whether the cow is cycling normally, as she should be. Most cows begin to cycle 2 to 3 weeks after calving, although they may not show standing heat. Examination at 30 days allows time for correction of any abnormalities before 60 days postcalving, which experience shows is about the best time to breed the cow again.

Complete information should be recorded for each individual in the herd. A variety of commercially prepared forms is available for the purpose, but human nature considered, the simplest is the most likely to be used. Reproduced here is a facsimile of a simple individual health and breeding record (Figure 4-13). It is based on one used by the author and further refined in collaboration with the late Professor A. M. Meek in the Department of Animal Science at Cornell University.

Reg. Name and Number		Ragapple Annie		516280								
		BREEDING HISTORY										
Birth Date 1-1-95	Year	1996	Sire	1997	Sire		Sire		Sire		Sire	
Sire Big Apple	Jan.			30								
Dam Maude	Feb.	28		20								
R. Ear Tag 21AN2146	Mar.	20		(13)	1005							
L. Ear Tag CV31850	Apr.	(11)	1153									
Purchase Date 3-1-95	May											
Purchased from John Doe	June											
	July											
VACCINATION DATE	Aug.											
Brucellosis 3-15-95	Sept.											
Leptospirosis 6-15-95	Oct.											
I.B.R. 6-15-95	Nov.											
B.V.D. 6-15-95	Dec.											
Other	Date due	12-26										
Barn Name or Number 98	Date fresh	1-1-97										

			GENITAL EXAMINATIONS				GENERAL HEALTH RECORD	
Date	Cervix	Uterus	Right Ovary	Left Ovary	Breeding Date or Treatment	Date		
1-1-96	N	N	CL	N				

Produced by Animal Science Extension, Cornell University, Ithaca, New York

Figure 4-13. Health and breeding record, front (top) and back (bottom).

The front has space for the identifying name and number of the individual cow, her sire and dam, and the dates of vaccination for the more common diseases. Dates are important for vaccines such as leptospirosis, which must be repeated annually. The remainder of the front has space for 5 years of breeding history in chart form.

To illustrate how the cards are used, the example Ragapple Annie was born on New Year's Day 1995 and purchased from John Doe on March 1 of that year. She was vaccinated on the dates indicated and was observed to be in heat on February 28, 1996, and again 20 days later. Her next heat period was on April 11, at which time she was bred to bull number 1153. Breeding is indicated by circling the date. She was examined for pregnancy by a veterinarian 50 days later and found to be pregnant. Her due date was recorded as 12-26-96, and she actually calved on 1-1-97. Due date is not entered until the pregnancy is confirmed. She came into heat again on January 30, and the condition of her reproductive tract was determined by veterinary examination on February 3. The cervix, uterus, and ovaries were found to be normal with a corpus luteum (CL) on the right ovary. Her next heat periods were on February 20 and March 13, at which time she was again bred. If any abnormalities had been found at the time of postcalving examination, these would have been noted together with the treatment given. Similarly, if she had failed to show a heat period after February 3, 1997, and a subsequent examination revealed a CL on the left ovary, this would be positive evidence that she had a heat period although it was not observed.

Most reproductive problems are hormonal in origin, and because there is no practical field test for hormone levels, diagnosis must be retrospective and based, to a considerable extent, on what changes have occurred. Without good records of reproductive history and results of prior examination, the diagnosis is frequently more difficult and less reliable. Although there are other systems equally good, none is more simple or economical than the health and breeding record shown on page 79. When coupled for barn use with a heat expectancy chart (available from many feed companies and AI organizations), it provides about all the information needed. Under general health, on the reverse side, there is space to record, in abbreviated form, any major disease episodes the animal experiences. While paper records are adequate for the small to medium-sized herd, computerized records are essential for the "mega" dairies that are becoming more common. In some herds, the cows now carry their own record with them in the form of a microchip embedded in a plastic tag or, in some cases, implanted subcutaneously in the neck. The microchips are then read by a scanner when the cow enters the milking parlor. The computer then tabulates lists of cows due to be bred or whatever else it is programmed to do.

The importance of management in cattle reproduction cannot be overemphasized, and the economic importance of reproduction is obvious. Unless the beef cow has a calf every year, her production is zero, and despite extensive research and some claims to the contrary, no feasible method has yet been devised to consistently induce dairy cattle to give a profitable quantity of milk without the stimulus of parturition.

Pregnancy Examinations

It behooves the cattle owner to learn as much as possible about reproduction and to apply this knowledge diligently. One management tool that should be used is pregnancy examination. An experienced veterinarian can diagnose pregnancy, or the lack thereof, with a high degree of accuracy beginning about 35 days after breeding, simply by rectal examination. With first-calf heifers, the diagnosis can even be made a few days earlier. Most theriogenologists, however, recommend that the examination be postponed until 45 days after breeding. Until that time, the placental attachment to the uterus is quite tenuous, and manipulation may induce abortion. This hazard is greatly reduced after 45 days, which is still early enough to initiate treatment of the nonpregnant cow to get her with calf in a reasonable length of time. The more advanced the pregnancy is, the easier and more accurate the diagnosis will be.

Early diagnosis is not made on the basis of palpating the embryo but rather on a combination of factors. Record of breeding is one, of course, but beyond that, disparity in size of uterine horns with a corpus luteum on the side of the larger is one indication of pregnancy. In addition, if an amniotic vesicle, the sac within which the embryo lies, can be felt, the pregnancy is confirmed. After 40 to 45 days, the fetal membranes can be "slipped" between the fingers, and after 60 days the fetus itself usually can be felt.

Cattlemen often ask if they can save some money by doing pregnancy examinations themselves. The technique can be learned by anyone of reasonable intelligence, but accuracy comes only with practice. Cattle owners simply don't have sufficient practical opportunity to become proficient, whereas a veterinarian in cattle practice may average more than one hundred pregnancy examinations in a week. Because accuracy of diagnosis is essential, it seems to me that the herd manager's time could be used more profitably in other endeavors.

Abortions

Once a viable pregnancy has been established and confirmed, it's just a matter of time until the calf is born — if an abortion doesn't occur. Abortion may occur at any time and there are many possible causes. If you have a cow that aborts, don't attribute it to bad luck and forget about it. There is always a reason, and any money and effort spent to find the reason can pay big dividends even if you only have one cow. At one time brucellosis was a major cause of abortion, and it still is in some parts of the world. It also causes undulant fever in humans and, therefore, diagnosis is doubly important. For the protection of the rest of the herd, it's vitally important that a diagnosis be made.

At the very least, segregate the aborting cow from the rest of the herd until a diagnosis has been made because her vaginal discharge may be teeming with pathogens. Put the aborted fetus in a plastic bag and hold it in a cool place until your veterinarian can get there to do a necropsy and collect samples for laboratory diagnosis. Last, thoroughly clean and disinfect the area where the abortion occurred to reduce the risk of spreading infection.

Calving

Where to have the cow calve often represents a dilemma. A 10-foot by 10-foot or larger box stall can be ideal — or it can be a disaster. If it is clean, well bedded, and left vacant for a couple weeks after the cow calves, it is ideal. But if it must be in constant use with one cow right after the other, it can be a disaster because the resulting buildup of pathogenic organisms will infect a majority of the cows and calves using it. This will show up as a frequently fatal septicemia in the calves, and metritis, mastitis, or both in the cows. The only way to break this cycle is to stop using the maternity pen — even if it means that the cows must calve outside.

The approach of parturition in the cow is characterized by udder enlargement and relaxation of the pelvic ligaments, giving the tail head a raised appearance. Frequently, the vulva lips become puffy and distended, and a string of gummy mucus will be seen extending from them. The cow will act restless and often will refuse feed for 12 hours prior to calving. Once true labor begins, the calf usually will be delivered within an hour or so.

Complications

The cow is unique from other species in the frequency with which parturition-associated complications occur. One of these is *parturient paresis,* or milk fever (see page 287). The other is *retained placenta,* which may affect 10 percent or more of the cows in the herd. Prolapsed uterus also is a common problem.

Retained Placenta

For a variety of reasons, some known and others not, in retained placenta the cotyledons and caruncles fail to separate as the calf is being born. Retained placenta is more frequent when twins are born and usually ensues when forced extraction of the fetus is necessary.

If infection is not present, retained placenta by itself is not a serious complication. The placenta will eventually loosen and fall out. Unfortunately, it acts as a wick along which bacteria can travel to set up a serious uterine infection called *metritis.* Also, once the calf is born, circulation to the placenta is cut off and the tissue dies and decomposes. Decomposing placenta has a very characteristic foul odor and it may be a month before all the bits and pieces have liquefied and been discharged. Medicating the uterus may help to prevent serious infection but does little to hasten placental expulsion.

If an unusually high percentage of retained placentas occurs in the herd, some attempt should be made to find the cause. This isn't easy and usually ends up as a trial-and-error procedure. Malnutrition and mineral imbalances are factors that can be eliminated by balancing the ration. Lack of exercise during the dry period also seems to play a role in all calving complications. Vitamin A deficiency has been considered a factor, although scientific evidence is lacking. Because the incidence of retained placenta is unpredictable, it's hard to design a controlled study. I do recall a herd in which administration of 1 million units of vitamin A intramuscularly during the dry period seemed to reduce the prevalence from over 30 percent to less than 5 percent.

More recently, selenium deficiency has been incriminated as a cause, and as with the vitamin A, injection during the dry period reduced the prevalence.

Selenium is known to be an essential trace element but in large doses it is also carcinogenic, so its availability is controlled by law. There are undoubtedly other factors such as hormone imbalances and miscellaneous infections that contribute to retained placenta. It's a problem that needs more study.

Prolapsed Uterus

The last major complication of parturition in the cow is prolapsed uterus. This condition, in which the uterus turns completely inside out, is one of the few true emergencies in farm animal practice. It is most prevalent in cows but certainly not rare in sheep and goats. This condition requires veterinary assistance without delay. It's a rare occasion when a prolapsed uterus can be replaced without medical assistance because it invariably swells. Attempts to push it back in stimulates a straining reflex, and in a contest of push against strain, the cow always wins.

The best thing to do is to restrain the cow so she can't walk around, thereby injuring the uterus. Then wrap it in a clean cloth such as a large towel or even a bedsheet and keep it moist with warm water until the veterinarian arrives. And in the interest of veterinarians everywhere, I would add, be prepared to help with the job at hand. Replacing a prolapsed uterus can be physically demanding work, taxing the strength of even the strongest individual.

Surprisingly, most cows survive the ordeal if the prolapse can be corrected before many hours elapse. Many will even become pregnant again. However, when it happens once, it is more likely to occur again at the next calving, and for that reason it is probably not advisable to keep the cow in the herd at the conclusion of that lactation.

Dehorning

Calves should be dehorned as soon as you can feel the horn buds, generally at 2 to 3 weeks of age. Horns serve no useful purpose on a cow and can be a hazard. The electric dehorner is the best implement for the purpose if properly used. Perhaps most important is selecting a dehorning iron that will maintain cherry-red heat throughout the procedure. The object is to destroy the cells that produce horn tissue. Generally, this means applying the hot iron to the horn bud for 15 to 20 seconds. When properly done, a leathery copper-colored ring will appear where the iron was applied. If not, reapply the iron because inadequate burning will lead to unsightly horn scurs.

Alternatively, a horn gouge such as the Barnes-type calf dehorner can be used, but it causes some hemorrhage and can lead to infection. Its advantage is that it can be used after the horn buds are too large for the electric dehorner.

The use of caustic paste is not recommended. It not only prolongs the pain but it also can be smeared, damaging other areas of skin or, even worse, the eyes. Dehorning is not essential, but for safety is strongly recommended.

Horses

The mare is classified as seasonally polyestrous — that is, she will show signs of heat on a regular basis only during certain seasons. This seems to be a function of hours of daylight, and the mare will usually cease cycling in late fall and early winter, beginning again as the days get longer. In the northern latitudes, the mare will usually begin to show signs of heat every 16 to 25 days in March and will continue on into fall if she is not bred.

The onset of estrus can be hastened by artificial light and by a management technique called *teasing,* or controlled daily exposure of the mare to the stallion without allowing direct contact. On breeding farms, mares and stallions are brought together this way once or twice daily but with a strong board fence between them and under hand control so injuries don't result. This procedure heightens libido in the stallion and markedly accelerates onset of estrus in the mare.

When to Breed

Breeding mares as early as possible in the spring has importance in the racing industry, but because it is counter to the normal reproductive pattern, it leads to more frequent reproductive failures than occur when mares are bred in May or June.

Early breeding is important in the racing industry because somewhere in antiquity it was decided that a horse's age would be decided by calendar year of birth rather than by date of birth. Thus, horses born on New Year's Day and those born on December 31 of the same year are reckoned to be the same age. Since the normal gestation period of the mare is 11 months, it is most desirable to get them bred in early February and to have them foal soon after January 1. From a physiological standpoint, this is the poorest time to breed mares. The advantages to the owner are obvious, however. In a race for 2-year-olds, for example, early in the season, a horse barely 2 years and one almost 3 years would qualify. Since the older horse is likely to be larger and stronger, the odds favor his winning the race. Don't bet on it, though, because genetics and training are still important factors.

The duration of standing heat in the mare is usually about 5 days and will be evident for the first time at around 18 months of age, although it may appear as early as 10 months and as late as 24 months, depending on such things as heredity, plane of nutrition, and season of the year. Unlike the cow, ovulation in the mare takes place about 1 or 2 days before signs of heat subside. The optimum time to breed, therefore, is generally about day 3 of estrus. The possibility of conception failure due to faulty timing can be reduced somewhat by breeding twice during the heat period if conserving the stallion is not important. The use of prostaglandin $F_2\alpha$ to induce estrus and ovulation in otherwise fertile mares has taken some of the guesswork out of timing the breeding. Use of hormones such as this should be considered a supplement to, and not a substitute for, good management. Careful rectal palpation and ultrasound will often detect imminent ovulation.

Detecting Estrus

Detection of estrus in the mare is not as simple a matter as it is in the cow because mares rarely exhibit the homosexual behavior of standing to be mounted by other mares. Daily teasing and noting changes in attitude toward the stallion are the most reliable means to detect estrus. The mare not in heat will resist the overtures of the stallion by squealing and kicking. The latter can cause serious injury if the stallion is not protected by a strong barrier. Gradually, as the heat period approaches, her attitude will soften and she will actually seek out the stallion, turning her hindquarters to him. Coincident with this, she may show other signs such as squatting, frequent urination, "winking" of the clitoris, and rapid tail switching.

Breeding Management

Conception rates can vary tremendously on different breeding farms due to season (lowest in February and highest in July) and management. Good managers provide mares and stallions with ample exercise and maintain them on a balanced, nutritious diet. They also start planning for the breeding season several months in advance by having mares and stallions examined for fertility in late fall by a veterinarian. Mares are particularly susceptible to uterine infections, which if detected early can be treated successfully by the time the mare is ready to breed.

Hygiene

Because of susceptibility to infection, good hygiene at the time of breeding is essential. The mare's tail should be bandaged and her hindquarters thoroughly scrubbed with soap and water and then rinsed. Similarly, the stallion's penis and sheath should be scrubbed and rinsed prior to breeding.

To prevent injuries, good restraint, depending on the dispositions of the mare and stallion, may be needed during breeding. To prevent injury to the stallion, breeding hobbles are often put on the mare (see page 117). These should be tight enough to prevent a well-directed kick but at the same time loose enough so she won't lose her balance and fall when the stallion mounts.

Some stallions have a habit of biting mares severely when they mount, necessitating use of shoulder pads on the mare. If the stallion is overly large for the mare he is breeding, possible vaginal injury can be prevented by placing a stallion-roll over the erect penis to control the depth of penetration. If necessary, one can be improvised by holding a roll of cotton between the penis and the belly wall as the stallion mounts.

Handling Precautions

Breeding should be done on ground where footing is good because concrete or plank floors are often dangerously slippery for horses. Both mare and stallion are restrained in halters, and the person controlling the stallion must be particularly alert to any untoward moves that might result in injury. The stallion is brought alongside the mare and, after a period of foreplay during which the penis becomes erect, the stallion mounts and intromission takes place. Manually directing the penis into the vagina precludes the possibility of false entry into the rectum. Copulation in horses lasts 5 to 7 minutes and terminates with ejaculation of 50 to 100 mL of semen. As with other species, volume is determined to a large degree by frequency.

When the stallion dismounts, he should be put back in the stall. Young, vigorous stallions may want a second chance but it serves no useful purpose at this time.

Some older mares have vulvae that tip inward, allowing fecal contamination of the vagina with subsequent extension of infection to the uterus, followed by early abortion. It has been shown in mares with this condition that suturing together the upper two-thirds of the lips of the vulva (a procedure known as a *Caslick operation*) immediately after breeding will improve conception rates. The vulva must then be surgically opened, of course, prior to subsequent breeding or foaling.

Artificial Insemination

Artificial insemination in the mare has had limited application for a number of reasons. First, fresh horse semen does not remain fertile much beyond 8 hours, although techniques have been developed for freezing it to keep it viable much longer. Second, the difficulty of detecting mares in heat makes the timing of artificial insemination too much a matter of luck. Third, the objections of several breed organizations have tended to discourage research. At present, the best application appears to be when two or more mares are to be bred to the same stallion on the same day. Semen can be collected using a "breeder's bag," or condom, or, preferably, an artificial vagina. The semen thus collected from a single ejaculate can be extended 1:1 and used to breed several mares.

Tests for Pregnancy

Pregnancy diagnosis is perhaps more important in mares than in cattle because of the relatively short breeding season. The teasing schedule should be maintained for at least 3 weeks after breeding to see if the mare returns to estrus. Failure to return to estrus is not positive evidence she is pregnant, although odds favor it, but it does provide a logical basis for a rectal examination for pregnancy a couple of weeks later. A small percentage of mares may show signs of heat 3 weeks after breeding, but it is usually of short duration and can be differentiated from a true heat period by rectal palpation.

Although several biological tests for pregnancy in mares are available, none is superior to or can be done earlier than rectal palpation by an experienced veterinarian. Those who do such examinations frequently become sufficiently skilled to detect pregnancy as early as 17 days after breeding, but 30 to 40 days after breeding is probably more realistic. In the hands of a skilled operator, ultrasonography is reliable for pregnancy diagnosis as early as 9 or 10 days after breeding. A diagnosis of pregnancy made very early during gestation should be confirmed by a second examination a few months later, because early embryonic deaths occur in about 5 percent of equine pregnancies. When this occurs, the mare may not return to heat that season and the breeder blissfully assumes that she is pregnant. It pays to confirm the pregnancy!

Biological Tests

The biological tests for pregnancy rely on changes in hormone concentration, especially in chorionic ganadotropin and estrogen, that occur during the pregnancy. They are rarely used today, however, as rectal palpation and ultrasonography are preferred.

Rectal Examination and Ultrasonography

Rectal examination of the mare is not a job for the novice, if for no other reason than that it can be dangerous. Some mares take violent exception to a hand in their rectum and will lash out with both hind feet with disastrous results if they are on target. Leave it to your veterinarian! He knows what to expect and what measures to take to prevent the worst from happening.

Ultrasonography, with good equipment and in the hands of an experienced operator, can provide accurate diagnosis of pregnancy in mares and in other species as well. Much like sonar used on boats and Doppler radar used to predict weather, ultrasonography relies on graphic depiction of electronic echoes created by electrical impulses transmitted by a transducer for diagnosis.

Outward Signs

The outward signs of pregnancy, in some cases almost right up to foaling, are not nearly as evident in the mare as they are in the cow. Some increased distention of the mare's udder may be noticed, beginning about 3 to 6 weeks before foaling. It becomes filled with colostrum about 2 days prior to foaling and some leakage called *waxing* may be noticed on the teat ends. None of these time estimates is absolute, but waxing of the teats is an indication that preparation for foaling should not be delayed. Mares prefer peace and quiet when they foal and seem to have an uncanny ability to delay parturition until no one is around. When foaling is imminent, they should be put in a clean, well-bedded box stall and watched discreetly. Sometimes observation through a knothole is the best way. It's not uncommon to have an anxious owner stay up all night watching a mare due to foal only to have the foal born while the owner is in the house getting some breakfast.

First Signs of Labor

Perhaps the first signs that labor is beginning are slight sweating in the flanks and refusal of feed. These are followed by restlessness and evidence of abdominal discomfort. The mare will get up and down frequently until finally she stays down and begins to start some straining. The *chorioallantois,* or water bag, usually breaks about this time, and the foal gets his first look at the world usually within the next half hour. Strenuous labor beyond that time with no apparent progress is a cause for concern and an indication that the mare needs some professional help. The foal can get into any of the malpresentations we described earlier, but because of the heavier abdominal musculature of the mare compared with other species, the mare's straining effort makes correction somewhat more difficult. Also, the uterine wall ruptures more easily and the uterus is more susceptible to infection than is the cow's. For these reasons, professional help is strongly recommended. If no veterinarian is available in a reasonable length of time, do the best you can, but remember that cleanliness and gentleness are essential.

The equine placenta differs from that of the cow. At the moment of birth, 10 to 15 percent of the foal's blood supply may be in the placental blood vessels. Don't be in a hurry to cut the umbilical cord. Wait 15 minutes or so, then tie the cord 3 or 4 inches from the belly, using umbilical tape or a piece of sterilized cotton string. Cut the cord on the placental side of the tie. Spread the placenta out and examine it to see that it is all there. Retained placenta is not as common in the mare as in other species, but sometimes torn pieces will be left in the uterus. Pieces or an entire placenta retained in the uterus is a complication that needs correction without much delay. This is not only an ideal medium for bacterial growth, but also decomposing placenta in the uterus can cause a severe endometritis and laminitis (founder).

Care of the Foal

After the umbilical cord has been cut, a few other procedures for the foal are recommended. The navel should be dipped in tincture of iodine. Unless the mare has been previously immunized, the foal should receive a dose of tetanus toxoid or antitoxin. Horses are very susceptible to tetanus and the stump of the umbilical cord is an ideal place for the bacterium *Clostridium tetani* to gain entrance.

Normally a foal will be on its feet within an hour after birth and looking for his first meal. He should be helped if necessary. If for any reason the foal can't get up to nurse, bottle-feed him with colostrum milked from the mare. Last, many foals require an enema within 6 to 12 hours after birth to remove the hard lumps of meconium that would otherwise cause constipation and all the complications that implies.

The majority of mares will come into heat within a week after foaling. This is the so-called foal heat, and if the delivery was uncomplicated and everything else is normal, they can be bred back at this time. Conception rates on this first breeding are generally not as good as they will be at the next heat period, however.

If you have gotten the impression that horse breeding is a complicated procedure with frequent disappointments, you are correct. And you might well ask why. Certainly bands of wild horses have no trouble reproducing themselves. The answer lies not with the horses but with the people who own them. Most wild mares are bred during June and July at the peak of fertility, and they foal late in the spring when there is ample grass for nourishment of mare and foal. If, instead of attempting to make nature conform to our needs through artificial birth dates and other means, we would adjust our breeding procedures to simulate those found naturally, I have no doubt that conception rates would improve markedly.

Swine

Gilts will generally start showing signs of estrus at about 6 months of age. However, unless they are especially well grown, it is advisable to postpone breeding another 3 months or until they reach 250 pounds of body weight. They are polyestrous, having heat periods about every 3 weeks throughout the year except when pregnant or lactating. The period of estrus will last 2 or 3 days and ovulation occurs a few hours thereafter. The duration of pregnancy averages 114 days. If you have trouble remembering numbers, think of it in terms of 3 months, 3 weeks, and 3 days. As with teasing the mare, the onset of estrus can be hastened by putting a boar in an adjacent pen.

Although the sow will cycle throughout the year, conception rates fall during periods of very hot weather. Hot weather also tends to lower the fertility of the boar. If sows must be bred when it's hot, some method of cooling the barn, such as evaporative coolers or foggers, will improve conception and litter size.

Impending estrus is usually evident a few days prior to standing heat. The vulva shows some swelling and reddening, and the sow becomes restless, utters typical grunts, and sniffs at the genitals of others in the pen. This is followed by mounting other sows and, finally, by standing to be mounted. During the period of peak fertility, most sows will stand for hand pressure on the rump and, of course, will be receptive to the boar. Best conception results when the sow is bred about 20 hours after the onset of standing heat and again 12 hours later. A second mating will increase litter size by about 10 percent. Since weaning a maximum number of pigs per litter, at least nine, is one of the keys to success in the swine business, this extra 10 percent becomes important.

Another management technique that helps to increase litter size in pigs is called *flushing*. Increasing feed intake of the sow by 6 or 8 pounds for 10 days prior to breeding will increase the number of ova released, thereby increasing litter size. Reverting back to the normal daily ration a few days after signs of heat have passed will keep the sows from getting too fat.

When to Breed

When to breed sows depends on many factors; market conditions, feed availability, housing, and, for those with only one or two sows, sometimes personal preference enters in. But for the commercial operator it is important from a disease-control standpoint to plan matings so that there will be a 2-week period every 6 months when there are no hogs in the farrowing house. This allows time for thorough cleaning, disinfection, and drying, which kills off populations of pathogens that otherwise cause a constant problem with such things as baby pig scours, metritis, and mastitis.

Availability of boars presents a problem for the person breeding one or two sows as a hobby. The economics of a swine enterprise that small is questionable at best, and if one must feed a boar all year to have him available to sire two litters of pigs a year, the enterprise certainly must be considered a hobby. As a way of saving money, some people either borrow a boar when needed or take their sow to a boar. This is an ideal way to spread contagious swine diseases and is certainly not recommended. Artificial insemination is much more preferable. The technique is successful and practical, although thus far it has not been possible even with a variety of extenders to keep boar semen viable much more than 36 hours. Frozen semen has not produced good conception rates.

Collecting Semen

Collection of semen and insemination are not difficult procedures, and once learned are probably no more time-consuming than transporting a sow or boar from one farm to another. Certainly there is less disease hazard involved, and the equipment requirements are minimal. The only real drawback is the availability of a sow in heat on the farm where the semen is to be collected to stimulate erection by the boar. Even this can be circumvented with electroejaculation.

To collect semen, when the boar mounts the sow, grab and hold the penis firmly in a gloved hand and direct it toward an opaque widemouthed, sterilized, and warm pint bottle. Firm hand pressure on the penis is sufficient to stimulate ejaculation, which usually takes 5 minutes or more for completion.

The ejaculate from a mature boar will just about fill the jar, but the first part of it is heavy gelatinous material that should be discarded. The balance of the semen containing the spermatozoa should be protected from chilling by wrapping the jar in paper or other insulating material. If used within an hour or so, the loss in fertility is not great and there's a good chance of conception.

Prior to use, the ejaculate is strained through sterile cheesecloth to remove any extraneous material. Although equipment has been designed for swine insemination and is undoubtedly preferable, insemination can be done by using a bulb syringe with about a half-pint capacity attached to a semi-flexible plastic pipette similar to that used for cattle insemination. The pipette is inserted carefully into the vagina and upward at about a 30-degree angle and gently worked through the cervix. Once the pipette is in place, the bulb is slowly squeezed until the semen has been expelled. This technique has some obvious disadvantages, but these are outweighed by the reduced risk of disease transmission inherent in transporting sows or boars from one farm to another.

The same technique is equally or more useful on the large breeding farms where there is a shortage of boar power. By extending the semen up to fivefold with commercially available semen extenders or even sterile homogenized milk, one boar can be used to breed several sows in a day, which would not otherwise be possible with any degree of success. Fertility of even mature boars declines if they are used more than twice a day or ten times a week. Boars less than a year old cannot be used successfully that frequently. Fertility of the boar has a noticeable effect on litter size, and to lessen the chance of breeding a sow to a boar of low fertility, it is common practice to breed sows twice during the heat period to different boars. This puts added demands on boar power and makes adequate care and management of boars as important as that of the sows.

Introducing New Boars

For genetic improvement, if nothing else, new boars with different bloodlines are frequently added to the herd. These boars should be purchased well in advance of anticipated need and, as a disease-control procedure, segregated from other swine for 30 days. If no health problems develop, they can then be placed in service, but it is good practice to first test-mate them to a couple of gilts to be sure they are fertile.

The sexual and social behavior of pigs seems quite different from that in other animals. A strange boar put in with a pen of sows or gilts may show more concern about his surroundings than about his love life. It helps to put him in an adjacent pen for a few days beforehand to get him acclimated. Similarly, a boar simply left in a pen of females sometimes gets bored with the whole procedure and ignores their overtures. Putting a second boar in the pen introduces an element of competition, and once they settle their differences, both boars will approach the situation with renewed vigor. Some young virgin boars put in a pen with a sow in heat will simply regard the sow's antics with amazement and not know how to proceed. A few have to be patiently coaxed to mount the sow until they learn their purpose in life. Once they get the idea, there is usually no further problem.

Copulation is a more protracted procedure in swine than in other species, lasting from 20 to 30 minutes. And also, unlike other species, the slim penis of the boar passes through the cervix, so ejaculation takes place directly into the uterus. The excitement associated with sexual activity in other species is generally absent, and once ejaculation begins, some boars actually give the impression they are going to sleep. The only indication of activity may be just an occasional soft grunt.

Diagnosing Pregnancy

Pregnancy diagnosis in the sow is accomplished with biological tests for blood progesterone or estrone sulfate, or the use of ultrasonography. Of these, real-time ultrasonography is the most accurate. Except in large sows, rectal palpation is more traumatic than useful. Changes in vaginal epithelial cells determined by biopsy and microscopic examination are a reliable indicator of pregnancy, but these procedures are not very practical on the farm.

Farrowing

A couple of days before the sow is due to farrow, she should be scrubbed clean with soap and water and put into a previously cleaned and disinfected farrowing pen or stall. These are described in the section on housing (pages 54–57). At the same time, the sow's diet should be changed to one containing more bulk. Sows tend to develop problems with constipation when they are confined in a farrowing pen. As a result, they go off feed and have a reduced milk flow when it is most needed. A diet high in fiber using more ingredients such as bran and even chopped hay helps prevent the problem.

Depending on litter size, farrowing may extend over several hours, taking longer as a rule for gilts than for older sows. Sometimes the first piglet in the procession will be larger than the others or malpresented and the sow will have to be helped. This usually can be reached by hand and removed with gentle traction. Remember to be clean and gentle. Anyone farrowing hogs regularly should have a set of pig forceps and/or an obstetrical snare available. When it appears that the last piglet has arrived, some swine growers routinely give the sow a dose of oxytocin. This is a prescription drug that stimulates smooth muscle contraction. It causes the uterus to contract, ideally expelling any additional pigs that are left, and it also helps to stimulate milk flow.

Care of Newborn Pigs

Unlike dairy cows or goats, the profit from a swine operation comes from the sale of market hogs, finished hogs, or breeding stock. It follows that raising as many pigs as possible to market age determines gross income. The suggestions in this section should enhance the survival of piglets.

Supplemental Heat

Supplemental heat from a heat lamp or a brooder is necessary for the newborn pigs except during hot weather. Chilling after birth not only predisposes piglets to disease problems such as scours and pneumonia but also can itself cause death. So place the piglets under the lamp as they are born and, at the same time, dip each navel in tincture of iodine.

Needle Teeth

This is also a good time to clip the needle teeth. Baby pigs have very sharp teeth that, when nursing, may irritate the sow to the point where she won't let them nurse. Only the tips of the teeth should be removed, as clipping them at the gum line may crush the teeth, leaving the piglet with a mouth so sore that he won't nurse. A Resco brand dog nail trimmer works well for the purpose.

Castration

Male piglets may be castrated at 2 to 3 weeks of age. By then they are strong enough and yet young enough that the procedure doesn't bother them too much. Because of their short spermatic cords compared to those of calves, lambs, and kids, piglets must be surgically castrated using an instrument such as White's emasculator, which cuts the cord and crushes the stump to reduce hemorrhage. A word of caution is in order. If you plan to castrate piglets yourself, be prepared to repair a hernia at the same time. Inguinal hernia with a loop of intestine in the scrotum is not uncommon in pigs. It's embarrassing, to say the least, to find when you incise the scrotum to get at the testicles that the intestines are also coming out.

Anemia

Iron deficiency anemia in baby pigs is a universal problem that is easily prevented. Several methods are commonly used. The oldest and simplest, which is still used by many swine growers, is to put a few shovelfuls of clean sod in the pen so the pigs can root around in it. Another, less certain, way to get iron into the piglets is to swab the udder of the sow with a saturated ferrous sulfate solution on the theory that the piglets will lick it off when they nurse. A more certain way is to drench the individual pigs with ferrous sulfate solution (about 1 teaspoon) or to give each an iron/copper tablet. But perhaps the best way is to inject each pig with iron dextran within 1 or 2 days after birth and again 3 weeks later. This injectable form of iron is available from several companies, and the dosage depends on the concentration of the product used.

Pigs can be weaned at 4 weeks of age, and the sow will usually come into heat and can be bred 5 to 7 days after weaning. Those piglets that are destined to become market hogs can be castrated at this time or earlier. Castration of males is essential for palatable meat, and the earlier this is done, the less traumatic it is.

Sheep

Sheep tend to be seasonal breeders with the onset of first estrus appearing in late summer or early fall and appearing about every 16 days thereafter until late fall unless pregnancy intervenes. Unlike other domestic animals, however, there is a noticeable difference among breeds. For example, the Rambouillet and Dorset may come into heat at any time of the year and usually always by June, whereas the Cheviot and Shropshire rarely show signs of heat before September. This difference is important when selecting a breed for commercial lamb production. A great deal of crossbreeding has been done in the sheep industry in an attempt to concentrate desirable traits, one of which is a short anestrus period.

The average gestation period is 147 days, with the onset of puberty ranging from 5 to 12 months depending on heredity, plane of nutrition, and when the ewe lambs are born. Those born early in the year will often come into heat that fall; those born later usually don't come into heat until the following year. Because it is economically desirable that a ewe produce as many lambs as possible during her lifetime, there is a distinct advantage in having lambs born early in the year. Unfortunately, lamb mortality due to inclement weather in the winter tends to be higher unless special care is taken. "Flushing" the ewes with extra feed a few weeks prior to breeding will improve conception rates and perhaps stimulate more multiple ovulation.

Ovulation takes place late in the heat period, but timing of mating is of little consequence because sheep are almost invariably pasture bred, and when sufficient ram power is available, copulation will occur several times during the heat period. Although libido and fertility of rams will vary, a mature ram should be able to breed twenty-five ewes during the season.

Fertility

Fertility is generally better in cool weather and when the rams are not constantly kept with the flock. As with the mare, sight, sound, and smell apparently play a role in the onset of estrus for ewes. More ewes will come into heat sooner when the rams are put with them a few weeks prior to the desired breeding season than when rams are left with them all the time. When the rams are left with the ewes all the time, the ewes become accustomed to their presence and the element of sexual excitement is lacking.

Artificial insemination of sheep, although technically feasible, has not become a common practice. It requires close observation of the ewe flocks, individual handling, and careful timing of insemination, which makes it less practical than for other species.

Estrus synchronization through use of hormones, on the other hand, is a useful management tool adopted by some shepherds. Use of synthetic or natural progesterone-type hormones given in feed or via a pessary placed in the vagina as the breeding season approaches will inhibit the onset of estrus in most cases. When the drug is withdrawn, the majority will come into heat during the space of a few days. This has the advantage of shortening the breeding season and subsequently the lambing season. It also has a disadvantage. Because all ewes come into heat at about the same time, it keeps the rams pretty busy, and for maximum conception rates, more rams will be needed.

Identifying Barren Ewes

Pregnancy diagnosis in sheep is important to good management. A barren ewe must be fed, just as a pregnant one must be, yet without one or more lambs she produces no income. The earlier that barren ewes can be identified and culled, the higher the flock productivity will be. Because the unit value of commercial sheep is low, biological tests based on hormone assay are not feasible, as the labor requirement in collection of blood samples and the cost of the test itself are prohibitive.

However, development of other techniques has accelerated in recent years. A few people have become adept in diagnosing pregnancy at about 90 days by digital palpation of the cervix through the vagina. In the pregnant ewe, the cervix generally cannot be reached with the fingertips, while in the barren ewe it will feel dense and almost cartilaginous.

In advanced pregnancy, of course, lambs can often be felt externally, but by that time parturition, or lack of it, is so near that examination is hardly worthwhile. External ultrasonography is the most practical pregnancy diagnostic tool for the commercial sheep grower. With experience, it is both fast and accurate.

Fitting a ram with a breeding harness and crayon helps to identify ewes that have not been bred because they will not have a crayon mark on their backs. Using a different-colored crayon at the end of the breeding season will identify nonpregnant ewes that have returned to heat.

Lambing Shed

Because of the desirability of having ewe lambs that will come into heat as early as possible and the better market for spring lambs in some areas, most shepherds prefer to have their lambs born as early in the year as possible.

Unfortunately, this coincides with cold weather in many regions, so a reasonably warm, protected lambing shed is a necessity. This can be the same building in which the ewes are housed, but if so, it should have a section reserved for lambing pens, holding no more than one or two ewes. When the whole flock is left together at lambing time, lambs and their mothers often get separated, and mass confusion results.

As lambing time approaches, watch the ewes carefully for signs of imminent parturition such as engorgement of the udder with milk, or "bagging." These ewes should be separated from the flock and put into the lambing area. At the same time or even sooner, it's good practice to "tag" the ewes — that is, to clip off the wool around the udder and perineal area. This keeps the udder and vulvar area cleaner, which makes lambing a more sanitary procedure and also makes it easier for the lambs to find their first meal.

Multiple Births

Twins and triplets are common in sheep, and multiple births are desirable. The flock that doesn't average at least 1.5 lambs per ewe per year is not likely to be profitable. One of the criteria used in select matings is twinning and mothering ability. Due at least in part to multiple births, sheep tend to have more difficulty at parturition and frequently require assistance. The good shepherd will check his lambing ewes every few hours, day and night throughout the lambing season, so he can help those in trouble.

Delivery

Normally the first lamb will be born within 1 or 2 hours after true labor begins. If nothing happens by then, a careful pelvic examination is in order. With an assistant holding the ewe, scrub the vulvar area thoroughly with soap and warm water and do the same with your hands and arms. The pelvic canal of a mature ewe will admit a well-lubricated, average-sized hand. If the problem is merely a cervix that is not fully dilated, wait a little longer and try again if nothing has happened. If the problem is a malpresentation, it must be corrected before the lambs can be delivered. The illustrations shown earlier in this chapter (see pages 68–69) should help in determining the position of the lamb and what must be done to straighten it out. Once it is straightened out, it can be delivered with gentle traction. An obstetrical snare or forceps, available from most instrument supply houses, is a valuable aid to grip the lamb.

Frequently when *dystocia,* or difficult birth, occurs, the ewe will be tired and her uterine musculature exhausted, or atonic, so any lambs remaining after the first will also have to be manually delivered. Injection of oxytocin may stimulate uterine contractions, but it is a powerful drug that can be dangerous. In most states it is available only by prescription. Use of oxytocin to stimulate uterine contractions without first ascertaining that the cervix is dilated and the lamb in a normal position can lead to a ruptured uterus and a dead ewe. Oxytocin is a useful drug, but it must be used judiciously.

Protect against Infection

Once the obstetrical operations have been completed, it's time to look toward the future. Any time an instrument or the hand is introduced into the uterus, infection called metritis is likely to ensue. This is especially true during obstetrical operations, because there is always some degree of injury to the uterine lining, making it more susceptible to bacterial invasion. A variety of antibiotic preparations are available to medicate the uterus, and most of them are effective when used as directed. In addition, it's a wise precaution to give the ewe 5 mL of penicillin intramuscularly. For a valuable ewe, a dose of tetanus antitoxin as an added precaution is indicated, because sheep are especially susceptible to tetanus.

Care of Lambs

The lambs need attention, too. They chill rapidly and need to be rubbed dry with a towel and kept warm. Rubbing them briskly but gently also helps to stimulate circulation and respiration. Once they appear to be breathing normally, the navel should be dipped in tincture of iodine to prevent infection. The next step is to induce them to nurse, which means patiently heading them in the right direction and sometimes stripping a little milk from the ewe into their mouths until they get the idea. If all else fails, lambs can be bottle-fed until they get a little stronger or a little smarter. An ordinary baby bottle and nipple will do, although commercially made lamb nipples will last longer. In any event, lambs need their first meal of colostrum within an hour after birth, and for the first few days they will take a little milk every few hours. As they get older, the frequency of feeding can be reduced.

Despite the best effort of the shepherd, there is usually some mortality of lambs and ewes during the lambing season, resulting in orphan lambs or ewes with milk and no lambs. It's worth the effort to try to get them together so the lamb can be raised without hand feeding. Unfortunately, most ewes will not accept nursing except by their own offspring, which they identify by smell. Sometimes they can be fooled by tying the skin of the dead lamb onto the orphan. Some ewes that are heavy milkers develop swollen, engorged, and painful udders from lack of milking, and mastitis may be an added complication. Milking will help, of course, but few people have the time and patience to milk a ewe regularly. Furthermore, milking actually increases the milk flow and once started will have to be continued. It's better to dry off the milk flow as rapidly as possible. Pressure in the udder helps, but contributes to the ewe's discomfort. Massaging the udder several times a day with camphorated oil relieves some soreness and suppresses milk flow.

Docking and Castrating

At 3 to 5 days of age, all lambs should have their tails docked and males should be castrated. At this age, the emasculatome is the most satisfactory instrument for castration. It crushes the spermatic cord, interrupting the blood supply to the testicles so they don't develop. It has the advantage of not cutting into the skin or causing any bleeding; thus, there is no danger of infection or hemorrhage. The instrument should be in good condition and should not be used for anything else that might spring the jaws. A small emasculatome suitable for one-handed operation is adequate for young lambs.

With an assistant holding the lamb, force the right spermatic cord to the outside edge of the scrotum with the left hand and with the emasculatome in the right hand, clamp it about halfway between the testicle and the body wall. Change hands and repeat on the left side. This technique crushes the spermatic cord without breaking the skin. By manipulating the spermatic cord on the testicular side of the instrument, a separation can be felt when the job is properly done. Then the blood supply to the testes is cut off and they gradually shrink and disappear.

Don't try to take a shortcut by clamping the entire scrotum, because with that amount of tissue to clamp, "skips" may occur. When carefully done as described, this method is as effective as the use of knives or elastrator bands and is safer. The same technique works well for calves, although a larger size emasculatome may be necessary.

The emasculatome is also a good instrument for tail docking, since virtually no hemorrhage results even though the tail must be snipped off where the instrument was applied. An application of antiseptic on the stump is usually the only aftercare required. Castration and tail docking should be done in a clean area. Docking tails of filthy lambs in a filthy place may lead to serious death losses from tetanus.

Lambing time is a busy time for the shepherd, but successful sheep husbandry is proportional to success of the lamb crop, and merits all the time the shepherd devotes to it.

Goats

Like sheep, goats are seasonally polyestrous, usually coming into heat from August through January, with the peak months of fertility being September, October, and November. During this period, does will cycle every 21 days, with each heat period lasting 2 or 3 days. Ovulation occurs late in the heat period; therefore, the day 2 is usually the best time to breed. Signs of impending estrus include uneasiness, tail shaking and frequent urination, some mucus discharge from the vulva, and receptivity to the buck.

Bucks: Smelly but Essential

The owner of one or two goats faces a problem in getting them bred. It's not economical to keep a buck for one or two does. Furthermore, the odor from their musk glands makes them socially unacceptable to all but a dedicated goat enthusiast — or another goat. This usually means that the doe must be transported somewhere to a buck when she is in heat. This transporting is often inconvenient and carries with it the risk of transmitting disease from farm to farm. Artificial insemination, therefore, is a logical and practical solution, but unfortunately its availability is limited.

Frozen semen is available from a limited number of sources, one of which is Central Ohio Breeding Association, Columbus, Ohio. Breed association secretaries maintain lists of semen sources, and perhaps the best solution for the owner of a limited number of goats is to arrange with a local AI technician to obtain and store frozen semen for use in the herd. With the rapid increase in popularity of the dairy goat, AI service will no doubt become more readily available. Until then, transporting the does or keeping a buck will be the only alternatives for some people.

The larger commercial goat dairies can justify a buck on economic grounds, but they still have to live with his odor, which permeates everything unless he has been successfully deodorized. Even then, bucks during the breeding season have a nasty habit of urinating on their beards and then shaking urine all over. Although undesirable from many standpoints, they are essential. Fortunately, only one is necessary for a doe herd of up to thirty head.

Diagnosing Pregnancy

As with sheep, ultrasonography is the most reliable method of pregnancy diagnosis in goats.

The duration of pregnancy averages 151 days, and since the breeding date for goats is usually known, the time of kidding is predictable. The pregnant doe should be put into a clean box stall, at least 5 feet by 5 feet, a few days ahead of time. Signs of impending parturition include udder enlargement; relaxation of the pelvic ligaments, giving the tail head a raised appearance; and a hollow appearance in the flank. Frequently there will be a thick white discharge from the vulva for a few days prior to kidding. As the time draws near, the doe will act restless, changing positions frequently. The majority give birth lying down, but some will remain standing.

Birth

Once labor begins, the sequence of events is the same as for other species. The water bag appears first, followed normally by the front feet and head. Parturition in the goat differs in only one respect from other species. It is usually accompanied by an excessive amount of bleating. This is not an indication that the doe is in trouble, only that she is not as stoic as other animals. If no progress is made on delivery in a reasonable length of time, she should be helped in the same manner as described for the other species. Retained placenta is not common in the goat, but when it occurs it should be handled by a veterinarian. Twinning is common.

As kids are born, clear any mucus from the nose and wipe them dry if the doe refuses to lick them off. They also need colostrum within the first hour, just like other animals, but feeding thereafter is a matter of choice. If the doe's milk is not to be used, it's probably best to begin hand feeding immediately. The longer the kids are allowed to nurse, the more traumatic the weaning experience is.

Disbudding

One thing that definitely should be done before kids are 1 week old is disbudding, unless you are dealing with a polled breed. Dehorning of adult goats is a major and often unsatisfactory procedure. It's much easier to do with a hot electric dehorning iron when they are young. A small dehorning iron — not the large size used for calves — is the most satisfactory. The horned breeds have a whorl of hair around each horn bud, but if you can't identify this, shaving the hair will expose the horn bud attached tightly to the skull. Generally it takes a 5- to 15-second application of a cherry-red dehorner to burn the horn bud adequately. This is not a job for the squeamish, and the burning must be thorough or unsightly scurs will grow at the site. On the other hand, excessive burning may cause brain damage.

Although it may seem heartless, using local anesthesia is of questionable value, because the kids object as much to injection of anesthetic as they do to the actual dehorning. While you are dehorning the males, slide the iron slightly to the rear and center of the horn bud. This will destroy the musk glands from whence comes the stink when they get older. When burning has been adequate, the skin will have a leathery, copper-colored appearance. A disbudding box makes restraint of the kid much easier.

Male kids not destined to become herd sires can be castrated at the same time using the emasculatome in the manner described for sheep. Don't neglect this important procedure because they are precocious, and some are fertile much earlier than you may realize. The result, if kids and doelings are kept together, may be doelings that are pregnant long before they should be. Unless they are unusually well grown, does should not be bred until they are at least a year old.

Restraint
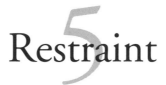

EVERY ANIMAL, regardless of species, has to be restrained for some purpose at some time. The degree of restraint depends on the reason for it. For some things a simple halter will suffice, but on occasion more severe measures are required. The important thing is to gear the degree of restraint to the need, using the minimum restraint necessary for protection of you and the animal.

Keep in mind that domestic animals are not far removed from wild animals and that in some cases, the more confining the restraint applied, the more they will struggle. I have seen beef calves just off the range struggle so hard to get out of a squeeze chute that they have collapsed from exhaustion. Being restrained can be a frightening experience for animals, and they remember it. The more traumatic their first experience is, the more difficult it will be to get them into a similar position the next time it becomes necessary. If you are dealing with just a few animals, get them accustomed to mild restraint such as a halter early in life, because it will make things much easier when they are older and larger.

Never forget that cattle, horses, and even mature pigs can hurt you badly. Much as we may love them, they are animals and their actions and reactions are unpredictable. Simply because a horse has not kicked you in the past does not mean he won't in the future.

Last, keep in mind that our primary advantage over animals is our capacity to reason. If you surrender that advantage and look upon restraint of the large farm animal as a contest of brute strength and determination, you will certainly lose and may get injured in the attempt. Be gentle and compassionate. Know what you want to do and how to go about it, and both you and your animal will fare much better.

Cattle

When it comes to restraint, dairy and beef cattle must be considered separately. Restraint of dairy cattle is much less of a problem because they are accustomed to being handled individually and being restrained for milking. Beef cattle, on the other hand, may be confined no more than once a year for vaccination and sometimes never. As a consequence, there is considerable difference in their attitude toward being individually handled.

Everyone who keeps more beef cattle than he can conveniently train to lead with a halter should have, at the very least, a chute and headgate to handle the herd. Too many owners of beef herds neglect this important management tool. They are also the ones who find veterinarians reluctant to work for them, since every call turns out to be a mini-rodeo and takes much longer than it should. Don't expect your veterinarian to play cowboy. He doesn't have the time and you can't afford it.

Construction plans for pen, chute, and headgate layouts are available at minimal cost from the department of agricultural engineering at all land-grant universities. Basically, the chute comprises two parallel plank fences or rail fences leading from the holding pen and terminating at a headgate or squeeze. The chute should be at least 5 feet high and no more than 28 inches wide inside. Although it may not seem so, that is adequate for a mature beef cow. Any wider than that and a few smart cows will manage to turn around and head the other way. In a chute designed for one-way traffic, this is frustrating because the cows behind the smart one have to be backed out and then all of them chased in again.

If you are using a rectangular holding pen or corral, it helps to have the entrance to the chute at one corner so that, as the cattle follow the fence, they can be directed into the chute with a crowding gate. In this regard, a circular holding pen works even better.

The length of the chute depends on how many cows you want to handle at a time, but plan on about 5 feet per cow. If the length of the chute warrants, it's helpful to build it in a curve so that when the cattle enter they can't see that the far end is blocked. For a procedure such as vaccination or application of insecticides, crowding cattle into the chute is all the restraint necessary.

Headgates and Steel Squeezes

For more detailed procedures, cows have to be held individually in the headgate. The headgate depicted in Figure 5-1 is simply a strong wooden gate with a stanchion built in that can be pulled shut quickly from the side. When the procedure is complete, the animal's head is released and the gate opened to let her go. When herd size warrants the investment, consider commercially available steel squeezes that serve the function of the headgate but, in addition, have sides that close in to hold the animal firmly in position. Smaller versions are available for calves. At least one manufacturer has modified the calf squeeze with a large hoop at each end so the whole unit can be rolled into any position, with the calf firmly fixed inside. Commercial squeezes may operate mechanically or hydraulically, the primary difference being price. The optimum for restraint is a hydraulic table to which the cow can be strapped and laid down flat. These are especially good for hoof trimming and surgical procedures.

Sooner or later, rope will be necessary for restraining cattle. I've found that 35 feet of ½-inch nylon rope, with a quick-release honda on one end, is the most versatile. Hard manila is better for throwing a loop, but it is too stiff for tying and doesn't have the tensile strength of nylon. Furthermore, manila is much more likely to cause rope burn.

MATERIALS

Full dimension oak
  2 x 4
  2 x 6
  2 x 8
  6 x 6
Bolts, ½" machine
Flat steel
  ¼ x 1 ½
  ¼ x 2
  ¼ x 3

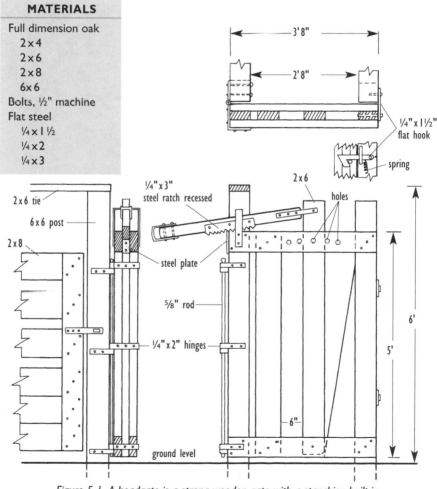

Figure 5-1. A headgate is a strong wooden gate with a stanchion built in that can be pulled shut quickly from the side.

Cow Halter

A halter is the mildest restraint commonly used on the cow. This is customarily made of rope, but leather or webbing is just as good. If none is available, a halter can easily be improvised with a lariat as shown in Figure 5-2. First, a noose is put around the neck; then a bight of rope is pulled through the noose and placed up over the muzzle and the running end of the rope drawn tight. With a flick of the quick-release honda, the animal can be immediately released. A rope with a ring on one end is also a very useful item, and its application as a halter is shown in Figure 5-3.

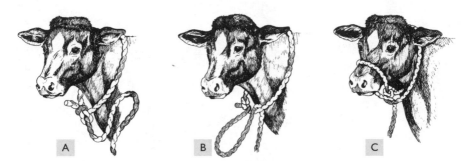

Figure 5-2. Steps in tying a rope halter: **A.** Place a noose around animal's neck. **B.** Form bight of rope. **C.** Pull bight through noose and over muzzle; draw the running end tight.

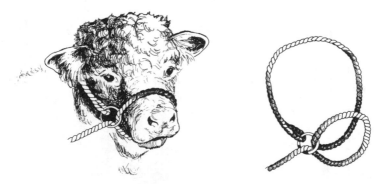

Figure 5-3. Rope halter with ring

One of the important things to remember when tying an animal with a halter is to use a knot that can be easily undone. If the head is tied and the animal struggles and falls, the animal may strangle unless the rope is untied immediately. Every stockman should master the halter tie shown in Figure 5-4. It's quick and easy, and a tug on the free end of the rope immediately unties the knot. While the knot shown in Figure 5-4C will hold, it can be untied by an animal that grabs the end and pulls. This can be prevented by passing the running end through the loop as shown in Figure 5-4D. If the knot is drawn tight in this position, however, it can't be untied easily.

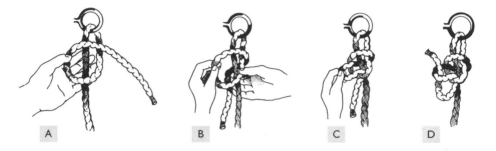

Figure 5-4. Steps in tying a quick-release knot or halter tie: **A.** Holding the standing part of the rope (attached to the animal) in your left hand, bring the free end over the standing part to form a loop. **B.** Make a second loop with the free end, and thread it through the first loop. **C.** Tighten the knot. **D.** To secure the knot, thread the tail end of the rope through the loop, as shown.

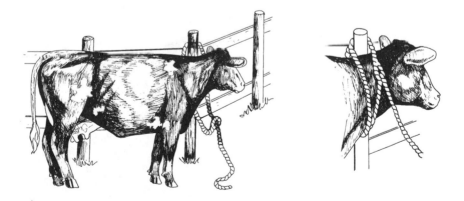

Figure 5-5. When a stanchion is not available, cattle can be restrained for minor procedures by immobilizing the head against a fence post, as shown.

Nose Lead

A more severe form of restraint for the head is the nose lead. This not only immobilizes the head, but it also causes sufficient pain that the animal hesitates to move in any direction. Properly used, it is quick and easy to apply, but there is a right way and a wrong way. I have seen people stand in front of the cow with one side of the nose lead in each hand, making passes at the cow's nose each time she swings it by. No self-respecting cow will stand still with head outstretched so you can put in a nose lead this way. The proper technique is to stand alongside the cow's head facing in the same direction. Grasp her head under your arm, and with the other hand put the nose lead in place. This technique serves two purposes: (1) it slows down head movement, and (2) it blocks her vision so she can't see what is about to be placed in her nose.

Figure 5-6 illustrates a common mistake people make, much to their later sorrow. A nose lead should never be tied in place but should be snubbed and held by an assistant. If the cow in the illustration were to struggle and fall to her knees, the nose lead would tear her nose, causing unnecessary pain and suffering until it healed. An assistant holding the rope can immediately slacken off if it looks as if the cow will fall. A nose lead will work more smoothly if, instead of passing a rope through the handles as shown, the rope is fastened to a ring that in turn is fastened to each handle with a few links of chain.

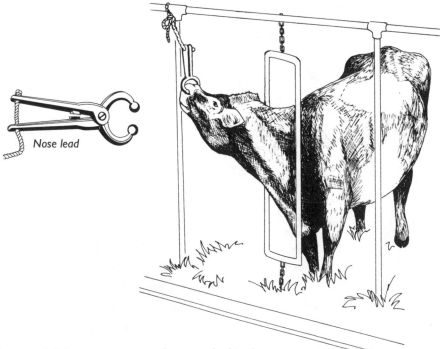

Nose lead

Figure 5-6. A common error — tying a nose lead in place

Bull Ring

A modification of the nose lead, permanently installed, is the bull ring, which is generally reserved, as the name suggests, for bulls. The dairy bull, as some people learn each year, is a dangerous animal, and his disposition doesn't improve with age. Up to the time they reach a year old, dairy bulls aren't too bad to handle, although they may play a bit rough. The best way to handle them after that time is to keep them in a facility constructed in such a way that you never have to be on the same side of the fence as the bull. Because this isn't always possible, have your veterinarian put in a good strong ring when the bull is 8 to 12 months old. At least the ring gives you a handle for restraint.

A bull staff, shown in Figure 5-7, can be attached to the ring for leading the bull. Several types are available, but essentially each is a 4-foot steel pole that attaches to the ring. With it not only can you lead the bull forward but also you can push back if he gets too friendly. And even if your back is turned, because a rigid pole is attached to the bull you can detect any movement he might make.

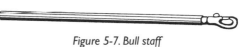

Figure 5-7. Bull staff

Another technique that increases the utility of the bull ring as a restraint device is to permanently attach a 3-foot length of chain to it. This is especially appropriate for bulls at pasture. Putting bulls in a pasture is not a good safety practice but if you do and he decides to run you out, the odds favor his stepping on the chain and being brought up short, giving you time to reach the fence or climb a tree.

The same precaution applies to bull rings as to nose leads. *Never* tie a bull solely by the ring. Use a halter, or if he has horns, put a rope around the horns, lead the running end down through the ring, and then tie it. I have seen a number of older bulls with their noses torn out because people failed to heed this advice. And once the nose is torn out, the most useful avenue of restraint is lost.

Kicking and Hind-Leg Restraint

Once the cow's head is secured by stanchion, halter, or nose lead, the only weapons she has left are the hind feet. Unlike the horse, she can kick forward and to the side as well as to the rear, almost with equal accuracy. It also seems necessary to do procedures on the cow within range of the hind feet more frequently than anywhere else. Hind-leg restraint is therefore often necessary, and there are several effective methods. If you have a willing assistant with a strong back, have him pick up the front leg on the same side on which you are working. The cow won't kick effectively unless she has the other three legs planted firmly on the ground.

Another method is to have an assistant push the tail firmly straight up over the back as shown in Figure 5-8. This throws the cow off balance, making her reluctant to move. For most cows, this alone provides sufficient restraint. Caution must be exercised, however, because excessive force may break the tail. A third method is to apply a squeeze just forward of the udder as shown in Figure 5-9. This works well on some cows, but others resist it and, while they can't kick, they will hop around, making it difficult to work.

I don't recommend the hobble restraint. Whether fashioned from rope or the commercial variety made of metal, hobbles tie the rear legs together at the hock. While some cows may tolerate this, others will not.

As a young practitioner more years ago than I care to remember, I bought a set of commercial hobbles that looked like a good idea at the time. These are

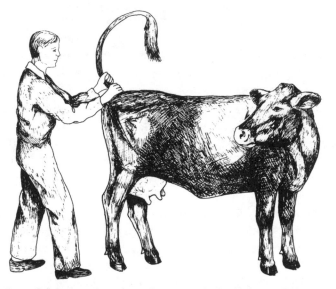

Figure 5-8. Pushing the tail straight up over the back prevents kicking.

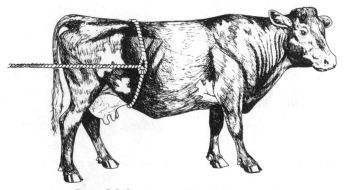

Figure 5-9. Some cows will resist this restraint.

still widely advertised and, I presume, sold. Basically they are two metal U straps that hook over the Achilles tendon above the hock, linked together by a chain that can be drawn tight and hooked. My first opportunity to use them came with a call requiring minor teat surgery. With pride and skill I put the new hobbles in place, intending to impress the client with my ability and the marvels of modern devices. All went well until I was about half done and struck a sensitive spot. The cow jumped into the air with both hind legs and, because they were locked together, lost her balance and landed on her side — with me underneath. After getting extricated, I removed the hobbles and, as far as I know, those shiny new hobbles are still at that farm. I never put them back in the car, deciding then and there that it's preferable to be kicked than crushed.

Rope Squeeze

As a last resort, the cow can be completely immobilized and laid down flat by applying a rope squeeze, as shown in Figures 5-10 through 5-12. The half-hitch method in Figure 5-10 seems to work a bit better, but with either method a cow can be gently laid down flat by pulling on the free end of the rope. The half-hitch method should not be used on bulls because of possible injury to the penis by the rear half hitch. Once the cow is down, an assistant sitting on her head can keep her that way. Needless to say, cows should not be cast in this manner on a hard floor or where the footing is likely to be slippery when they get up.

This technique is *not* recommended for general use because it can cause complications such as torsion of the uterus during advanced pregnancy and displaced abomasum. Furthermore, when cows are kept flat on their side very long, there is a risk of bloat, regurgitation, and inhalation pneumonia.

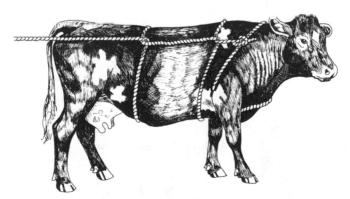

Figure 5-10. Getting a cow off her feet — first method. The rope is passed around the neck and behind one leg and tied. The long end is then passed around the body in two half hitches, and the free end is pulled back straight.

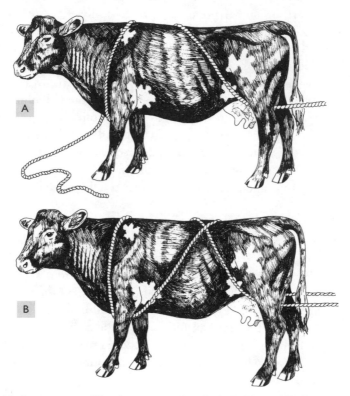

Figure 5-11. Getting a cow off her feet — second method. **A.** The middle of the rope is draped over the withers and the free end brought back between the forelegs. **B.** The ends are then crossed over the back and pulled straight back between the rear legs. In either method, pulling on the rope causes the animal to fall. An assistant should hold the animal's head down as soon as the animal is down.

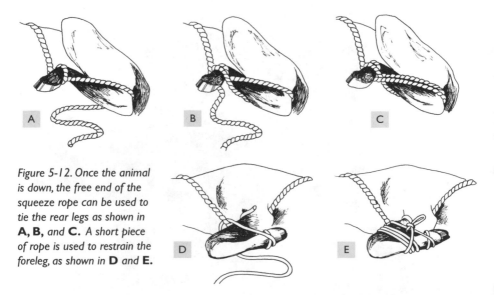

Figure 5-12. Once the animal is down, the free end of the squeeze rope can be used to tie the rear legs as shown in **A, B,** and **C.** A short piece of rope is used to restrain the foreleg, as shown in **D** and **E.**

Foot Restraint

The frequency with which cows' feet need to be examined and trimmed presents a physical challenge. They simply don't stand well on three legs, as a horse will. Some type of mechanical aid is usually necessary. The front feet are generally no problem; Figure 5-13 shows a method of supporting the front leg. The hind legs are a different story. Not only are they more mobile and lethal, but also the cow resists having them picked up because they must be drawn backward and upward in order to work on the sole.

One effective method is shown in Figure 5-14. A loop, preferably with a quick-release honda, is placed around the pastern (A). The running end is then put through a ring or over a beam or over whatever is handy; brought back to

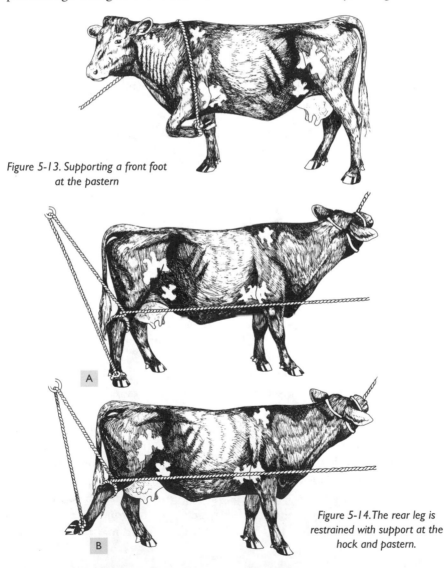

Figure 5-13. Supporting a front foot
at the pastern

A

B

Figure 5-14. The rear leg is
restrained with support at the
hock and pastern.

form a half hitch around the hock; and then passed forward and snubbed around something solid and held by an assistant. As the foot is picked up, the rope is tightened so that the leg is suspended with support at the hock and pastern (B). Once the leg is elevated to the proper position, the rope should be held in place by the assistant. It should never be tied, because some cows will resist the procedure and struggle until they fall. If they fall from this position, a broken hip is a common sequel. Always be ready to release animals from potentially dangerous restraint instantly.

Tail Tie

Although it restrains nothing but the tail, the tail tie shown in Figure 5-15 is simple and frequently useful. If nothing else, it will keep a manure-soaked tail out of your face while you are milking.

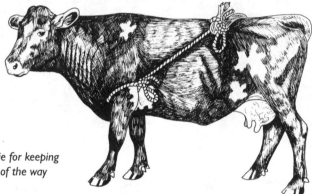

Figure 5-15. Tie for keeping the tail out of the way

Calf Restraint

As a part of good dairy herd management, extra teats should be amputated from the heifers when they are 2 to 3 weeks old. For this operation, the heifers must be restrained on their backs. Depending on the technique used, this posture may be necessary for castration of bull calves as well. Calves at this age can be pretty frisky, but it isn't hard to lay them down if you go about it in the right way. Figure 5-16 shows the preferred method. Standing alongside the calf, bend over and grasp the front and rear legs nearest you and lift. This tips the calf toward you and allows her to gently slide down against your legs. You are then in position to put your knees on the calf to hold her down, while you tie the rear legs as shown in Figure 5-17. Tipping the calf the other way, away from you, not only causes the calf to fall with a jarring thump but also puts you on the side where the legs will be flailing until and if you can get them under control. Never try to throw a calf by grabbing the front and rear legs and twisting until the calf falls. This is painful for the calf and may be for you, too.

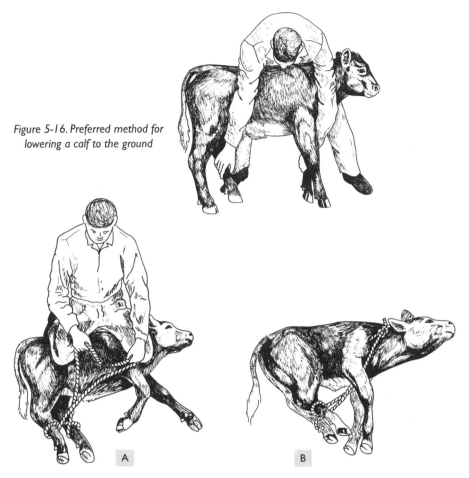

Figure 5-16. Preferred method for lowering a calf to the ground

Figure 5-17. **A.** Rest your knees on the calf to hold her down. Tie the rear legs as shown. **B.** Secure rope around calf's neck.

Horses

Although comparable in size and weight to cows, when it comes to restraint, horses are much different. By nature they are much less phlegmatic and more responsive to pain. Their movements are quicker, and in addition to kicking with the hind legs, they will rear and strike with the front legs and may bite when you least expect it. They are also much stronger, and the potential for injury from an obstreperous horse is considerably greater than from a cow.

On the plus side, most horses today are what must be classed as companion animals. They are brushed, petted, and pampered daily to the point where a few are just plain spoiled. The frequent attention does accustom them to handling, although when the discomfort of some necessary veterinary procedure is a factor, their response may be totally unexpected.

Once I was called by a woman who wanted her horse vaccinated for sleeping sickness. She had a beautiful 2-year-old Morgan filly, born on the farm and never handled by anyone other than herself. When I approached the filly, syringe in hand, she literally went wild. I couldn't even get into the box stall with her. After a few futile attempts, I handed the syringe to the owner and told her how to give the injection while I got out of sight. Then she proceeded to go into the box stall with no restraint whatever. That's how that horse was vaccinated every year thereafter. Strange as it may seem, it turned out that the filly had never seen a man before and was simply terrified by the sight or smell or both. She just didn't like men. Horses are different from other livestock.

Approach Quietly

Because horses are different, a little "horse sense" and judgment go a long way in preventing injury to them and to you when restraint is necessary. Approach the horse quietly and confidently but never sneak up on him. Let him know you are there by a quiet word or two. Then put a hand on him, starting at the shoulder and working toward the area you want to reach. To avoid serious injury from a kick, incongruous as it may seem, stand in close. That way a suddenly raised leg may push you away rather violently, but you won't get the full force of the kick. Don't make the mistake of thinking you can avoid injury by standing as far away as possible and reaching to touch a sore spot or whatever. This leaves you off balance, and because the horse's leg is longer than your arm, you are certain to get hurt if the horse should kick.

Halter

The most universal restraint device for horses is the halter, and horses should be introduced to it early in life. If the halter is to be used as a restraint device for a procedure the horse doesn't like, however, the lightweight show-type halter will not be strong enough. Most show halters can be easily broken. A heavy leather or web halter will do a better job. In an emergency, a halter can be improvised with a lariat as shown in Figure 5-18. A strong lead shank with a snap is fastened to the halter ring. A piece of ½-inch nylon rope about 6 feet long does a good job if properly used. The novice will often hold the lead shank near the end with one hand and try to lead the horse like a dog. This method doesn't really provide any control because with slack in the rope, if your back is turned, the horse can reach out and bite or strike with a front foot before you realize what happened.

The proper way to use a lead shank is to stand on the left side of the horse's head facing the same direction. Grasp the shank firmly in the right hand about 6 inches from the halter, and hold the other end in the left hand. By holding the shank close to the halter, you can detect the slightest movement of the horse and do something about it if his intentions appear hostile.

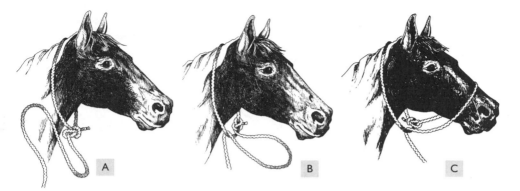

Figure 5-18. Three steps for quickly tying a lariat into a halter. **A.** *Slip a noose over the horse's head and form a bight.* **B.** *Slip bight through noose.* **C.** *Lift bight over horse's nose.*

Cross-Tying

Cross-tying, illustrated in Figure 5-19, provides added restriction of movement. This may be all that is needed to restrain the animal for common procedures such as shoeing. Cross-tying is strongly recommended for horses being moved in trucks or trailers because it helps the animal maintain his balance when the vehicle sways and also prevents head injuries.

A variety of further restraints can be used in addition to cross-tying. Picking up one foot sometimes helps to ensure that the other three will remain on the ground. Twisting an ear may provide sufficient distraction to take the animal's mind off what is being done to him somewhere else.

Twitch

When these mild measures fail, a twitch may have to be used. A typical commercial chain twitch is shown in Figure 5-20. To put this on, assuming you are right-handed, put the finger-tips of your left hand through the chain loop and spread your fingers to hold the chain near your fingertips. Then grab the horse's nose with your left hand and maintain the hold while you

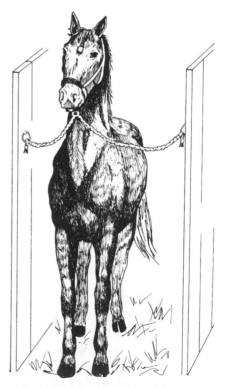

Figure 5-19. Cross-tying is used for many common procedures.

slide the chain loop down on the horse. Still holding the nose in the left hand, twist the twitch handle with the right until the chain tightens up, then hold the handle with both hands. While a few horses will fight a twitch, most will give up in response to the pressure applied. Use

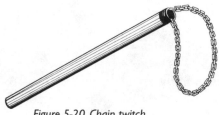

Figure 5-20. Chain twitch

only the degree of twisting pressure required because the twitch is painful, and there is no need for cruelty. Although the commercial twitches shown in Figures 5-20 and 5-21 will do, they are too short to provide the leverage and control sometimes needed. I prefer the homemade variety, using a 36-inch hickory pick handle because it gives a little more mastery of the situation and permits you to maintain a grip and still avoid flying front feet.

In an emergency, twitches can be improvised with rope and a piece of wood or claw hammer as shown in Figure 5-22, but these have limited value. Although some people do it, a twitch should *never* be put on a horse's ear. Not only is it acutely painful, but it also may rupture a blood vessel in the ear, causing a hematoma that almost invariably ends up as an unsightly scar.

Other Restraints

Various other restraint techniques can be used as the situation requires. Some stallions, for example, can be difficult to control when teasing or breeding mares. A helpful technique is to use a lead shank that has a foot or so of chain interposed between the rope or strap and the snap. The snap is threaded

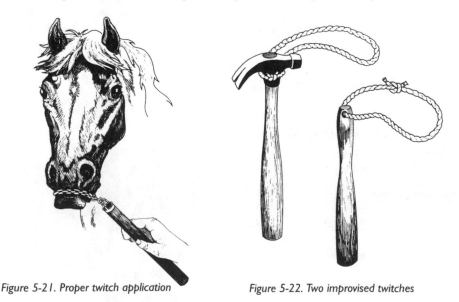

Figure 5-21. Proper twitch application

Figure 5-22. Two improvised twitches

through the left side ring of the halter, over the
bridge of the nose, and attached to the corre-
sponding ring on the right side of the halter
With this arrangement, the stallion more interested in his sex life than in his behavior can be
brought back to reality by a sharp tug on the
lead shank. The discomfort of the chain pressing
on the bridge of his nose will give him something else to think about. If that is inadequate, a
war bridle applied as in Figure 5-23 may help.
This is simply a slip noose passed back of the
poll and under the upper lip where it puts pressure on the gums of the upper incisors when

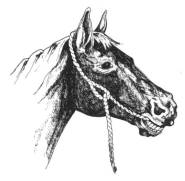

*Figure 5-23. A war bridle can be
used on an unruly stallion.*

tightened. It hurts, and most horses develop a healthy respect for it.

To protect the stallion from the kick of a reluctant mare during breeding,
it's sometimes advisable to use breeding hobbles. Figure 5-24 shows a method
of applying rope breeding hobbles; Figure 5-25 shows how to tie rope breeding hobbles. (Rope breeding hobbles should never be left untied, unless there
are two reliable assistants on either side of the horse holding the rope.) Some
mares may need similar restraint for rectal palpation or pregnancy examination. The best rope to use in this manner is ⅝-inch or ¾-inch cotton, which is
preferable for horses. Manila and even nylon may cause rope burns, which are
slow to heal and may leave a scar. As a word of caution, hobbles should not be
so tight that the mare's movement is unduly restricted. If they are, she may lose
her balance and fall, causing injury.

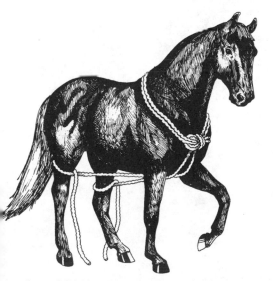

Figure 5-24. How to apply rope breeding hobbles

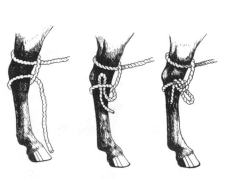

Figure 5-25. How to tie the breeding hobbles

The tail tie shown in Figure 5-26 is sometimes useful to stabilize or control lateral movement of the rear end. It's a simple method of tying the switch to a rope that can be quickly released. Although it usually isn't necessary, a rope tied to the tail can be used to help support the rear leg, as shown in Figure 5-27.

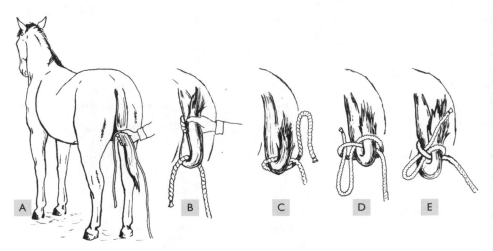

Figure 5-26. How to apply the tail tie

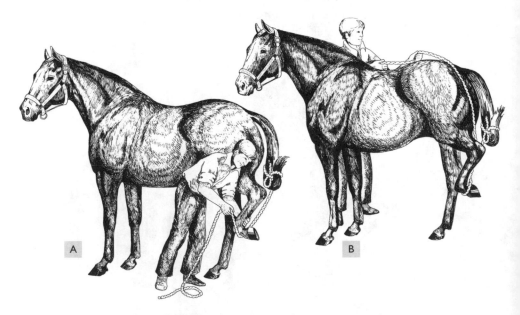

Figure 5-27. The tail tie can be used to support a rear leg.

Figure 5-28 illustrates the use of a rope to support the foreleg. Occasionally it's necessary to carry or restrain a young foal. Figure 5-29 shows the preferred method, which provides restraint yet is comfortable for the foal.

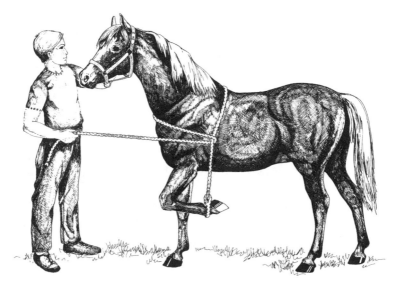

Figure 5-28. A rope tie can be used to support a front foot.

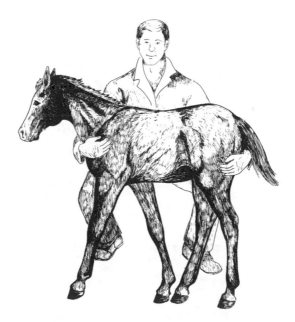

Figure 5-29. A comfortable, secure method to restrain or carry a foal

Sheep, Goats, and Swine

With the exception of mature swine, these species are much more manageable than horses or cows because of their smaller size. Nevertheless, a few tips may be helpful.

The most difficult part about restraining a sheep is catching it. A flock of sheep will run at the slightest pretext, and it's difficult to separate a single one from the flock. The only practical method is to drive the entire flock into a pen or corral to limit their movement. Then, with an assistant and a couple of portable crowding gates, you can isolate the one you want to catch. For the purpose, light gates 3 feet high and 6 to 8 feet wide are very useful. When you have your sheep separated, hold it with one arm under the neck and the other under the tail. Never grab a sheep by the wool because it breaks the fibers, making the fleece less valuable. Once caught, sheep seldom struggle. Goats, too, are not much of a problem and can be restrained easily with a collar or halter.

Pigs, however, are a whole different matter. Once a pig reaches 100 pounds or so, there is nothing much more difficult to hold than a frightened, determined pig. There are no good handles to grab, and they are all muscle. Once they are cornered together, piglets and goats can be held by the hind legs for vaccination, castration, and other procedures, but larger pigs require a different technique. For oral administration of drugs or examination of the pig's mouth, a speculum, as shown in Figure 5-30, is very useful.

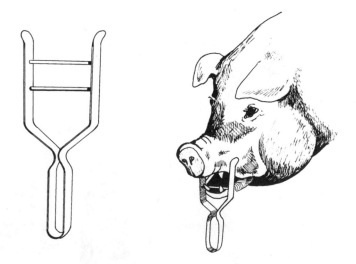

Figure 5-30. This swine mouth speculum is used to hold the mouth open for examination or to give oral medication. The same instrument can be used on sheep and goats.

Bucket and Rope Halter

The only real defense a pig has is his very sharp teeth, which he doesn't hesitate to use. But he can also knock the legs out from under you if he runs into you with his solid bulk, so approach with some care.

A common challenge is to move a pig from one pen to another when gates are not available. When you are trying to drive a pig, he always seems to get his head on the wrong end. A good way to take advantage of this propensity is illustrated in Figure 5-31. Put a bucket over the pig's head and with an assistant pulling on the tail as a tiller, back the pig wherever you want him to go. A second method of dubious value is to put a noose around the neck supplemented by a half hitch around the middle and to lead — or more likely drag — the pig where you want him to go. Figure 5-32 shows the technique.

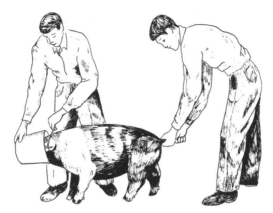

Figure 5-31. A bucket over the head and a tug on the tail is the preferred method for moving a pig backward.

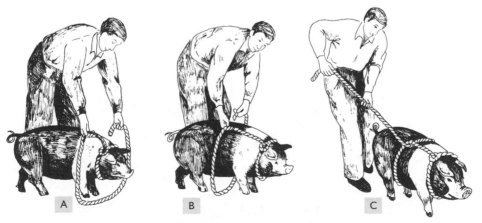

Figure 5-32. This roping method may also work for moving a pig.

Pig Snare

The most useful instrument for catching and holding a large pig is the snare, shown in Figure 5-33. This is basically a 4-foot length of pipe through which a

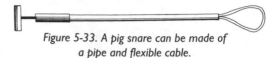

Figure 5-33. A pig snare can be made of a pipe and flexible cable.

flexible cable is threaded with a loop formed in the business end. By holding the pipe in one hand and pulling the handle with the other, the loop is tightened. Characteristically, a pig trying to avoid capture in a pen will back into a corner and keep his myopic eyes on you. With a pig in this position, it's easy to put the snare loop over his snout and draw it tight. Once it is tightened, he usually just pulls back and squeals. The same thing can be done with a rope, but it is a bit harder to manage (Figure 5-34). With a rope, however, you have the advantage of a free end that can be tied around a hind leg, as shown in Figure 5-35, to immobilize the pig. When restraining pigs, especially piglets, for any purpose wear some type of ear protection. Their high-pitched squeal, an expression of fear as well as pain, is deafening.

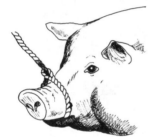

Figure 5-34. Rope can be used as a snare.

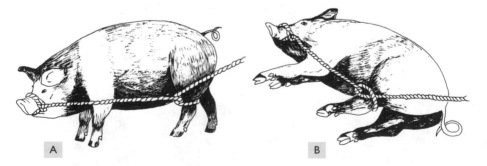

Figure 5-35. A rope snare looped around back leg will immobilize a pig.

Summary

Most of the restraint techniques described here, as well as others not described, have evolved since man first domesticated animals — a period during which there was no alternative to physical restraint. But during the past 50 years, veterinary research has developed techniques and drugs for sedation, tranquilization, and anesthesia that have made major physical restraint unnecessary in most cases. These techniques are safer for the animal and for the operator.

Now a word on behalf of veterinarians everywhere: If you have a cow or horse that you know has an inclination to kick, tell the veterinarian before he gets in range so he knows what to expect. There are few things more maddening than the phrase all of us have heard after the fact, "I meant to tell you — she kicks." Similarly, if your veterinarian asks you to hold an animal while he works on her, do so with undivided attention. I still have a scar from a kick received when the client dropped a twitch and ran the first time the horse jumped a bit.

Finally, remember that within the context of this book on animal health, you will often be restraining an animal that is sick. Be as gentle and quiet in your handling as possible because excitement and exertion will only make a sick animal worse. If the cure is worse than the disease, nothing is accomplished.

Physical Examination 6

ONE OF THE MOST FRUSTRATING and discouraging aspects of large-animal practice for a veterinarian is the frequency with which he is called at the last moment when little to nothing can be done. Many reasons are given. "I didn't realize she was sick until this morning," or "I thought she might get better." One of the most maddening is, "Well, Doc, I knew she was a little off so I gave her penicillin, some sulfa pills, and a good laxative last week but that didn't help, so I thought I'd give you a chance to see what you can do"!

All too often the animal is so far gone by then that poor Doc has no chance at all, and neither does his patient. Too often the end result is that death terminates the animal's suffering and Doc gets the blame. The only benefit, if there is one, from this kind of situation is that the owner can ease his or her conscience by proclaiming to all who will listen, "Well, I called Doc to look at her but it was a waste of money because she died anyhow. I guess he isn't too sharp."

Every veterinarian has found himself in this position many times. But the owner is right; employing veterinary service in this manner is a waste of money. The earlier a disease is recognized and properly treated, the more probable a satisfactory outcome will be.

Most diseases are preventable, and if you follow the advice in this book, serious illness will be minimal. But despite everyone's best efforts, problems will occur occasionally. The effect of these can be minimized if they are recognized early and if an intelligent judgment is made as to what the condition may be and what degree of treatment may be required. If it looks as though a veterinarian may be needed, don't delay calling. The oldest drug in history is tincture of time, but it's not foolproof.

Observe Your Animals

Briefly defined, *disease* is any departure from normal function. It follows, then, that before you can recognize a disease problem, you must be thoroughly familiar with the normal behavior and function of the animals in your care. Spending a few minutes every day watching your animals is time well spent. This is the only way you can learn their normal behavior and attitude, and unless you know that, you won't be able to recognize anything that may be wrong. This knowledge marks the difference between the animal husbandryman and the less experienced animal owner.

For example, are you always greeted by a whinny when you first enter the horse barn in the morning? This is typical of most horses, but suppose you don't hear that whinny some morning? What does it mean? Perhaps nothing, but it certainly merits further investigation. You can be sure your horse's whinny isn't broken, but he may be sick. Take time to observe his attitude. Does he hang back in the stall with head down or ears drooping? Does he seem interested in feed or not? Is he sweating or salivating? These are the kinds of things to look for and investigate further.

Observe the herd at pasture for signs of unusual behavior. Cattle, sheep, and — to a lesser degree — swine tend to be gregarious and will usually stay close together when grazing. Horses are a little more independent and goats are even more so, but they all tend to congregate. The animal that stays off in a corner by itself usually does so for a reason. That reason may be nothing more than aberrant social behavior if it does so consistently. But if an animal normally found with the herd seeks solitude, it is usually for a reason. It may be a normal function such as imminent parturition, but it could be illness and needs to be investigated.

Common sense, a little knowledge, and your physical senses applied to examination will often reveal the problem. The important thing is to apply these in a systematic manner and not jump to conclusions.

Things to Look For

In physical examination, the first thing to do is observe the animal from some distance. Look for such things as symmetry of conformation. Swelling, depending on location, may indicate an infection, an abscess, a tumor, a hernia, a hematoma, a fracture, or just a bruise.

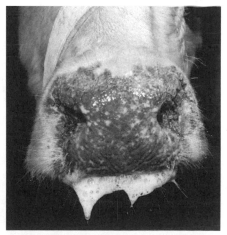

Note the crusty muzzle and slobbering, suggestive of bovine virus diarrhea or malignant catarrhal fever.

Look at the head. Does one ear droop or is one eye partially closed? Is the animal drooling or making aimless movements with its tongue? Are the eyes bright or do they lack luster and appear dull? Are they sunken, indicating dehydration? Although nonspecific, the luster of the eye is a good measure of an animal's well-being.

Does the abdomen have a "tucked up" appearance? Note the character and consistency of the manure. Is it abnormally hard or soft? Does the animal make straining movements? Is the urine of

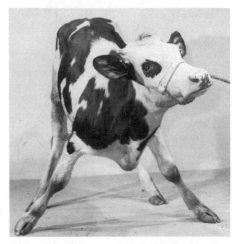

An unusual posture like this is indicative of a lesion in the brain or upper spinal cord.

normal color or is it coffee-colored or bloody? In male animals, does the urine flow in a normal stream, does it just dribble, or is there none at all? Is the animal thin, its hair coat rough? Is hair falling out or being rubbed off?

Watch how the animal moves. Is its gait normal, stilted, staggering? Is it reluctant to move or is it lame? A keen observer can learn a lot by systematic observation of an animal from a distance. Once this part of the examination has been completed, the next step is to zero in at close range on those concerns noted by visual examination.

Preliminary Examination

Be methodical by not overlooking anything or jumping to conclusions. Where a problem is not obvious, the possibilities can be narrowed down by recording temperature, pulse, and respiration rate before the animal gets excited from handling. The normal ranges are given in Table 6-1. Measuring temperature, pulse, and respiration helps to narrow down the possible causes of illness. It even gives some indication of what the final outcome may be.

Take the Temperature

The most useful diagnostic instrument an animal owner can have is a 5-inch ring-top rectal thermometer. These are available at almost any instrument supply house and drugstore. A word of advice from one who has been there: tie a string on the thermometer, unless you want to hold it in the rectum for the required 3 minutes or so. In the cow, especially one with a relaxed anal sphincter, the deeply inserted thermometer may slip in and be out of sight by the time you are ready to retrieve it. The only recourse then is to go in after it —

TABLE 6-1	NORMAL VITAL SIGNS		
SPECIES	TEMPERATURE (°F)	PULSE/MINUTE	RESPIRATION/MINUTE
Cow	100.4–102.8	60–70	18–28
Horse	99.1–100.8	32–44	8–16
Pig	101.6–103.6	60–80	8–18
Sheep	100.9–103.8	70–80	12–20
Goat	101.7–105.3	70–80	12–20

or to pull the string. To prevent loss of the thermometer, tie the free end of the string to a spring-type clothespin and clip it to the tail fold. When the thermometer is attached in this manner, you can proceed with the rest of the examination while the temperature is being recorded. For a little more money, instant reading electronic thermometers are available; these are more convenient.

The body temperature of animals is not nearly as consistent as that of humans. Their heat regulatory mechanism is not as efficient. On a cold day the body temperature will be at the low end of the range, and on a hot day at the high end or even higher. Excitement will also raise body temperature, possibly leading to an erroneous interpretation. Pigs are particularly vulnerable to hot weather and may suffer heatstroke, with body temperatures sometimes exceeding 108°F. Therefore, one must use judgment in interpreting the reading on a thermometer. On a hot day, a reading slightly above the normal range does not necessarily indicate fever.

Aside from weather influence and excitement, an elevated temperature may indicate viral or bacterial infection or occasionally severe pain. Temperature will be subnormal in the cow with milk fever, for a transitory period following high fever, and prior to death. A normal temperature at initial examination of an animal off feed suggests some type of digestive, metabolic, or functional disorder. Much can be learned with the aid of a thermometer.

Pulse and respiration rate generally but not always parallel body temperature. Both go up, of course, in response to excitement or exertion; therefore, it's important to handle sick animals quietly and carefully. The added exertion of being chased around the pen can kill an animal with pneumonia. Heart and respiratory rates will be elevated without fever in cases of anemia due to iron deficiency, blood loss due to parasitism or hemorrhage, red blood cell destruction as occurs with anaplasmosis or piroplasmosis, and in some types of poisoning, as well as in response to pain or fear.

Check the Pulse

The pulse is the surge of blood through the arteries immediately following contraction of the heart ventricles. It normally parallels the heart rate, and its character reveals much about an animal's condition. Pulse rate may be variously classified as regular, irregular, weak, strong, or thready. Except for regularity, these nuances will not be detected by the layperson, and, for our purposes, need not be.

In cows, the pulse is most easily detected by palpating the middle coccygeal artery on the underside of the tail, about 6 inches down from the tail head. The easiest site to detect the pulse in horses is where the facial artery crosses the underside of the jawbone, just in front of the large muscle that forms the cheek. In goats and sheep, the heartbeat can usually be felt directly, but the pulse can easily be felt over the femoral artery, about a third of the way down on the inside of the thigh. The same location is satisfactory for young, thin pigs, but in most pigs the fat thickness precludes palpation of an arterial pulse. Practice taking the pulse on several healthy animals until you can do so readily and with confidence.

Check Respiration

Increased rate of respiration with fever and coughing is frequently indicative of pneumonia. Without fever, it reflects anemia or impaired lung function, such as pulmonary edema due to allergy, organophosphate poisoning, or circulatory collapse.

Check the Rumen

For ruminant animals — cows, sheep, and goats — a fourth measurement can be added, and that is rate of rumen contraction. The rumen can be likened to a mixing vat that churns periodically to stir up the ingested feed. In the healthy animal, rumen contractions occur two to four times a minute. By pressing firmly on the left flank, one can feel this movement when it occurs. Contractions will be slower than normal or absent with some types of indigestion, in the cow with traumatic gastritis or displaced abomasum, during milk fever, as a result of dehydration, and in conditions affecting the vagus nerve. Contractions may be faster than normal in the animal that has or is about to have diarrhea.

The examination so far, whether the illness is due to infectious or noninfectious causes, permits some tentative conclusions, and this helps to narrow the possibilities considerably. A preliminary judgment whether to call a veterinarian can even be made at this point. If you decide to call, tell your veterinarian what you have observed. He will appreciate it because what you describe will help him to decide whether he should drop everything else and come right out (often at added cost to you) or whether it is safe to wait until later when he will be in the area. As the veterinarian develops confidence in your ability at preliminary evaluation, you may find that he takes less time to make a final diagnosis. Because the veterinarian's time is worth money — yours — ultimately you save.

Further Examination

If you still don't know what to do, start methodically examining the accessible organ systems, paying particular attention to the presence or absence of fever and lameness.

Ailments Causing High Fever

If there is high fever, the odds favor disease involving the respiratory tract, the reproductive organs including the mammary gland, or the urinary tract.

For the respiratory tract, look for nasal discharge, coughing, labored breathing, and in extreme cases flaring of the nostrils during inspiration. In his examination, your veterinarian would also add careful auscultation of (or listening to) the lungs with a stethoscope and percussion. In the case of such diseases as infectious bovine rhinotracheitis and influenza, samples also may need to be taken for virus isolation or serological work in the laboratory before a final diagnosis can be made.

If nothing is obviously wrong with the respiratory tract, the next good possibility is the mammary gland. Acute mastitis with fever is common in dairy cattle. While mastitis is less common in beef cattle and other species, the udder should not be overlooked in any species as a possible site of infection. The infected udder with acute mastitis will feel hot and swollen to the touch and will usually be very sore for the animal. The color and consistency of the milk will be abnormal. It may be watery and have clots, flakes, or pus in it. These abnormalities can best be detected by squirting some milk on a black strip plate. The type of strip cup employing a fine mesh screen will reveal clots and flakes but will not identify milk that is off-color or watery. Most farm-supply stores stock some satisfactory type of black strip plate. Acute mastitis is a serious disease that requires prompt and appropriate treatment locally and systemically.

Urinary tract infections such as leptospirosis and pyelonephritis may be difficult to diagnose based on physical signs alone. This is a job for the veterinarian unless you happen to see coffee-colored urine, which is typical of leptospirosis.

Obviously, there are many more diseases causing fever in domestic animals, but the foregoing discussion illustrates some of the steps taken to arrive at a diagnosis.

Disease without Fever

Disease conditions not associated with fever are many and varied. Some are accompanied by loss of appetite but others are not. If appetite is lacking, think first of indigestion. Is there history of recent diet change, a common cause of indigestion? Is rumination slow and are feces scanty? Is there evidence of abdominal cramps and pain such as restlessness; kicking at the belly; stretching and standing in a stretched-out, "saw-horse" attitude? All are indications of indigestion. Indigestion is a common cause of colic in the horse and is accompanied by rapid pulse, sweating, marked pain, and sometimes infection of the sclera. The latter is merely dilation of the blood vessels supplying the white part of the eye.

If there is no fever and no evidence of indigestion, yet the animal refuses feed and water, look in the mouth for swellings, ulcers, and, in the horse, sharp teeth. One word of caution — if you live in an area where rabies is endemic, don't put your bare hands in the mouth of an animal that is not eating for an unknown reason. Wear leather or rubber gloves.

Sharp teeth or malocclusion may be a cause of failure to eat. The inside edge of the lower molars and the outside edge of the upper molars of the horse become very sharp and sometimes abrade the cheek and tongue. The resulting soreness leads to inadequate chewing, which in turn contributes to indigestion. Check, too, for tongue paralysis, a principal sign of botulism and a common finding with listeriosis in cattle, sheep, and goats. Listeriosis also usually causes a unilateral facial paralysis and an inclination to walk in circles.

Lameness

Other nonfebrile disease conditions will usually be obvious at least insofar as the affected area is concerned. One that commonly causes confusion is lameness. Lameness is common in all species, and generally the trouble is in

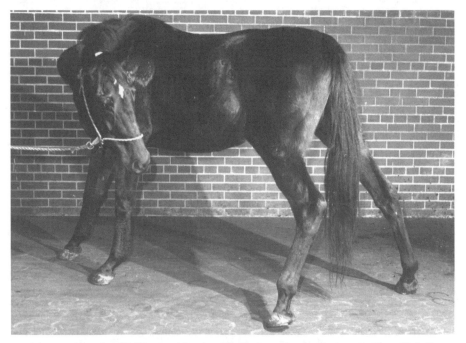

A horse with colic will often stand in a stretched-out position and look anxiously at his belly.

the foot itself. Every careful physical examination where lameness is a factor includes picking up the foot and examining it carefully. With a hoof pick, clean away all dirt and debris, and with a hoof knife pare away all dead-appearing tissue. Cleaning frequently reveals puncture wounds, embedded nails and stones, stone bruises, and infections. Sometimes trimming a badly overgrown foot is all that is required.

Foot rot is a specific disease in cattle, sheep, and goats that is recognizable by swelling, exudate, and a characteristic foul odor.

Aside from fractures, joint lesions are the next most common cause of lameness in species other than the horse. Except where there is obvious swelling, diagnosis of these is best left to the veterinarian.

Years ago a common cause of lameness in cattle was rubber canning-jar gaskets encircling a single claw or the entire foot. When these were carelessly discarded, cattle would step on them and they would work up higher on the foot. The pressure they exerted caused impaired circulation, and they cut into the skin, causing swelling and infection. As home canning became less popular, this type of injury almost disappeared.

Lameness in the horse has a variety of causes other than injuries to the foot. These are so varied, and four sound legs are so important to the horse, that diagnosis and treatment should be left to the veterinarian.

Consider Other Factors

When attempting to arrive at a diagnosis, consider extraneous factors as well as the clinical signs observed. Environmental factors influence the prevalence of some diseases. Pneumonia, for example, is relatively rare in summer but common in winter, from October through March, when rapid weather shifts occur. Conversely, labored breathing due to pulmonary edema is more common when animals are exposed to allergenic grasses at pasture. Internal parasitism with stomach worms in sheep, goats, and cattle is rarely a problem in winter but is serious on some farms during the pasture season. The onset of acute haemonchosis in sheep can be dramatic a few days after a rain following a prolonged dry period, because the moisture fosters maturation of the infective stage of the worm ova that have accumulated. Pregnancy disease or ketosis in the ewe, and ketosis and milk fever in the cow, is always associated with parturition. Similarly, metritis does not occur when the animal is pregnant but appears after parturition.

Regional Diseases

Some diseases occur only in certain regions. For example, winter dysentery in cattle occurs primarily in the northeast United States. Piroplasmosis in horses is limited mostly to the Gulf Coast states because that's where the tick that transmits it lives. The strains of virus causing equine encephalomyelitis tend to be regionally specific, identified as eastern, Venezuelan, western, and so on.

As you learn more about the pathogenesis of disease and take all factors into account, the problem of diagnosis — at least of the common diseases — becomes somewhat easier.

The previous discussion by no means covers all misfortunes that can befall animals, and it will not make you an accomplished diagnostician. It does outline a procedure for preliminary examination that, when coupled with the specific disease information that follows, should allow you to distinguish between those things you can handle on your own and those things for which veterinary assistance is required.

Once the physical examination has been completed and the animal has been evaluated, the following tables may help to suggest some possible causes for the illness. These include most but certainly not all of the specific disease entities afflicting animals. This is essentially the procedure every veterinarian goes through in reaching a diagnosis — complete history, careful physical examination, evaluation of clinical findings, differential diagnosis, and final diagnosis. The veterinarian, of course, by virtue of training and experience will have a much greater depth of knowledge about the physiological and pathological processes involved, as well as the advantage of a battery of diagnostic tests when necessary.

Except in the most obvious conditions, it will always be to your advantage to have diagnosis and therapeutic recommendations made by your veterinarian. I am always amazed at how many people who wouldn't think of attempting to repair their television sets don't hesitate to use a variety of potions and remedies on a valuable sick animal before calling a veterinarian. *Remember:* Nothing is absolute in medicine, and there are many variables to consider.

Although we may list and classify diseases and symptoms in a convenient manner, in reality medicine is not this orderly. Not all diseases produce all the clinical signs listed all the time, and there are varying degrees of disease severity. Nothing precludes the possibility of more than one disease affecting an animal at the same time. In fact, malnutrition and some types of internal parasitism frequently coincide. A good example of disease interaction is the MMA syndrome in sows. Predisposing factors for this condition are lack of dietary roughage, lack of exercise, unsanitary surroundings, and constipation. The clinical signs include metritis (uterine infection), mastitis, and agalactia, hence the acronym MMA. The implications for the sow are serious, but they are even worse for the piglets, which, because there is no milk, die of hypoglycemia or starvation.

The moral, if there is one, is that it is always better to prevent disease than to treat it, no matter how prompt the diagnosis and therapy. A better understanding of animal disease and its diagnosis will assist in the development of appropriate programs for disease prevention.

TABLE 6-2	**COMMON LIVESTOCK DISEASES CHARACTERIZED BY FEVER**		
DISEASE	SPECIES	PRIMARY SITE	REMARKS
Anaplasmosis	Cattle, sheep, goats	Red blood cells	Insect borne, anemia, southern states
Anthrax	Cattle, sheep, goats, horses, pigs	Generalized	High mortality, limited distribution
Babesiosis (piroplasmosis)	Horses	Liver, spleen	Insect borne, anemia, southern states
Bacillary hemoglobinuria	Cattle	Liver	Western and southern US
Blackleg	Cattle, sheep, goats	Muscle	Young cattle, 6–12 months, usually acute
Bluetongue	Sheep, cattle, goats	Generalized	Western states
Bovine virus diarrhea (BVD, musocal disease)	Cattle	Alimentary tract	Yearlings
Calf diphtheria	Cattle	Pharynx, larynx	2–6 months of age
Contagious ecthyma (sore mouth)	Sheep, goats	Lips, udder	Contact transmission
Enzootic pneumonia	Pigs	Lung	3 weeks and older
Eperythrozoonosis	Pigs, sheep, cattle	Red blood cells	Southern and midwestern states
Equine encephalomyelitis	Horses	Brain	Several viral strains
Equine infectious anemia (EIA)	Horses	Generalized	Acute, chronic, inapparent
Equine influenza	Horses	Upper respiratory tract	Clinical signs during inclement weather
Equine rhinopneumonitis (virus abortion)	Horses	Upper respiratory tract	Abortion follows
Erysipelas	Pigs	Generalized	Red blotches on skin
Heat stroke	Pigs, horses	Generalized	Weather influence
Hog cholera	Pigs	Generalized	High mortality
Infectious bovine rhinotracheitis (IBR, rednose)	Cattle	Upper respiratory tract	All ages, highly contagious, low mortality, early abortion
Infectious polyarthritis (Glasser's disease)	Pigs	Generalized	2–4 months of age
Leptospirosis	Cattle, pigs, sheep, goats	Kidney	Any age
Listeriosis	Cattle, sheep, goats	Brain	Silage thought to predispose
Lyme disease	Horses, cattle	Lameness	Northeast, north-central states
Malignant catarrhal fever	Cattle	Mouth, pharynx, generalized	Sporadic

TABLE 6-2   **COMMON LIVESTOCK DISEASES CHARACTERIZED BY FEVER** (continued)

DISEASE	SPECIES	PRIMARY SITE	REMARKS
Malignant edema	Cattle, sheep, goats, swine	Local, generalized	Wound infection, acute
Navel infection (navel ill)	Horses, cattle, sheep, goats, pigs	Navel, joints	1–3 weeks of age
Necrobacillosis	Cattle, sheep	Liver	Feedlots
Parainfluenza	All species	Lungs	Low mortality
Pasteurellosis	Sheep, pigs, goats	Lungs, generalized in swine	Very contagious
Pasteurellosis (shipping fever)	Cattle	Lungs	All ages, highly contagious
Polyarthritis	Sheep	Joints	Feedlot lambs
Potomac fever (ehrlichiosis)	Horses	Large intestine	Acute diarrhea equine
Pseudorabies	Pigs	Brain, nerves	Severe pruritus
Pyelonephritis	Cattle	Kidney	Sporadic
Salmonellosis	Cattle, sheep, pigs, goats, horses	Intestine	Young more severely affected
Shigellosis (sleepy foal disease)	Horses	Generalized	1–3 days of age
Strangles (distemper)	Horses	Pharynx	Young horses
Swine dysentery	Pigs	Intestine	8–12 weeks of age
Swine influenza	Pigs	Upper respiratory tract	Clinical signs during inclement weather
Tetanus	Horse, sheep, goats, pigs, cattle	Nerves, brain	Wound infection
Thromboembolic meningoencephalitis (TEME)	Cattle	Brain	Feedlot cattle
Toxoplasmosis	Sheep, goats, cattle	Generalized	May cause abortion
Transmissible gastroenteritis (TGE)	Pigs	Intestine	1–4 weeks of age
Tularemia	Sheep, pigs, horses	Generalized	Northwest US
Vesicular stomatitis	Cattle, horses, pigs	Mouth	Resembles tooth-and-mouth disease in cattle and pigs
Viral arteritis	Horses	Generalized	Easily confused with rhinopneumonitis and influenza
Viral encephalitis (Teschen disease)	Pigs	Brain	1–2 weeks of age

TABLE 6-3	COMMON LIVESTOCK DISEASES NOT CHARACTERIZED BY FEVER		
DISEASE	SPECIES	PRIMARY SITE	REMARKS
Acetonemia (ketosis)	Cattle	Liver, generalized	1–4 weeks after calving
Actinobacillosis	Cattle	Soft tissue, tongue	Sudden onset
Actinomycosis	Cattle	Bone, jaw	Chronic
Allergy	Cattle, horses	Skin, lungs	Weeds, drugs, sprays
Anaphylaxis	Cattle, horses, sheep, goats, pigs	Lungs, general	Vaccine injection
Anemia	Cattle, horses, sheep, goats, pigs	Red blood cells	Variable causes
Aneurysm	Horses	Mesenteric artery	Follows strongyle infestation
Bloat	Cattle, sheep, goats	Rumen	Lush wet legume pasture; chronic in some individuals
Botulism	Cattle, horses, sheep, goats	Nerve endings	Paralysis
Brisket disease	Cattle	Heart	High altitudes
Brucellosis	Cattle, pigs, goats, sheep	Genital tract	Abortion, infertility
Cardiac anomalies	Cattle, horses, sheep, goats, pigs	Heart	Congenital, young animals
Caseous lymphadenitis	Goats, sheep	Lymph glands	Chronic abscesses
Coccidiosis	Cattle, sheep, goats, pigs, horses	Intestine	Bloody diarrhea
Colibacillosis	Cattle, horses, sheep, goats, pigs	Intestine, general-ized	Young animals, sudden onset
Contagious equine metritus (CEM)	Horses	Genitalia	Chronic, venereal
Displaced abomasum	Cattle	Abomasum	Mature cows; easily confused with ketosis
Enterotoxemia	Cattle, horses, sheep, goats, pigs	Depends on type	Young, well-fed animals
Grass tetany (hypo-magnesemia)	Cattle	Generalized, neu-rological signs	Lush grass pasture
Greasy pig disease	Pigs	Skin	Easily confused with parakeratosis
Gut edema	Pigs	Intestine, general-ized	Thrifty feeder pigs
Indigestion	Cattle, horses, sheep, goats, pigs	Stomach	Feed change, overeating
Infectious keratitis (pink eye)	Cattle	Eye	Highly contagious

TABLE 6-3	COMMON LIVESTOCK DISEASES NOT CHARACTERIZED BY FEVER (continued)		
DISEASE	SPECIES	PRIMARY SITE	REMARKS
Internal parasitism	Cattle, horses, sheep, goats, pigs	Variable depending on parasite	Variable causes
Interstitial pneumonia (lungers, fog fever)	Cattle	Lungs	Variable causes
Iron deficiency anemia	Pigs	Blood	1–4 weeks of age
Isoimmune hemolytic anemia	Horses	Blood	Foals after nursing
Jowl abscess	Pigs	Throat	6 weeks and older
Laminitis (founder)	Horses, cattle, sheep, goats	Foot	Sequel to overfeeding on grain or other disease
Lead poisoning	Cattle, sheep, goats, pigs	Generalized	Paint, old motor oil, sprays, etc.
Lymphomatosis	Cattle	Lymph nodes	Chronic
Mammillitis	Cattle	Teats, udder, skin	More severe than pseudocowpox
Myoclonia congenita (shaker pig disease)	Pigs	Brain	Baby pigs, congenital
Necrotic pododermatitis (foot rot)	Cattle, sheep, goats	Foot	Sporadic in cattle, contagious in sheep
Neoplasms	Cattle, horses, sheep, goats, pigs	Variable	Slow onset
Nitrate poisoning	Cattle, sheep, goats	Blood	High nitrate forage
Nutritional deficiencies	Cattle, horses, sheep, goats, pigs	Variable	Develop slowly
Osteodystrophic fibrosis (big head)	Horses, pigs	Bone	Adults
Osteomalacia	Cattle, sheep	Bone	Adults
Papillomatosis (warts)	Cattle, goats, horses, pigs	Skin	Unsightly
Parakeratosis (zinc deficiency)	Pigs, cattle, goats	Skin	Aggravated by excess dietary calcium
Paratuberculosis (Johne's disease)	Cattle, goats, sheep	Intestine	Chronic
Parturient paresis (milk fever)	Cattle, goats	Metabolic, generalized	Associated with calving
Polioencephalomalacia	Cattle, sheep, goats	Brain	6–24 months of age
Porcine parvovirus	Pigs	Embryo, fetus	Reproductive failure
Pregnancy disease (ketosis)	Sheep	Liver, generalized	Occurs at lambing
Pseudocowpox	Cattle	Teats, udder	Transmissible by milker's hands

TABLE 6-3 **COMMON LIVESTOCK DISEASES NOT CHARACTERIZED BY FEVER (continued)**

DISEASE	SPECIES	PRIMARY SITE	REMARKS
Pulmonary emphysema (heaves)	Horses, cattle	Lungs	Chronic
Purpura hemorrhagica	Horses	Blood	Sequel to other illness, sporadic
Rabies	Cattle, horses, goats, sheep, pigs	Nerves, brain	Endemic areas, human health hazard
Ringworm	Cattle, pigs, horses, goats, sheep	Skin	Human health hazard
Salt poisoning	Cattle, pigs	Brain	High salt and low water intake
Spastic syndrome	Cattle	Rear leg muscles	Adults, hereditary
Sporotrichosis	Horses	Skin	Wound infection
Streptotrichosis (mycotic dermatitis)	Cattle, sheep, goats, horses, pigs	Skin	Chronic
Swine pox	Pigs	Belly, snout	May be transmitted by biting lice
Tuberculosis	Cattle, pigs, goats	Generalized	Human health hazard
Urea poisoning	Cattle, sheep, goats	Generalized	Acute; excess urea or inadequate mixing in feeds
Urethral calculi	Sheep, cattle, goats	Urethra	More common in castrated males
White muscle disease (stiff lamb disease)	Sheep, cattle	Muscle	Young thrifty animals; exercise accentuates
Winter dysentery	Cattle	Intestine	Highly contagious

TABLE 6-4 **COMMON LIVESTOCK DISEASES CHARACTERIZED BY DIARRHEA**

DISEASE	SPECIES
Bovine virus diarrhea	Cattle
Coccidiosis	Cattle, sheep, goats, pigs, horses
Colibacillosis	Cattle, pigs, sheep, goats
Indigestion	Cattle, horses, sheep, goats, pigs
Internal parasitism (some types)	Cattle, horses, sheep, goats, pigs
Malignant catarrhal fever	Cattle
Paratuberculosis	Cattle, goats, sheep
Salmonellosis	Cattle, horses, sheep, goats, pigs
Swine dysentery	Pigs
Transmissible gastroenteritis	Pigs
Winter dysentery	Cattle

TABLE 6-5   **COMMON LIVESTOCK DISEASES CHARACTERIZED BY NEUROLOGICAL SIGNS**

DISEASE	SPECIES
Acetonemia (occasionally)	Cattle
Botulism	Cattle, horses, sheep, goats
Equine encephalomyelitis	Horses
Grass tetany	Cattle
Lead poisoning	Cattle, sheep, goats, pigs
Listeriosis	Cattle, sheep, goats
Myoclonia congenita	Pigs
Polioencephalomalacia	Cattle, sheep, goats
Pseudorabies	Pigs, cattle
Rabies	Cattle, horses, goats, sheep, pigs
Salt poisoning	Cattle, pigs
Teschen disease	Pigs
Thromboembolic meningoencephalitis (TEM)	Cattle
Urea poisoning	Cattle, sheep, goats

TABLE 6-6   **COMMON LIVESTOCK DISEASES CHARACTERIZED BY RESPIRATORY DISTRESS**

DISEASE	SPECIES
Anaphylaxis	Cattle, horses, sheep, goats, pigs
Brisket disease	Cattle
Calf diphtheria (advanced)	Cattle
Equine influenza	Horses
Heatstroke	Pigs, horses
Infectious bovine rhinotracheitis	Cattle
Iron deficiency anemia	Pigs
Malignant catarrhal fever	Cattle
Nitrate poisoning	Cattle, sheep, goats
Parainfluenza	Cattle, horses, sheep, goats, pigs
Pneumonia (all types)	Cattle, horses, sheep, goats, pigs
Pulmonary emphysema	Horses, cattle
Strangles (advanced)	Horses
Urea poisoning	Cattle, sheep, goats

PART TWO

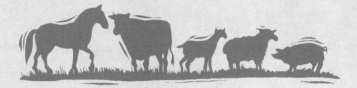

ANIMAL DISEASES

Part Two of this book is devoted to a brief discussion of the diseases affecting livestock, with suggestions for their prevention. Not every possible disease is covered, and the reader should keep in mind that two or more diseases can affect the same animal concurrently.

Familiarity with this section will not make the reader an accomplished diagnostician; that comes only with training and experience. It *will* help promote understanding of the many ills that can befall livestock, however, and should help the livestock owner to better understand the diagnosis and recommendations made when veterinary service becomes necessary.

Although most of the major disease entities affecting livestock in the United States are described in this section, little is said about treatment for several reasons. Effective treatment is contingent on accurate diagnosis and selection of the most effective drugs available. Drugs for use on livestock are widely advertised, but, unfortunately, the best advertisement and the best drug don't always coincide. For the novice, making the appropriate choice is difficult. In addition, where food-producing animals are concerned, government regulation is a factor. Some effective drugs that were once on the market have been removed from the market by law because of prolonged residue problems. Drug residues in meat or milk are considered adulteration, and adulterated food products are illegal. To prevent adulteration, there are legally specified withdrawal times (the interval between administration of the drug and the time of slaughter for meat or sale of the milk) for all of the drugs available for food animals. This withdrawal time varies for different drugs, and sometimes even for the same active ingredient in different vehicles. Last, what might be recommended for treatment today could become obsolete tomorrow. For all these reasons, definitive diagnosis and treatment recommendations for major problems are best left to your veterinarian. Indiscriminate use of drugs may only confuse the diagnosis and may create violative residues, leading to fines for you and bad publicity for your industry.

In keeping with the book's focus, although specific treatments for diseases are deemphasized, general recommendations for disease prevention through management and immunization appear throughout. The diseases within each chapter are ordered alphabetically. If you are unfamiliar with some of the terminology used in these chapters, consult the glossary, which begins on page 332, or a good medical dictionary.

Diseases 7 Caused by Bacteria

BACTERIA HAVE long been recognized as a cause of disease in humans and animals, and as a result have collectively received more study than any other class of pathogen. It is not surprising, therefore, that because of intensive study and the nature of the organism, bacteria as a group are more amenable to treatments than are some other pathogens, especially viruses.

Also, bacteria tend to be less host-specific than viruses, some readily infecting humans as well as animals.

Actinobacillosis

This disease of ruminants is closely related to actinomycosis in some of the lesions it produces, although in cattle it primarily affects the tongue, hence the name *wooden tongue*. Onset of infection with *Actinobacillus lignieresii* is usually rather sudden, with swelling particularly at the base of the tongue and of the adjacent lymph nodes. Affected cattle refuse feed, drool excessively, and make licking or chewing movements as though a foreign body were present in the mouth. The base of the tongue becomes hard and swollen, and ulcers may be present on the surface.

In sheep and goats the tongue is usually not affected, but lesions develop in the soft tissue of the lower jaw, face, and nose. These discharge a greenish yellow pus, and as the lesions progress, extensive scar tissue develops that may interfere with eating or breathing. Lymph nodes in the area commonly become enlarged.

Because it is primarily a soft tissue rather than a bone disease, actinobacillosis responds better to treatment than does actinomycosis. Sodium iodide, penicillin, streptomycin, and the tetracyclines have all been used effectively, usually bringing relief in 24 to 48 hours.

Like actinomycosis, the infection probably occurs via abrasions in the mouth. Coarse forage should be removed from the diet, but prompt treatment and segregation of infected animals are essential to control spread.

Actinomycosis

This disease sporadically appears in a few cattle in the herd to cause a rarefying osteomyelitis, especially of the facial and jaw bones. In cattle it is a disease of bone, and the bony enlargement it causes gives it the common name *lumpy jaw.* Although other species are recognized, *Actinomyces bovis* appears to be the principal cause of the infection in cattle, and it can infect people as well.

A. bovis has been reported to cause a serious granulomatous mastitis in sows and, with *Brucella abortus,* plays a role in poll evil and fistulous withers in the horse. Generalized actinomycosis has been reported involving the lungs and abdominal organs, but this form of the disease is uncommon.

Economically, the lumpy jaw syndrome is the most important form of the disease. Typically, this begins as a painless lump on the jaw or cheek. It can be distinguished from abscesses or other swellings by the fact that it is hard as bone and is, in fact, a part of the bone, although there may be some soft tissue swelling around it as the disease progresses. The disease is chronic and may extend over a period of several months to a year. Infection in the bone causes erosion of bony tissue with deposition of new bone surrounding the site, so enlargement occurs. Eventually tracts, which discharge a yellowish pus, develop to the outside. These heal, leaving an indented scar, and new tracts develop elsewhere. Abscessation and rarefaction of bone cause difficulty in chewing and swallowing. In advanced cases, molar teeth in the affected area may loosen and fall out. Affected animals die because they can't eat.

Diagnosis

Diagnosis of lumpy jaw can generally be made on the basis of physical examination and location of the lesion. If there is doubt, the diagnosis can be confirmed by finding minute granules in the pus typical of actinomycosis. Great care should be taken in handling infective material from the lesion because it is heavily laden with the organism, which can infect humans. For the same reason, animals with a discharging lesion should be segregated from all others to reduce the risk of spread.

Treatment

Treatment of lumpy jaw leaves something to be desired because the infection is in bone, where it is hard to establish therapeutic levels of drugs. In the early stages, surgical removal of the diseased area is probably the most satisfactory. Prolonged therapy with penicillin has some value. All things considered, however, except for very valuable animals, the best solution is probably to remove the infected animal from the herd. This is also the most effective control method. The disease is more likely to occur when cattle are grazing coarse stubble or fed coarse forage that may cause abrasions in the mouth. It is through these abrasions that infections occur.

Anthrax

This disease affects all species, including humans, and in its most common form is a highly fatal *septicemia,* or blood poisoning. It is caused by *Bacillus anthracis,* the spores of which are resistant to heat, cold, drying, and most disinfectants, and persist in the soil for years. Anthrax spores on hides and wool have been responsible for many cases of the disease in humans. Similarly, contaminated feedstuffs, especially bonemeal, have been the source of outbreaks in animals. There are areas of known soil contamination in some of the central and western states, and a few other states as well, where vaccination must be done regularly to prevent death losses. Outbreaks are more common in hot weather in animals grazing on alkaline soils. Outside those areas infection is rare, resulting only from contaminated feed or materials brought in.

The peracute, or more acute, form of anthrax generally seen early in new outbreaks may cause death of cattle, sheep, and goats in as little as 2 hours. Swine and horses tend to be more resistant, generally showing clinical signs over a period of 1 or 2 days. In fact, in swine the infection may be limited to the throat area, and some may survive. In animals that live long enough for clinical signs to be observed, there will be high fever, muscle tremors, abdominal pain, respiratory distress, staggering, and convulsions prior to death. Blood discharges from all body openings just prior to death and after death are common. Recovered swine may develop chronic abscesses in the lymph nodes of the cervical region.

With such a rapid, violent, and fatal syndrome, it isn't hard to understand why, historically, anthrax was such a feared disease. It still causes serious losses in many parts of the world, but vaccination and quarantine procedures in the United States have made it much less of a concern than it once was.

Diagnosis

The initial cases of anthrax can easily be confused with other diseases causing sudden death such as blackleg, poisoning, and lightning strike. There are, however, some distinguishing characteristics. Unlike blackleg, anthrax occurs in animals of all ages. The blood is very dark and does not clot, which is unique, and blood discharges from mouth, nose, and rectum are a fairly constant finding. These factors, plus the lack of rigor mortis and the disease's limitation almost entirely to known areas, tend to clinch the diagnosis. It can be confirmed by microscopic examination of a stained blood smear, culture of the organism from body fluids, or injection of body fluid into guinea pigs in the laboratory.

Necropsy of suspected anthrax cases should be avoided for two reasons. First, all body tissues are loaded with the organism, and human infection can occur through minute scratches or abrasions, by inhalation, or by ingestion. Second, *B. anthracis* from the carcass that get onto the ground will sporulate, or become resistant spores, on exposure to the air in just a few hours. These spores will then contaminate the premises almost indefinitely. Anthrax is a serious, dangerous, reportable disease that when suspected should be brought immediately to the attention of your veterinarian.

Vaccination

Anthrax is preventable by vaccination, but many states limit the use of vaccine to those areas where, through prior experience, anthrax is likely to occur. This precaution was made necessary by the type of vaccine in use for many years. It was, and is, an attenuated spore vaccine. Although the earlier vaccine produced a reasonable degree of immunity most of the time, individual and species differences in resistance caused some animals to develop the disease as a result of vaccination. More highly attenuated spore vaccines reduced this risk but did not provide as good an immunity. As a consequence, several vaccines with varying degrees of attenuation were marketed. These have been largely superseded by an avirulent attenuated vaccine that is safer but, nevertheless, frequently causes fever, drop in milk production, and abortion in swine.

Treatment of anthrax usually isn't possible because of its acute nature, but the organism is sensitive to penicillin, streptomycin, and the tetracyclines. Use of one or more of these on all animals in the herd when the disease is diagnosed may forestall additional cases. Given in large doses early in the disease, antibiotics will save some animals.

Much has been written about anthrax in recent years because of its potential for use as a germ warfare agent. It could wreak havoc on the unprepared human and animal population depending on mode of delivery. For that reason, a vaccination program for military personnel has been implemented.

Blackleg

On some farms blackleg is the most common of a group of diseases caused by spore-forming, soilborne organisms belonging to the genus *Clostridium*. It occurs most frequently in well-nourished cattle of the beef breeds in the range of 6 to 26 months old. It also occurs in sheep and goats, but in these species the disease is more commonly associated with wound infection such as occurs in sheep following docking, castration, or shearing. The mechanism by which infection occurs in cattle is less clear.

The spore form of the organism persists in the soil for many years, and is very resistant to environmental changes such as drying, high temperatures, and freezing. The organism can commonly be found in the digestive tract of normal cattle. Once contaminated, a pasture will remain that way for years; in floodplain areas, pastures downstream from the originally infected pasture will also become contaminated. The disease is primarily seasonal and is seen most frequently in late spring and summer when animals are at pasture.

Blackleg in cattle is a dramatic disease. Dead animals will be the first indication that the disease is present. Typically, one or two animals will be found dead in the pasture without any evidence of their having died other than suddenly and quietly. In fact, the disease at first glance could easily be confused with lightning strike. However, with blackleg, decomposition of body tissues occurs very rapidly and the dead animals will invariably be found lying on their sides, extremely bloated with the upper legs rigidly extended. Similar sporadic losses will continue if nothing is done.

Diagnosis

Although the mechanism by which infection occurs in cattle or why it occurs is not really known, it is apparent that the organisms in the digestive tract become vegetative (that is, they grow and multiply) and migrate through the intestinal wall to the bloodstream, where they are carried to all parts of the body, resulting in a bacteremia. *Clostridium chauvoei* in infected cattle can readily be isolated from the blood and vascular organs such as the liver and spleen, but its most pronounced effect is in the heavy muscles. Toxin produced by the organism produces severe muscle inflammation and death of muscle tissue with gas formation. Muscles in the hip area and loin are most commonly affected. Running your hand over the back and hips of the dead animal will often give a clue to the cause of death. If it is blackleg, gas produced during muscle necrosis gravitates upward under the skin to cause a palpable crepitation. At necropsy the affected muscles will be dark, hemorrhagic, and visibly necrotic. Because the carcass will be teeming with the organism, to avoid further pasture contamination, dead animals should be deeply buried right on the spot.

Once the diagnosis of blackleg has been made, careful examination of other animals in the herd may reveal a few in the early stages of the disease. It causes a very high fever, complete lack of appetite, depression, and lameness. These signs are generally not observed in the initial cases because the disease will be fatal in 12 hours or less. Given very early in the course of the disease, large doses of penicillin may prevent death of the animal, although, depending on the degree of muscle damage done, lameness may persist if the animal survives.

Prevention

Blackleg is readily preventable by immunization with bacterin. Because mixed infection is a common occurrence, the bacterin usually used contains *C. chauvoei* and *Clostridium septicum* antigen. A single dose provides reasonably good protection, but a second dose a month later is even better.

On farms where the infection is known to exist, this should be done with calves beginning at about 6 months of age, and they should have another dose a year later. In the face of an outbreak, further losses can be minimized by vaccinating all animals in the susceptible age range immediately, giving them a large dose of penicillin to provide some protection in the interval required for immunity to develop, and then putting them in another pasture. Most people experienced with blackleg routinely immunize susceptible animals yearly in early spring.

Blackleg in Sheep

The disease in sheep is somewhat different from that in cattle, although the end result, death, is usually the same. In sheep it is almost invariably a wound infection, either through a mechanical procedure such as docking, castration, or shearing or via vulvar lacerations incurred during lambing. If the lesion is in the leg muscles, the animal will walk with a stiff gait, if it walks at all. But the extreme swelling and gaseous crepitation found in the lesions in cattle are not nearly as apparent in sheep. The early stages of the disease are always associated with high fever, complete lack of appetite, and depression.

In sheep, as in cattle, the disease is readily preventable by vaccination, although sheep vaccinated under 1 year of age do not develop as solid an immunity as those vaccinated later. Vaccination of ewes 3 to 4 weeks prior to lambing not only will provide protection to the ewe but also, because of colostral antibody, will afford some protection to the newborn lamb. In areas where the disease is prevalent, injection of penicillin following surgical procedures or difficult lambing may prevent infection from occurring.

Although the diagnosis of blackleg on the basis of history and necropsy alone is generally not difficult, it can be confirmed by isolation of the organism from infected tissues or by fluorescent antibody test in the laboratory.

Botulism

This is not a common disease in farm animals, but it must be considered when signs of progressive paralysis of unknown origin are seen. It is not an infection but a toxemia caused by ingestion of the neurotoxin produced by *Clostridium botulinum*. Spores of the organism are widespread in nature and under favorable conditions of warmth, moisture, pH, and low oxygen tension multiply rapidly in decomposing animal and plant material. Several types of toxin are recognized and all are quite stable, persisting for long periods of time even when the organism is no longer present.

Causes and Diagnosis

The clinical signs are those of progressive paralysis, with the muscles of the tongue and throat being affected first. Tongue paralysis is considered one of the early specific signs. Death usually occurs in a few days due to respiratory paralysis.

The disease is common in wild waterfowl and is often called *limber neck* because of the neck muscle paralysis. It has been reported in horses, cattle, sheep, and goats, and less frequently in swine. In range animals it is more likely to occur during periods of drought or when, as a result of phosphorus deficiency, animals are more likely to chew on carrion.

These are not the only circumstances, however. Improperly stored and cured silage can be a factor. I recall one instance when a dairyman had put oat silage on top of corn in a conventional wood silo. Several months later as he was feeding from the interface of the corn and oats, cows began to die from botulism. Apparently there was sufficient spoilage at the interface for *C. botulinum* to proliferate. After he removed and dumped about 3 feet of stored silage from that point, no further cases occurred. Silage stored in airtight silos has also been incriminated in at least two outbreaks of botulism in dairy cattle.

Botulism from spoiled canned food is hazardous to humans, and spoiled food should not be fed to animals, as it's equally hazardous to them.

Antitoxin is the only specific treatment for botulism, and the amounts required for animals are usually too costly to be of practical value. With good nursing care, some animals recover if the dose of toxin consumed is small.

Brucellosis

Brucellosis is a disease of great economic significance that occurs principally in cattle, swine, sheep, and goats. Three distinct species of *Brucella* are responsible. *B. abortus* (cattle), *Brucella suis* (swine), and *Brucella melitensis* (sheep and goats) tend to be host specific. The principal and usually only clinical sign they produce is abortion, typically during the last third of gestation.

All three cause a serious, generalized febrile disease in humans called *undulant fever*. In animals, however, the infection is concentrated in the reproductive organs, where it localizes in the uterus, udder, and placenta of the female and in the testicles of the male. A fourth species, *Brucella ovis*, causes ram epididymitis, although ewes tend to be resistant, so ram infertility, not abortion, is the principal sign. Infected cattle, goats, and sheep shed the organism in milk, and drinking raw milk from infected animals is a public health hazard. The organism is readily killed by pasteurization. *B. abortus* was the cause of the suppurative diseases poll evil and fistulous withers in horses when draft horses were

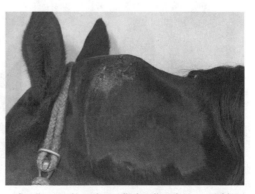

Swelling such as this, called poll evil, *is caused by* B. abortus *infection in the horse.*

kept in close association with infected cows. With the decline in draft horses and the much lower infection rate in cattle, these diseases are now rare.

Treatment of brucellosis in animals is generally unsatisfactory because of inconsistent results and cost. Ram epididymitis has been successfully treated with high levels of antibiotics over a long period of time, but the total cost of drugs usually exceeds the value of the ordinary commercial ram.

Eradication Program

Because of the economic and public health significance of brucellosis and because treatment is of little value, the state and federal governments many years ago adopted a policy aimed at total eradication. Basically this involves identification and slaughter of infected animals, with indemnity paid to owners to offset the difference between meat price and appraised value. Meat from infected animals is not a health hazard.

During the early stages of the eradication campaign in cattle, when infection rates ranged up to 25 percent or more, vaccination of calves was a useful adjunct. The vaccine used is a live modification of *B. abortus,* designated strain 19, which reduces the rate of spread and number of abortions; however, it does not provide complete protection. Two other vaccines used in Europe, 45/20 and H38, are currently being evaluated in the United States. Another vaccine, designated RB51, has proved useful to protect adult cattle from abortion and is used in calves as well. It is less likely to cause false positive blood test results compared to strain 19.

Vaccines for *B. suis* and *B. melitensis* are not available, but a vaccine is being used to control ram epididymitis.

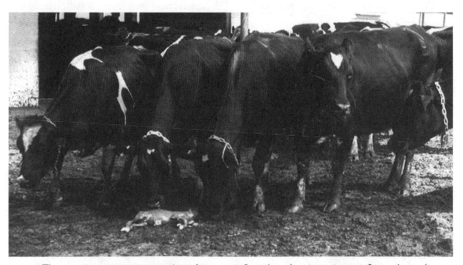

These curious cows are certain to become infected as they investigate a fetus aborted due to brucellosis. (Photo courtesy of Dr. Paul Nicoletti)

Diagnosis

Brucellosis is readily identifiable by several serological tests as well as by the milk ring test for dairy cattle. Diagnosis is sometimes handicapped, however, by a long interval between exposure and having the infection show up in the test. This may take up to 60 days. Therefore, a negative test on a recently exposed animal may be misleading. The significance of this delay will become apparent when we discuss ways of preventing infection.

In species other than sheep, spread of infection is primarily oral. Infection of rams occurs primarily during mating, particularly when the ewe has recently been bred by an infected ram. The vaginal discharges of infected animals and especially aborted fetuses are teeming with the organism. Although *B. abortus* has the capacity to penetrate the unbroken skin and infection caused by a droplet of infective material in the eye has been recorded, it's probable that most infections occur via the oral route because of the propensity of animals to sniff one another's genital areas.

Abortion is the primary evidence of infection with brucellosis, and infection apparently produces some degree of immunity, because typically animals that abort will conceive again after a time and carry subsequent fetuses to term. Nevertheless, the infection persists in a latent form, and these infected animals remain a source of infection for others.

Vaccination vs. Eradication

Because of its economic importance and the test-and-slaughter eradication program in effect for cattle, brucellosis often becomes an intensely emotional issue. The question most often asked is, "Won't my herd be protected if I vaccinate every calf?" The answer is no. The strain 19 or RB51 vaccine used will immunize only about 65 percent of those calves to which it is given, and the immunity produced lasts only about 5 years. So despite an intensive vaccination program, new infections will continue to occur. Experience has shown that, in the long run, the cheapest way to control a disease like this is to eradicate it. There is ample evidence to indicate that this can be done. Vaccination has value only in areas where the infection rate is so high as to make a test-and-slaughter program prohibitively expensive. Nevertheless, legislatures of a few states, responding to strong political pressure based on misunderstanding of the disease, have mandated compulsory calfhood vaccination.

Eradication of brucellosis depends on identification and slaughter of infected animals, quarantine of infected herds, and restriction on movement of animals. It also requires accurate identification of animals and good records of acquisition and disposition, so that when a reactor is found, she can be traced back to the point of origin and all contact animals individually tested to detect any spread of infection. Finally, it requires understanding and cooperation on the part of livestock owners, veterinarians, and regulatory program officials.

At the end of the year 2000, there were no known infected commercial herds of cattle, goats, or bison in the United States. This is the culmination of an eradication program begun in 1934 and intensified since 1954. Now we need to intensify the surveillance program to detect new infections before they spread through market cattle testing and the milk ring test. This is an effort in which producers and veterinarians as well as regulatory officials should be involved.

Prevention

There is much that the livestock owner can do to ensure that his herd does not become infected. Follow these recommendations.

■ If an animal aborts, don't ignore it and write it off as bad luck. Have your veterinarian examine the fetus and collect samples from fetus and dam for laboratory analysis. Brucellosis is readily identifiable at the time of abortion. Then segregate the dam from all other animals in the herd until the cause is determined, and thoroughly disinfect the area where the abortion occurred.

■ Remember that brucellosis does not appear in a herd by spontaneous generation. Almost without exception, when the disease appears in a previously clean herd, it was bought along with replacement animals. Be selective in your source of replacements, buying only from known clean herds whenever possible. If there is any doubt about the status of an animal, insist that it have a negative blood test within 30 days of the time you bring it home. And for added insurance, keep the animal separated from the main herd for at least 30 days until it is tested again and found negative.

■ As a general disease control procedure, ask visitors to stay out of the stable area. Keep buyers, trucks, and trailers away from areas that are accessible to your herd.

Following these few simple rules will do more than a vaccination program, at less cost, to keep brucellosis out of your herd.

A reservoir of *B. abortus* exists in bison and elk herds in Yellowstone National Park and perhaps in other areas as well. This is a concern primarily to ranchers whose rangeland adjoins the park, and the situation periodically generates much publicity nationwide and highly charged emotions at the scene.

Brucellosis in Goats

The disease in goats closely parallels that found in cattle, and control measures are basically the same. In fact, regardless of some species differences, the prevention recommendations listed for cattle are equally applicable for all species. Vaccination of goats is not done in the United States but is common in countries where the disease is more prevalent. Worldwide, the most common cause of undulant fever in humans is *B. melitensis,* contracted primarily by consuming raw milk or soft cheeses made with raw milk from infected goats.

Brucellosis in Sheep

B. melitensis occasionally causes brucellosis in sheep, but infection with *B. ovis,* causing ram epididymitis, is more common. Ram epididymitis is unique in that ewes, although they may become infected and occasionally abort, tend to be resistant and recover spontaneously. It is primarily a disease of the ram and is detectable by palpation of the testicles and a blood test. One or both testicles may be involved. The affected testicle, especially the epididymis, will feel swollen and even fibrous in the later stages. The first intimation of infection is usually a gradually reduced fertility. Susceptible rams become infected when they breed a ewe recently bred by an infected ram. The rate of spread therefore is greatest during the breeding season, particularly when young rams are placed with a flock along with older rams, which are more likely to be infected.

Control can be achieved through vaccination and by splitting the ewe flock into two or more groups. Only young rams are kept with one group and the older rams are kept with the other. In this manner a clean and an infected, or suspect, flock can be maintained separately. Rams known to be infected should be slaughtered.

Brucellosis in Swine

Brucellosis in swine more closely resembles undulant fever in humans, in that it frequently causes a systemic infection with bacteremia. Because, in the early stages, *B. suis* can be found in all body tissues, infected swine present a special hazard to packinghouse workers. Transmission in swine, as in cattle and goats, occurs via the oral route and also during mating. Infected boars may have a swollen testicle and impaired fertility. Palpation of the testicles and examination of the semen, coupled with serological testing, will identify infected animals. In an infected herd, low fertility, abortions, stillbirths, and weak piglets are common. Neither vaccination nor treatment is effective in swine, and eradication through depopulation or a testing program with total segregation of positive and negative animals is the control method used. Brucellosis is endemic in the wild pig population in the southern states, but this does not present a major problem for hog producers using modern methods of swine husbandry. It should be of some concern, however, to hunters handling the tissue of feral pigs.

Brucellosis in Exotic Species

Unfortunately, the disease is transmissible to other species such as bison and llamas. While the latter are sufficiently docile to be blood tested, feral bison present a different challenge. These animals provide a reservoir of infection that is of concern, primarily to cattle ranchers on the borders of parks where bison roam.

Campylobacteriosis (Vibriosis)

Bovine genital campylobacteriosis is a true venereal disease of cattle being spread at the time of coitus or by breeding cows artificially with untreated semen from infected bulls. Generally, the only evidence of infection is infertility and irregular heat period intervals. Early embryonic death is an important feature of the disease, but passage of the embryo in cervical and vaginal mucus is rarely observed. Abortions later in gestation due to *Campylobacter (Vibrio) fetus* var. *venerealis* occasionally occur.

When the disease first appears in the herd, there is usually a history of recent additions to the herd, a new source of untreated bull semen, or a new bull bought or borrowed. The disease is particularly troublesome in range cattle, where natural service is commonly practiced. Because there are no clinical signs, several months may go by before it becomes apparent that cows are not conceiving. The resulting delay in the calf crop can be disastrous. The prudent manager not only will do everything possible to prevent the disease but also will have the cows examined for pregnancy 60 days after the bulls are put with them to be sure that conception rates are satisfactory.

Bovine campylobacteriosis is self-limiting in the cow if the source of infection is removed, with the infection in a majority of cows clearing up in 2 to 3 months. Most cows develop sufficient immunity to conceive in about 4 to 6 months, but a few carry the infection through a normal pregnancy and remain carriers and a source of new infections. A mild endometritis may result from the infection, which responds reasonably well to infusion of the uterus with streptomycin. Young bulls tend to be resistant to infection but, nevertheless, mechanically carry the organism from an infected cow to others in the herd. Bulls 5 years of age and older are more likely to become infected and to remain carriers for life. Treatment of these bulls is not consistently satisfactory, and following a course of treatment, they should always be test-mated to a couple of virgin heifers and the heifers then examined by the mucus agglutination test.

Diagnosis

Diagnosis presents a challenge to the veterinarian and cattle owner. The history when infection is first introduced is one of greatly reduced conception rates and prolonged calving interval, without other clinical signs and with occasional abortions. This tends to set the disease apart from others affecting reproduction, assuming the bull is fertile or the semen of good quality. Diagnosis is more difficult in subsequent years when most of the herd has become resistant, and the problem is limited to susceptible older cows and those added to the herd. The disease must be distinguished from others causing infertility or abortion such as trichomoniasis, IBR, bovine virus diarrhea (BVD), and leptospirosis.

Several diagnostic tests have been developed, all of which require the services of a veterinarian and a good diagnostic laboratory. Among these are the mucus agglutination test; culture of cervical mucus, preputial washings, or an aborted fetus; fluorescent antibody test; and test-mating of bulls to virgin heifers. Where the history indicates campylobacteriosis as a possibility, a single negative test may be misleading, and in these cases the testing should be repeated. The laboratory must be careful to distinguish between *C. fetus* var. *venerealis* and *C. fetus* var. *intestinalis*. The latter is a common fecal contaminant that rarely produces abortion in cattle. A laboratory report, therefore, of "*C. fetus* positive" is not sufficiently specific for diagnostic purposes.

Control

Campylobacteriosis will not appear in a herd where all breeding is done artificially with properly antibiotic-treated semen, and artificial insemination is a strongly recommended control procedure. An alternative with slightly more risk is to use only virgin bulls on the herd, but this may limit herd improvement since the genetic potential of virgin bulls is not proved. A vaccine is available that, when given about a month prior to and again halfway through the breeding season, produces a reasonably good immunity. Its use is more practical in the beef herd where artificial insemination is not feasible. Annual booster vaccination about a month prior to the breeding season is recommended. Vaccination and treatment with dihydrostreptomycin are useful to treat infected bulls.

Campylobacteriosis in Sheep and Goats

While *C. fetus* var. *intestinalis* is insignificant for the cow, it is a cause of abortion in sheep and goats, but unlike campylobacteriosis in cattle, transmission is by ingestion. Abortion late in pregnancy or birth of weak lambs is the principal sign. There are usually no other clinical signs and no warning an abortion is about to occur. Lesions are confined to the fetus and consist of edema and necrotic areas in the liver. Other diseases can produce similar lesions, however, so definitive diagnosis is by culture of the organism from the fetus.

Because the infection spreads orally, it is important to isolate all aborting animals and promptly dispose of any aborted fetuses. Infection produces immunity lasting several years following the initial abortion. Administration of penicillin and streptomycin, incorporating tetracycline in the feed, and repeated vaccination with bacterin have all been used with some success to control outbreaks.

Colibacillosis

Colibacillosis is a major disease of the young, encountered primarily in calves, pigs, and lambs. It also affects foals and kids, although less frequently. The disease takes two primary forms: *enteric,* involving the intestinal tract and causing profuse diarrhea, and *septicemic,* involving the bloodstream, which may cause sudden death with no premonitory signs. Colibacillosis is the leading component of the neonatal diarrhea complex commonly called *scours*.

The causative organisms, *Escherichia coli* and, to a lesser extent, *Salmonella* species, are common environmental contaminants found universally in manure. Of interest, the count of *E. coli* per milliliter is the standard for potability of public water supplies, and a particular serotype, *E. coli* 0157:H7, has been responsible for a number of human infections, most of which have been traced to consumption of contaminated meat. A vaccine is currently being evaluated that, it is hoped, will reduce the prevalence of the 0157:H7 strain in cattle. Human infection can generally be prevented through proper cooking of meat.

There are many different strains of *E. coli,* some relatively innocuous and others highly pathogenic. A few of the highly pathogenic strains produce an endotoxin that accounts for their detrimental effect. Experimentally, minute quantities of *E. coli* endotoxin given intravenously have been shown to produce circulatory collapse and death in a matter of minutes. Lesser quantities perfused into an isolated loop of intestine will cause complete paralysis and dilatation of the loop. This effect is undoubtedly a factor complicating the enteric form of the disease. Colibacillosis is more frequent when large numbers of young animals are housed in close confinement.

Enteric Form

The enteric form is most common in dairy calves, pigs, and lambs, probably as a reflection of intensified husbandry methods. The route of infection is primarily oral, making sanitation an important factor in control. Typically, it appears within the first week after birth. Although there is usually a moderate fever at the outset, the first sign noted may be a pasty or watery, yellowish diarrhea that has a foul odor. There is some abdominal pain and frequent defecation and straining. Affected animals refuse feed, and, because of tremendous fluid loss from the diarrhea, rapidly become dehydrated. Without treatment, the disease usually terminates in coma and death within 3 to 5 days. In some dairy herds calf mortality from this disease may approach 100 percent. In piglets, perhaps because they are weaker at birth than calves, the disease is more acute. Although the symptoms are quite similar, onset in pigs is usually within 12 hours after birth and they will die a day later.

A specific enteric colibacillosis called *gut edema* occurs in pigs 2 to 4 months old and occasionally earlier. Evidence to date indicates that this disease is not due to the infection itself but is a reaction to endotoxins produced by several strains of *E. coli.* The condition occurs at any time of year and on a given farm will appear only in pigs in the same age range. It is most likely to appear during the interval between weaning and establishment on full feed.

Septicemic Form

The other major form of colibacillosis is septicemia with generalized infection. This is an acute disease of the very young that frequently causes death with no warning signs. Septicemic colibacillosis is the most common form of colibacillosis in lambs and foals. When the syndrome is less acute, meningitis commonly occurs, causing a variety of central nervous system disturbances. Animals that recover from the acute disease often develop arthritis due to localization of the infection in the joints. A common route of infection for septicemia is via the navel.

Treatment

Treatment of the enteric disease in all but baby pigs is reasonably successful. Newborn pigs die so quickly and there are usually so many of them that treatment is not very satisfactory, but nevertheless should be attempted. Use of antibiotics and antidiarrheal oral medications alone, however, may not do the job. The effects of endotoxin produced by some strains will linger after the bacteria have been destroyed. Furthermore, in many cases the enteric disease is compounded by the loss of tremendous volumes of fluid and electrolytes, resulting in dehydration. For best results, this loss must be replaced by equivalent quantities of electrolyte solution given intravenously and orally. Good results have been reported in calves when no milk at all is given for 24 hours. Instead, a simple homemade electrolyte formula is given (see box on page 156).

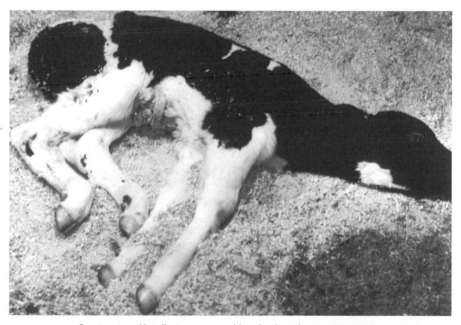

Septicemic colibacillosis causes sudden death, with no warning signs.

HOMEMADE ELECTROLYTE FORMULA

Table salt — 1 heaping teaspoon

Baking soda — 1 heaping teaspoon

Water — 1 gallon

While commercially prepared electrolyte solutions are more complete and better balanced, this simple, readily available formula, which is given instead of milk for 24 hours, will help to relieve the diarrhea by reducing the number of organisms present. At the same time, it will counteract loss of sodium and chloride ions as well as correct the acidosis that occurs with dehydration. The calf with diarrhea but not yet severely dehydrated will need 2 quarts of this warmed solution every 8 hours for the first day. After that, milk or milk replacer diluted with the same solution to 50 percent of normal concentration can be fed. Gradually increase the percentage of milk until it is back to normal at the end of the third day. This procedure alone will save many calves that otherwise would die.

If the dehydration is severe, regardless of species, electrolyte solutions will need to be administered intravenously in addition to being given orally. Although it is time-consuming, for the animal that is seriously ill with either the septicemic or enteric form of colibacillosis, nothing is better than a blood transfusion. This, however, is a job for a veterinarian.

Antibiotics in injectable or oral preparations are routinely given to control or treat scours in farm animals, with variable results. Because of its acute onset, antibiotic therapy for septicemic colibacillosis is only moderately helpful, although for the animal that survives the acute phase, antibiotics help to prevent secondary complications. Treatment of the enteric form must include fluid replacement and good nursing care for satisfactory results.

Prevention

Clearly, colibacillosis is a serious and complex disease that must be prevented by whatever means are possible. The single most effective method is to ensure that all newborn animals receive colostrum as soon as possible after birth. The majority of older animals, through prior exposure to pathogenic strains of *E. coli,* will develop protective antibody that is transferred in colostrum. To ensure exposure, some hog farms make it a practice to feed some manure to the sows during the last month of gestation. While this may increase the sow's *E. coli* antibody level, it also may expose her to other pathogens that can cause abortion, such as enteroviruses, so it isn't a practice that can be universally recommended.

Overeating is a common predisposing factor for all types of gastrointestinal disease and is a frequent cause of nonspecific diarrhea in dairy calves. Restricting milk intake to 10 percent of body weight daily for the first 7 to 10 days will help to prevent trouble. And, of course, sanitation is important. Animals born in a filthy environment are certain to be exposed to overwhelming numbers of *E. coli.*

There is a direct correlation between concentration of animals in the susceptible age range and the prevalence of colibacillosis. The rate of infection accelerates either when animals are all born in the same pen or area, without adequate intervals for thorough cleaning, or when they are all grouped together in the same pen after birth. Many dairy farmers have been able to almost eliminate the enteric form of the disease by rearing calves in isolated hutches, referred to in the section on housing (see page 51). Dipping the navel in tincture of iodine is strongly recommended to prevent infection via that route.

Numerous attempts have been made to prevent colibacillosis through immunization of the dam or the offspring immediately after birth. None has been very successful because of the number of antigenically different strains of the organism involved. Autogenous bacterins incorporating strains found on the farm may be helpful when other methods fail. Genetically engineered vaccines that incorporate only specific antigenic components of the organism are the most effective. Continuous low-level administration of antibiotics in the feed or drinking water may also be helpful. But *E. coli* is not only widespread; it is also very adaptable and readily develops antibiotic resistance. Constant low-level feeding of the same antibiotic promotes resistance and is therefore self-defeating. Administration of antiserum or antibody concentrate to valuable newborn animals may be worthwhile if the pathogenic strains of organism present on the farm are present in the product.

The really important thing is to prevent the disease from occurring in the first place. The following suggestions have all proved helpful:

■ Keep the calving pen, farrowing house, lambing shed, and other facilities as clean and sanitary as possible.

■ Insofar as possible, isolate newborn animals from one another.

■ Don't overfeed. Although it may seem heartless, keeping newborn animals on the hungry side for the first few days helps to ensure their survival.

■ Thoroughly scrub and sanitize feeding equipment after each use.

■ Provide supplemental heat, especially for piglets and lambs.

■ Be *certain* newborn animals get adequate colostrum as soon as possible after birth. If there is doubt whether a newborn animal has nursed colostrum, the zinc sulfate turbidity test can be applied to a small amount of blood serum. This gives a rough estimation of the amount of globulin absorbed. Your veterinarian can do it for you. Colostrum can be frozen in plastic zip-seal bags and kept almost indefinitely. It's a good idea to keep some colostrum on hand to feed an animal that becomes an orphan soon after birth.

■ Routinely use an oral *E. coli* monoclonal antibody product or *E. coli* dry cow vaccine.

Dermatitis, Exudative

The most obvious effect of this disease affecting pigs up to a month of age is the appearance of moist, crusty, weeping skin lesions that sometimes combine to cover the entire body. The appearance of the skin gives the disease its common name, *greasy pig disease*. Although sporadic occurrence is more common, possibly because of colostral immunity, up to 90 percent of a litter may become infected, and mortality ranges from 5 to 90 percent. Very young pigs are more severely affected and are less responsive to treatment than those in the older age range. At first glance, the condition closely resembles parakeratosis due to zinc deficiency, but the latter disease is rarely, if ever, seen in pigs as young as a month old. The lesions of greasy pig disease are caused by *Staphylococcus hyicus,* which gains entrance to the skin via cuts or abrasions. Resistance increases with age, and older, inapparent carriers are a source of infection.

Symptoms

The first indication of imminent greasy pig disease is listlessness, then dullness of the skin and haircoat. Depression and complete lack of appetite follow, but fever is not common. Concurrently, the skin thickens and reddish spots appear on the ears, back, and belly. Serum exudes from these, providing a

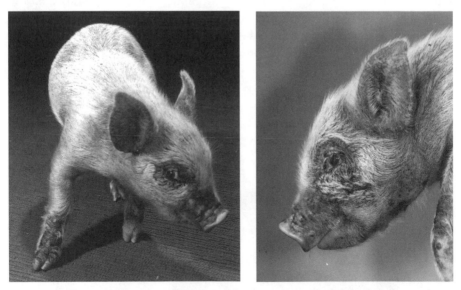

"Greasy pig" disease is characterized by moist, crusty, weeping skin lesions.

medium for secondary infection, which contributes to the obnoxious odor characteristic of piglets with this disease. Conjunctivitis is common, as is a purulent inflammation of the external ear. Frequently, blisterlike lesions develop on the snout and heels. These rupture, and the resulting infection leads to erosions and occasionally sloughing of the hoof. This type of vesicular lesion is characteristic of some viruses, leading to the belief that greasy pig disease may not be solely a staphylococcal infection but instead may be triggered by an as yet unidentified virus.

Treatment

The disease is contagious, and infected piglets and litters should be immediately segregated from others in the farrowing house. However, it is basically a wound infection disease, with the organism gaining entrance through skin abrasions. Occasionally the urinary tract as well as the skin is involved, and such cases terminate fatally.

Given early, antibiotics are helpful in relieving the clinical signs, but as a group the staphylococci develop antibiotic resistance quite readily, so several different antibiotics may have to be tried. Severely affected piglets can be bathed in warm soapy water to remove the crusts and debris, and then antibiotic ointment can be applied to the skin. These measures will help to save many piglets that would otherwise die.

Prevention

Skin abrasions are the primary route of infection. Scraped knees from rough concrete floors and bites and scratches incurred in the daily struggle for a place at the dairy bar are the common source of wounds that subsequently become infected. Reducing the level of environmental contamination through good sanitation will help to prevent infection. Abrasions from rough floors can be prevented by covering the floor of the pen with rubber mats or even indoor-outdoor carpet. Very smooth concrete floors, although good from the standpoint of reducing knee abrasions, are undesirable because they are slippery and contribute to the functional problem known as *spraddle-leg*. On farms where greasy pig disease is a major problem, extreme sanitary precautions must be taken. When outbreaks appear, giving antibiotics to all pigs in the litter, even before they show signs of disease, may be helpful.

Diphtheria, Calf

This disease occurs sporadically on some farms in calves under 6 months of age, although occasionally older calves may develop the disease as well. It is encountered most frequently when calves are penned together where the principal causative agent, *Fusobacterium necrophorum,* is likely to be present in large numbers. This is the same organism that causes foot rot, and conditions favoring development of one disease also favor development of the other. Although *F. necrophorum* can consistently be isolated from calf diphtheria lesions, it is quite probable that other organisms play some, as yet undefined, role.

Types

Two types of the disease may be encountered, *necrotic stomatitis* (inflammation of the mouth) and *necrotic laryngitis* (inflammation of the larynx), but the pathogenesis is the same. Necrotic stomatitis occurs more frequently in younger calves and involves the tongue; inside of the cheeks, especially at the angle of the lips; and the soft palate. Fever and refusal to eat are the earliest signs noted, followed by drooling and swelling of the tongue and cheeks. The breath has a foul odor identical to the smell of foot rot. Mouth lesions, consisting of deep ulcers of the cheek and sometimes of the area adjacent to the tongue, filled with necrotic tissue debris and food particles are readily apparent. The lesions are painful, and affected calves generally refuse feed and water of any kind.

Diagnosis

The clinical signs of necrotic laryngitis are more pronounced and severe, with fever of 106°F; moist cough; labored breathing, especially on inhalation; complete lack of appetite; and painful swallowing movements. External swelling in the laryngeal area may be evident and will be sensitive to the touch. Nasal discharge may be present, and the breath always has the typical odor of foot rot. Necrotic laryngitis can occur as a primary disease, concurrently with necrotic stomatitis or secondary to it. In any case the infection may extend to the lungs, causing severe pneumonia.

Calf diphtheria is unrelated to diphtheria in humans and is not a contagious disease in the usual sense. It is primarily a wound infection, with the organism gaining entrance through mouth abrasions caused by coarse feed or erupting teeth. More than one calf in the pen may be infected, however, because infection is more likely when the environmental contamination level is high. Affected calves dehydrate rapidly because of fever and failure to drink. Without treatment, the disease is usually fatal in a week or less. Fortunately, the disease responds well to treatment with several of the sulfa drugs, penicillin, and tetracycline. The sooner treatment is started, the better the response will be.

A similar condition, *necrotic rhinitis* ("bull-nose"), is occasionally seen in young pigs. Swelling of the face, nasal discharge, sneezing, nasal hemorrhage, lack of appetite, and emaciation are typical of the disease in pigs. The infection may be severe enough to cause erosion of the nasal turbinate bones and facial distortion. Generally, only a few pigs in the herd are affected, and infection is generally thought to be a sequel to clipping needle teeth too close to the gum line. The disease can be confused with atrophic rhinitis, but the latter affects more pigs, is more chronic, and causes a lateral deviation rather than a bulging distortion of the face.

The only effective means of preventing these diseases lies with good management and sanitation. Keeping the pens clean and dry will make their occurrence a rarity.

Dysentery, Swine

There are many causes of diarrhea in pigs, including salmonellosis and colibacillosis to name two. But the term *swine dysentery* is reserved for a specific severe mucohemorrhagic diarrhea complex due primarily to *Serpulina hyodysenteriae*. It is often referred to as *vibrionic dysentery,* although the role *Campylobacter coli* plays in causing it is unclear. Other names are *black scours* and *bloody scours.*

The disease is most prevalent in young growing pigs, although it can affect piglets and adult hogs as well. Up to 90 percent of the weanling pigs on a farm may be affected at one time, and reports of 30 percent mortality are not unusual. The disease is spread by ingestion of feces from sick pigs or from recovered or unaffected carriers. Initial outbreaks are most common in late summer or fall and can usually be correlated with addition of pigs to the herd. Once it appears, recurrences tend to be cyclical, with new cases occurring every month or so. Many, but not all, recovered pigs become resistant to further infection. Severity of the disease is related to the size of the infecting dose, stress, and the age of the pig. Swine are the only known reservoir of *S. hyodysenteriae,* and carrier swine are the source of infection. Once infection appears in a herd, recurrences can be expected.

Symptoms

Diminished appetite and soft mucoid feces are the first signs of infection. Body temperature may rise slightly in the early stages but more often is normal. The diarrhea rapidly becomes worse and frequently bloody. Dehydration and weight loss accompany the severe diarrhea. Mucus and bits of intestinal lining tissue often appear in the feces as the disease progresses. The course is variable, ranging from 2 days to a month. In some cases it looks like the animals are recovering, but in a few days or weeks they are as bad as ever. Recovered pigs are frequently stunted and unthrifty, making this one of the economically most important diseases of swine.

Control

Control of the infection is difficult because carrier swine cannot readily be identified with currently available methods. Certainly, additions to the breeding herd of pigs of unknown origin or pigs from herds where the health status is unknown should not be made. This admonition is not so easy to follow for the feedlots, where feeder pigs commonly come from random sources. Hygiene, sanitation, and isolation are all important to reduce fecal contamination and spread of disease. The disease can be transported from one pen to another or one farm to another on dirty boots and feeding utensils. The risk of spreading this and other diseases is the reason most swine growers prefer not to receive visitors in the barns.

Where the infection is present on the farm, a degree of control can be achieved by adding medication to the feed or drinking water. A variety of antibiotics, sodium arsenilate, and carbadox have been used with success. However, *S. hyodysenteriae* develops antibiotic resistance quite rapidly; therefore, medication must be changed frequently. The same drugs can be used for treatment but must be given individually where possible or in drinking water, because sick pigs won't eat.

Control through medication alone is not only a continuing expense but is also rarely successful. It must be coupled with sound hygienic husbandry practices. A vaccine for control of this disease has recently been developed.

Edema, Malignant

This is an acute, commonly fatal disease of cattle, horses, sheep, goats, and swine that in some respects resembles blackleg. It is caused by *Clostridium septicum,* and in cattle and sheep mixed infection with *C. chauvoei* is not rare. Like the other clostridia, *C. septicum* is a soilborne, spore-forming organism that can survive for long periods of time under favorable conditions. Infection when it occurs is usually through contamination of wounds, particularly bruising-type injuries where there is considerable damage to tissue. The organism is anaerobic, and deep puncture wounds provide a favorable site for its rapid multiplication. Although *C. septicum* is the principal organism causing malignant edema, other species of clostridia can be involved. For example, the swelled-head condition sometimes seen in rams as a result of post-fighting infection is usually due to *Clostridium novyi.*

C. septicum is a potent toxin producer that causes profound, rapidly fatal clinical signs. The first indication of its presence is generally soft swelling in the area of the wound that extends very rapidly because of exudation and infiltration of the surrounding area. The adjacent muscle will become dark brown to black in color, but without the gas production and subcutaneous crepitation commonly seen with blackleg. There is always high fever, and affected animals are depressed, weak, and may show muscle tremors and lameness before they die. Death may occur in 24 hours or less.

At necropsy there is usually gangrene of the skin overlying the infected area, and the subcutaneous and intramuscular connective tissue around the site will be very edematous, or filled with fluid. Small hemorrhages and blood-tinged edema fluid will be found in all of the body cavities.

Because of the similarity of malignant edema to blackleg and especially to anthrax, diagnosis based on postmortem examination alone is sometimes difficult. A fluorescent antibody test in the laboratory is helpful in distinguishing between these clostridial infections and anthrax.

Malignant edema is preventable by vaccination, as outlined for blackleg (see page 145), but because of its acute nature and rapid progression, treatment of infected animals is generally not satisfactory. The organism is susceptible to penicillin and broad-spectrum antibiotics if they are given early enough. Antitoxin used to treat the toxemia caused by the disease in humans is too costly to be of practical value for use in animals.

Other clostridial infections, such as *Clostridium sordelli* on the West Coast, have been incriminated as a cause of sudden death in feedlot animals. They are controllable by use of specific bacterin.

Edema, Udder

Udder edema may be associated with mastitis, but more often it is not. Still, it is appropriate to discuss it here. Edema is an excessive accumulation of body fluid outside the body cells and vascular pathways. Swelling is a form of edema in response to infection or injury. A physiological edema in the absence of udder infection is rather common, particularly in animals lactating for the first time. It generally disappears a few days after parturition and causes no problem. But a few dairy heifers develop a severe and persistent edema that requires some care.

Testing for Edema

Physiological edema can readily be distinguished from swelling caused by acute mastitis. Edema, on the one hand, is usually symmetrical, involving the lower third of the entire udder and extending forward sometimes to the belly wall. Mastitis, on the other hand, usually affects only one-fourth or one-half of the gland. Furthermore, edema does not produce heat as infection does. As a further test, press a finger into the swollen area. If it is edema, pressure will force extracellular fluid out of the compressed area, leaving a pit that will last for several minutes. This is a good diagnostic test for edema.

The causes of udder edema are probably multiple, although there is some hereditary predisposition. Lack of exercise prior to parturition is certainly a factor, and there is some evidence that a high-protein diet or excess salt during the weeks preceding parturition contributes to the problem.

Generally, the swelling will gradually subside following parturition and milking or nursing, and no special care is necessary. But in a few animals it may be severe enough to interfere with milking and even walking. The objective is to get the excess fluid absorbed back into the general circulation, and anything that stimulates blood circulation will help. Exercise and massage are particularly helpful. Frequent application of alternate hot and cold packs will also help, as will massage with a mild liniment. If these measures don't improve matters, your veterinarian can give oral or intravenous diuretics that will. In a few individual cows, slight edema will persist for several weeks or months, particularly on the lower and posterior aspects of the rear quarters. It will appear quite firm to the touch and will resist most efforts to remove it, but fortunately it does no harm and has little significance.

Enterotoxemia

This is an acute, highly fatal disease most commonly encountered in lambs and calves, although it is occasionally seen in kids, piglets, and foals. It is the result of toxins produced by *Clostridium perfringens*. Several toxins are recognized, each producing a slightly different but overlapping clinical pattern. Types B, C, and D are the most frequently seen in the United States, although type A has been reported to cause colitis in horses and diarrhea in pigs. Enterotoxemia is most frequent in young animals, but it can cause sudden death in adults as well.

Regardless of toxin type, onset is sudden and mortality is high. Type A in lambs causes severe depression, pallor, jaundice, hemoglobinuria, and rapid breathing. It is a hemolytic disease that, in some respects, resembles leptospirosis in calves. Type B enterotoxemia is responsible for the severe enteric disease often called *lamb dysentery*. It usually occurs in lambs less than 2 weeks old and may cause death without any premonitory signs. Less acute cases will demonstrate severe abdominal pain; failure to nurse; and profuse, often bloody, diarrhea. The disease rapidly progresses to coma and death in 24 hours or less.

Type B generally affects calves 7 to 10 days old, but occasionally older calves will be affected. The symptoms in calves are similar to those in lambs, but calves that don't succumb in a few hours may develop central nervous system signs as well. The disease in piglets, foals, and kids is essentially the same as that seen in lambs. Because of its very acute nature, diagnosis of enterotoxemia is generally based on postmortem lesions. Hemorrhagic enteritis with ulcers and peritonitis is a common finding. Laboratory examination of a portion of intestine and intestinal contents will confirm the diagnosis.

Type C causes similar lesions, and typing of *C. perfringens* exotoxin in the laboratory gives a definitive diagnosis. Type C is responsible for the disease known as *struck* in adult sheep in Great Britain and occasionally seen in this country.

Type D enterotoxemia is a major problem in feedlot lambs, although it can affect those under 2 weeks of age. Characteristically, those in the best nutritional state will be the first of the group affected. Because the disease is usually seen in well-fed animals, it is commonly referred to as *overeating disease.* Sudden death may be the only sign. Those that live a little longer may exhibit excitement, incoordination, and convulsions. Depending on how soon the animal dies, postmortem lesions may range from almost none to hemorrhages of heart muscle, abdominal muscle, and the surface of the intestines. Rapid postmortem decomposition of the kidneys is the basis for its other common name, *pulpy kidney disease.*

Control

Regardless of type, the various forms of enterotoxemia share some common characteristics and control methods. *C. perfringens* is a common soil-borne inhabitant of the intestinal tract of animals. Although the exact mechanism is obscure, it's apparent that under some conditions the organism produces exotoxin, a poison, in excess of an animal's capacity to cope with it. Excessive consumption of milk or grain is a known predisposing factor. As evidence of this, the fattest animals are usually the first affected, and the disease is rarely seen in nursing twin lambs because they simply don't have much milk available to them. Similarly, in the feedlots, outbreaks are most common a few days after the animals are put on full feed.

Regardless of type, a standard recommendation for control of enterotoxemia is to reduce feed intake, whether it be milk for the very young or grain for the older groups. Unfortunately, in the feedlot, reduced grain feeding is inconsistent with rapid rate of gain. Some feedlot operators have successfully reduced the incidence through continuous low-level feeding of broad-spectrum antibiotics, such as tetracycline, to reduce the bacterial population.

These antibiotics and immunization are the most effective means of controlling the disease. Several types of biological products are available, including toxoid, antitoxin, antiserum, and bacterins. Each is type specific. Polyvalent products are available and recommended, even though they are more expensive, unless the specific type of toxin causing the problem has been identified. The choice of product to use depends on circumstances, and advice from a veterinarian is highly recommended.

Generally speaking, antitoxin and antiserum are used to provide immediate protection, such as when animals are first put in the feedlot or during an outbreak. If antiserum is used, animals should be carefully watched for a few hours afterward for signs of anaphylactic shock. Some protection can be provided to the newborn through colostral antibody when the dams have been actively immunized with bacterin or toxoid. When using these products, be sure to follow the manufacturer's recommendations for dose, site, and route of inoculation, because tissue reactions from these products are not unusual.

Erysipelas

The organism causing this disease, *Erysipelothrix rhusiopathiae*, is widespread in nature and persists for long periods of time in soil and water. It is resistant to freezing and drying, and can tolerate most common disinfectants. It is capable of infecting a wide variety of animal species including humans, fish, and birds. It is an infectious disease in swine, turkeys, and fish, but in other species it is generally a wound infection disease.

Except for the individual turkey grower who experiences an outbreak, the disease is most significant economically in pigs. The disease may range from inapparent to acute, subacute, or chronic in pigs. The organism can readily be isolated from the tonsils of many apparently normal pigs. It is excreted in the manure, and infection in pigs occurs primarily via the oral route. Stress seems to be a factor in the development of the clinical disease, and it frequently occurs following farrowing. It is usually not seen in suckling pigs under 3 weeks of age.

Diagnosis

Acute septicemic erysipelas produces fever ranging up to 108°F, lack of appetite, and a reluctance to move. The organism becomes generalized and, among other things, produces painful arthritis. Although they don't always occur, the disease typically produces characteristic skin lesions on the neck, ears, shoulders, and belly. These are raised, reddened areas that take a definite diamond or trapezoidal shape. Because of this, the disease has been referred to as *diamond skin disease.* The coloration ranges from pink to an angry purple, and as the disease progresses the skin lesions may coalesce to form a large discolored area. The skin lesions usually appear within 24 hours and are a good diagnostic sign. Death may occur 2 to 4 days later.

Mortality with the subacute form is lower, and the skin lesions are the most prominent sign. Fever is not as high and although appetite may be depressed, affected pigs will usually eat. Depending on the severity of the lesions, affected patches of skin may become necrotic, dry, and peel off. Occasionally the tips of the ears and tail will slough off. The underlying surface after the skin peels is raw and should be treated with antiseptics as you would treat any open wound.

The acute or subacute forms of the disease may lead to the chronic form. The chronic disease is characterized by arthritis, especially of the hip, hock, stifle, and elbow and knee joints, which at first is hot and painful. In a few weeks the active inflammation subsides and pain is no longer a factor, but the joints are stiff. A more significant lesion for the life of the pig with chronic erysipelas is vegetative endocarditis, especially involving the heart valves. This is a frequent complication that may be inapparent at first but may result in sudden death due to pulmonary embolism or cardiac infarct. More extensive endocarditis causes unthriftiness and labored breathing. Affected pigs have a poor rate of gain and are unprofitable to keep.

Treatment

Erysipelas responds well to treatment with penicillin, and the earlier treatment is started, the better. This disease has important implications for the productivity of the swine herd, and prompt professional diagnosis based on clinical signs, necropsy, or culture of the organism from tonsils or blood is important. Biannual vaccination with bacterin is reasonably but not entirely effective in preventing it.

Erysipelas also can cause problems in sheep flocks as a result of wound infection following castration or docking. Arthritis is the principal sign in lambs, and the resulting production loss can be severe. Performing these operations in clean surroundings with instruments disinfected after use on each lamb will minimize the problem.

Flock outbreaks of laminitis due to *E. rhusiopathiae* 2 to 3 weeks after dipping sheep have been reported. Infection in these cases occur via skin abrasions if the dip water is heavily contaminated with the organism. Addition of a suitable germicide to the water helps to minimize the problem.

Fever, Potomac

More properly called *equine ehrlichial colitis,* this disease causes an acute diarrhea in horses. The causative organism, *Ehrlichia risticii,* is a member of the rickettsiae group, most of which are transmitted by insects. Occurrence sporadically and primarily in summer and early fall indicates that this disease is carried the same way, although a specific vector has not been identified.

Symptoms

Lack of appetite, depression, fever, and increased intestinal motility are followed in 24 to 48 hours by profuse watery diarrhea in many but not all cases. The disease closely resembles acute salmonellosis. It may be complicated by colic and laminitis. Severity varies, and only one or two horses in a herd may be affected, though mortality may reach 30 percent. The symptoms, coupled with a positive enzyme-linked immunosorbent assay (ELISA) or fluorescent antibody test, generally provide a positive diagnosis.

Prevention

Prevention includes protection of horses from biting insects and vaccination early in spring and again 4 months later. Fortunately, only a few will be affected at a time, and it doesn't seem to spread from horse to horse. Nevertheless, affected horses should be isolated until Potomac fever is positively identified. Rapid favorable response to oxytetracycline therapy helps identify the disease. Intravenous fluid therapy is important for horses with severe diarrhea.

Fever, Shipping

The respiratory disease complex is probably the most important faced by the cattle feedlot operator and is the greatest source of economic loss in feedlot cattle, not only because of significant mortality but also because of unthriftiness and decreased rate of gain. There are several factors known to make up the respiratory disease complex and some that are probably unknown as well. But one of the most significant is the disease called *shipping fever,* or *pasteurellosis.* It is caused by a bacterium, *Pasteurella multocida,* and a virus, such as *parainfluenza-3* (PI-3), working together at a time of stress. Recent work has incriminated bovine respiratory syncytial virus (BRSV) as an additional factor. Although each of these viruses may cause infection by itself with mild clinical signs, it is when *P. multocida* or *P. haemolytica* appears as a secondary invader that serious disease results.

The most common stress is that of moving animals from one location to another, sometimes over great distances, hence the name *shipping fever.* It is not limited to feeder cattle, and can be equally disastrous in the dairy herd. Shipping fever differs somewhat from a simple pneumonia in that it tends to be quite contagious. These organisms apparently increase in virulence as the disease becomes active in animals under stress, and their invasiveness increases so even animals not under stress soon fall victim to the disease.

Shipping fever in cattle is basically a severe contagious bronchopneumonia. The earliest sign is a high fever ranging up to 106°F and occasionally higher, with lack of appetite, coughing, and nasal and occasionally ocular discharge. As the disease progresses, respiration becomes rapid and shallow, eventually with an accumulation of fluid and cellular debris, and occasionally outright pus, in the smaller air passages that restricts air flow. Consolidation of lung tissue will become so severe that cyanosis results from lack of oxygen. Animals in this extreme condition will be reluctant to move and will stand with head and neck outstretched, sometimes with tongue protruding, actually gasping for air. Some outbreaks of pasteurellosis in cattle are characterized by diarrhea as well as the respiratory signs. Because of the respiratory distress, the clinical signs are greatly aggravated by exertion. It's extremely important, therefore, that animals with pneumonia be handled quietly and gently. If you have to chase them around the pen to treat them, they may be better off untreated.

Related Factors

Although, as the name implies, pasteurellosis is commonly associated with shipping, this is not the only factor that can trigger an outbreak of the disease. Because many healthy cattle harbor the organisms responsible, it requires only a lowering of resistance from any cause to induce an outbreak. The stress of a radical change in diet if the animals don't eat well for a day or two has occasionally been incriminated as a factor. The disease is seen more commonly in fall and winter months during or following periods of inclement weather, but cold does not seem to be an important factor provided the animals have at least a windbreak or some sort of minimal shelter. In fact, it occurs more frequently during winter in herds that are stabled in enclosed barns where ventilation is poor. The buildup of ammonia fumes from decomposing manure and high humidity provides sufficient stress. Also, of course, in an enclosed barn lacking frequent air change, the concentration of infective moisture droplets in the air will be considerably more than it would be outside.

Last, it appears possible, circumstantially at least, that shipping fever can be spread from farm to farm on boots and clothing, because it is not unusual to find the disease appearing sequentially on adjacent farms where there has been traffic in and out.

Treatment

Fortunately, *P. multocida* often responds well to proper treatment that is initiated early. Treatment has no effect on the virus components of the complex. Several antibiotics, penicillin and others such as tetracycline, tylosin, erythromycin, and cephalosporin, can be reasonably effective. The key is to start treatment early before too much damage is done to the lungs, using an antibiotic to which the bug is sensitive, and to continue it long enough so the last vestiges of infection are removed. The longer treatment is delayed, the less likely a successful outcome will be.

Advanced cases generally result in impaired lung function and walled-off abscesses of the lung that make the animal unthrifty and unprofitable, even if it survives. The latter is a common complication in the feedlot where hundreds, and sometimes even thousands, of animals are kept, making it difficult to observe them individually to detect early signs of pneumonia. Furthermore, treatment of animals under these conditions is difficult on an individual basis because of the time and labor involved. Medication of drinking water or feed with a broad spectrum antibiotic is helpful, but unfortunately the really sick animals usually don't eat or drink as much as they should, and the problem of regulating drug dosage is almost insurmountable when it is administered in this manner.

Prevention

The key is to do everything possible to prevent this disease from occurring in the first place. It goes without saying that you should start with healthy cattle insofar as possible. The best way to do this when you are buying replacements is to buy directly from the farm where the animals have been raised, rather than through a commission sale. While the sales managers do the best they can to provide you with healthy cattle, it is not at all unusual for cattle going through commission sales to have been en route from the farm of origin for 2 weeks or more, often traveling through several commission sales before they reach their final destination. This kind of stress almost ensures that they are going to have disease problems of some kind.

Second, regardless of the source and whether you are dealing with dairy cattle or beef cattle, it's effort well spent to keep the replacement animals separated from the main herd for at least 2 weeks when you get them home. In that way, if they do develop shipping fever or some other disease, at least they won't endanger your other animals.

If you are dealing with feeder calves, remember that these are usually right off the range and rather unaccustomed to being handled, and equally unaccustomed to anything but grass to eat. Therefore, they should be segregated in clean surroundings and left alone with hay and clean water so they can rest and become acclimated to their new environment. Similarly, avoid the temptation to put them on full feed immediately in hopes of getting a faster rate of gain. This is usually self-defeating because they aren't accustomed to grain and frequently will get a digestive upset, which is sufficient added stress to contribute to the onset of shipping fever.

With dairy cattle, the same general recommendation holds true. Buy them from the source least likely to contribute to disease, and segregate them from the main herd for a minimum of 2 weeks.

The same precaution should be observed for your own animals that you may be bringing back from a fair or show. There is no way of knowing what diseases they have been exposed to when mixed in with other animals at a show; therefore, they can be just as dangerous to bring directly back into the herd as are entirely new replacements. These management procedures will do much to prevent shipping fever from appearing in the herd. In addition, vaccine given early enough can be helpful.

Vaccines

There are several vaccines available singly or in combination that will help to prevent shipping fever, but none is 100 percent effective. The simplest of these are bacterins for *P. multocida* and *Pasteurella haemolytica*, which are moderately effective for a short period of time. Vaccines are available for protection against PI-3, BRSV, *P. multocida, P. haemolytica,* and infectious bovine rhinotracheitis (IBR), all of which contribute to the respiratory disease complex. These are available singly or in various combinations and, depending on formulation, are given subcutaneously, intramuscularly, or intranasally, so the choice can be quite confusing. Your veterinarian can best advise you as to what vaccines should be used in your area and under your conditions. But in any case, remember that although intranasal IBR/PI-3 vaccine produces local cellular immunity in the upper respiratory tract in 48 hours, it takes at least 2 weeks for solid immunity to develop following administration of vaccine.

Vaccine given the day the animal was shipped or the day it arrives will be of very questionable value in preventing disease outbreaks.

If you are in the business of finishing beef cattle, whenever possible buy feeder calves that have been preconditioned. These will have been weaned, castrated if necessary, vaccinated, and accustomed to grain well before their shipping date. Experience has shown that conditioned feeder calves arrive in better condition with fewer problems than those taken directly off the range.

Hemoglobinuria, Bacillary

This disease of cattle and sheep, sometimes called *redwater,* is caused by *Clostridium haemolyticum* and occurs primarily in the western states in animals on irrigated pastures. The organism appears to produce two toxins, one causing tissue destruction similar to other *Clostridium* species and the other causing destruction of red blood cells. The result is severe anemia and loss of hemoglobin from red blood cells through the kidney, which gives the urine a dark red color, from which the disease gets its common name.

The organism is a soilborne spore-former, and where the disease is prevalent spores are commonly found in the livers of normal cattle and occasionally sheep and goats. Liver damage, as from flukes, is apparently necessary before the spores become vegetative and start producing toxin. Initial infection occurs orally in animals grazing contaminated pasture or forage. Losses may begin 7 to 10 days after susceptible animals are put into the pasture. Sudden death may be the only clinical sign, but more often there is evidence of acute abdominal pain, fever, rapid respiration, and reluctance to move. Profound anemia with hemoglobinuria and edema of the brisket is a common finding. Anoxia attributable to the anemia occurs late in the disease, which is frequently fatal in 4 days or less.

Diagnosis is based on history, symptoms, postmortem examination, and serologic testing. The blood test is not completely specific, however, and blood or tissue cultures are more positive.

Treatment

Early treatment with penicillin or broad-spectrum antibiotics, coupled with blood transfusion, good nursing care, and antiserum, if available, will save some animals. Annual subcutaneous vaccination with *C. haemolyticum* bacterin provides a fair degree of control, although in high-risk areas a second dose during the pasture season may be necessary.

Hepatitis, Infectious Necrotic

This is a highly fatal disease of sheep caused by *C. novyi* and occasionally seen in cattle and pigs. It occurs, like bacillary hemoglobinuria, when liver damage from any cause creates an environment in which the organism already present can proliferate. The toxin it produces causes extensive tissue destruction, disrupting capillaries and causing hemorrhagic areas in many body organs. Small subcutaneous hemorrhages give the underside of the skin a black appearance when observed at necropsy, hence the common name, *black disease.*

Normal animals harbor the organism in areas where it is found, and fecal matter from them further contaminates pastures. In sheep, the primary triggering factor is migration of immature flukes through the liver. They provide sufficient liver injury for *C. novyi* to multiply, which in turn causes more liver destruction, making conditions even more favorable. Flukes can be a factor in cattle, too, although other liver disease may be more significant. Liver abscesses commonly encountered in feedlot cattle and pigs on high-concentrate diets may account for the greater frequency of the disease in these species in feedlots. In sheep the disease is more prevalent from midsummer until early fall when the snail population — the intermediate host for liver flukes — is at its peak. High moisture conditions that favor snail growth make the disease more prevalent on irrigated pastures. Adult sheep are most commonly affected, and with few exceptions those affected will go from an apparently well-nourished, healthy state to death in a few hours. Mortality is 100 percent, and anywhere from 5 to 30 percent of the flock may be affected.

Diagnosis

At necropsy the dark areas under the skin, coupled with necrotic areas in the liver and accumulation of blood-tinged fluid in body cavities, help to distinguish this from other diseases causing sudden death. The fluorescent antibody test applied to liver tissue in the laboratory confirms the diagnosis.

Control

While immunization with toxoid will control the disease even during an outbreak, control of the fluke population should be attempted as well, either by fencing sheep out of wet areas or by using a molluscicide where this is legally permissible, because heavy fluke infestations can cause serious primary disease without bacterial complications. Feeding some hay in addition to concentrates to feedlot cattle helps to reduce the incidence of liver abscesses that predispose the animals to black disease.

Jowl Abscess

Although they have little relevance for the life or productivity of the pig, jowl abscesses due to *Streptococcus* species are a common cause of partial carcass condemnation at slaughter. This adds to the cost of pork, and annual losses are as great as millions of dollars.

The condition is endemic on some farms, with recovered animals acting as carriers and infecting every new pig brought to the farm as well as a high percentage of those born on the premises. The organism colonizes in the tonsils and extends from there to the cervical lymph nodes, where abscesses develop. Abscesses may be as large as 5 to 6 cm in diameter and contain a greenish yellow pus. Most abscesses ultimately rupture and drain on the outside. Healing takes place after several weeks, but fistulous tracts often remain. Initial infection is usually accompanied by mild fever of 2 or 3 days' duration, but this is rarely observed.

The first indication that anything is wrong is usually swelling at the site of a developing abscess. Unfortunately, by then it's too late for treatment to have much value. Streptococcal abscesses develop a thick wall or capsule, with little if any blood supply to the interior. Because antibiotics are transported in the bloodstream, they can't reach the site of infection.

Prevention is by far the best course to take. Your veterinarian can help you to design a control program that may include vaccination and/or incorporation of low levels of antibiotics in the feed. While reasonably effective, legal constraints on the type and level of antibiotics used make the latter procedure less effective than it could be.

Keratoconjunctivitis, Infectious

This disease, commonly called *pink eye,* occurs frequently in young cattle and less often in sheep and goats. It is most common during the summer months, although sporadic cases occur in the other seasons.

Clinical Signs

Onset of the disease is sudden, and it spreads rapidly. The first indications of the disease are usually an excessive flow of tears and a tendency to hold the eye partially closed. Bright sunlight increases the pain of the disease, and affected animals usually seek a shaded area. Within a short time an ulcer develops, almost always in the central part of the cornea. Infiltration of leukocytes and swelling of the ulcerated area cause the cornea to become opaque and milky in appearance. At first this is limited to a ring around the ulcer, but in 24 to 48 hours the entire cornea becomes opaque. The animal is then blind. In a majority of cases only one eye is affected, but involvement of both eyes is by no means rare. The elapsed time from onset to total corneal opacity may be no more than 48 hours.

Without treatment the corneal ulcer may heal spontaneously, but more often it gets progressively worse. As the ulcer gets progressively deeper, the strength of the cornea is diminished and pressure within the eye causes the front part of the eyeball to assume a conical shape. Concurrently, blood vessels extend from the periphery into the cornea in an attempt to speed the healing process. In a few days, the ulcer may extend completely through the cornea, resulting in loss of fluid and collapse of the front chamber of the eye. Blindness is then permanent.

Adjacent structures of the eye are also involved. The blood vessels in the sclera, the white fibrous covering of the eyeball, become enlarged, and there is inflammation of the lining of the lids that causes a mucopurulent discharge and conjunctivitis.

For some reason, at least in my experience, pink eye seems to be more prevalent in some years than in others. This may be related to climatic conditions and fly population. I recall very vividly seeing more than two hundred beef calves on one farm at one time with varying stages of the disease. It was a heartbreaking sight, and many of them never recovered.

The most common causative organism in cattle is *Moraxella bovis,* and in all probability it is carried from one animal to the next by flies, especially face flies. Irritation by dust and tall grass increases susceptibility of the eye to infection. In sheep, *Chlamyida psittaci* is the common cause, but species of *Mycoplasma* and *Neisseria* may also be involved.

Diagnosis

Diagnosis is not difficult, although the condition must be distinguished from the eye lesion caused by IBR virus. Almost invariably the corneal opacity of pink eye extends from the center of the cornea outward, whereas that of IBR extends from the periphery inward. Also, with pink eye there is usually no adverse symptom other than the eye lesion, whereas with IBR some animals in the group will usually have fever and respiratory involvement.

The most important thing is to recognize the disease and start treatment early before too much damage is done. It responds well to antibiotic ointment instilled onto the eye and to small amounts of antibiotic injected into the conjunctiva.

Too many people turn young stock out to pasture in spring and forget about them until fall. In the interim, some may get pink eye and become blind. It pays to check them at least once a week. Incipient pink eye isn't hard to spot because there will always be the evidence of tears streaming down the cheek.

Affected animals should be put in a darkened stall and treated immediately. Where this isn't feasible, as with range cattle, at least one manufacturer makes an eye patch that is fastened over the eye with adhesive after treatment with antibiotics.

As a result of considerable research, there is now a bacterin for the prevention of the disease in cattle caused by *M. bovis.* Vaccination, fly control, isolation of infected animals, and reduction of dusty irritating conditions, insofar as possible, are the best means of prevention. Early treatment of affected animals is essential to recovery. Topical application of antibiotics is effective if applied several times daily. Alternatively, drugs such as oxytetracycline can be used parenterally. The cause of pink eye in animals and pink eye in humans is entirely different, and there is no known relationship between the two.

Leptospirosis

This disease is seen in all species but is most frequently reported in cows, pigs, goats, sheep, and horses, in that order. It is also transmissable to humans, and human cases are not rare. It is caused by several species of *Leptospira* including *Leptopsira pomona, Leptospira hardjo, Leptospira grippotyphosa,* and *Leptospira icterohaemorrhagiae. Leptospira canicola,* a species affecting dogs, rarely is found in livestock other than swine.

Clinical signs of the disease are variable, and diagnosis may be difficult. It tends to be much more acute in young animals, resulting in high fever, complete lack of appetite, hemoglobinuria, jaundice, anemia, and death. Calf mortality, for example, may range up to 15 percent. Although a few adult animals may show similar clinical signs, the infection is often inapparent. In milking cows or goats, there may be a sharp drop in production, and a few may produce thick, ropy, blood-tinged milk without evidence of udder inflammation. Abortions several weeks after the infection passed through the herd or flock may be the only evidence that the infection was there. Serologic testing or identification of the organisms from the stomach contents of an aborted fetus will confirm the diagnosis. There is strong evidence linking prior leptospirosis infection with recurrent iridocyclitis (recurrent uveitis, periodic ophthalmia, moon blindness) in horses.

Kidney Involvement

The primary site of infection is the kidney. Many recovered animals will continue to shed the organism in their urine for considerable periods of time without themselves showing any clinical signs whatsoever. Such carrier animals are an obvious hazard to other susceptible animals in the herd. The organism survives well in water such as in ponds or potholes. Water from these sources, when contaminated by urine from infected animals, or the urine droplets themselves are the primary source of infection. Although most infections are probably acquired orally, the organism is quite invasive, and infective urine droplets splashing into the eye can result in infection. For this and other reasons, people handling aborted fetuses should wear gloves and wash thoroughly afterward.

Leptospirosis occurs in wild as well as domestic animals, and it is probable that many swine herds become infected through contamination of feed by carrier rodents. Similarly, the infection occurs in deer, and it has been postulated but not proved that the initial infection in some cattle herds occurs when carrier deer and cattle share the same pasture.

Vaccination

When treated early, animals with the acute infection respond well to antibiotic therapy, but because the most important economic effect is abortion following acute or inapparent infection, prevention is much more desirable.

Several steps are effective. One is to ensure that purchased replacements test negative for leptospirosis in a blood test conducted by a reliable laboratory. Protecting the feed supply from rodent contamination and fencing animals away from potentially contaminated water supplies are also helpful strategies. But routine vaccination is by far the most effective approach.

Although *L. pomona* is the most common serotype affecting livestock, there are farm and regional variations. Bacterins are available that incorporate antigens to stimulate immunity against all common types of the organism. Depending on the manufacturer, these are available in several combinations or as *L. pomona* bacterin alone. The latter is relatively inexpensive and will provide good protection for almost a year. All animals on the farm should be vaccinated annually, especially when the possibility of carriers from prior infections exists in the herd.

Listeriosis

Despite rapid progress in animal disease research, the development of some diseases remains mysterious. Listeriosis, commonly called *circling disease* and caused by *Listeria monocytogenes,* falls into that obscure category. Although it occurs primarily in cattle, sheep, and goats, the organism has been isolated from a wide variety of domestic and wild animals, birds, fish, and humans. Many normal animals carry the organism, and the clinical disease occurs sporadically for reasons not well understood.

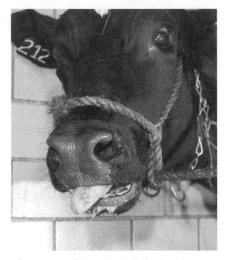

Symptoms of listeriosis include drooping ear, sunken eye, and tongue paralysis.

In ruminants, there appears to be a causal relationship with corn silage feeding, particularly if the silage is not well preserved and has a pH above 5.5. In sheep, outbreaks commonly occur about 3 weeks after they are started on a full feed of silage and terminate when silage is withdrawn from the diet. It can and does occur, however, in animals that have never been fed corn silage.

The organism is extremely hardy, surviving in manure for a year or more and readily withstanding repeated freezing and thawing. Its distribution is limited primarily to the colder-climate areas, and the disease is rarely seen in the South. The route by which infection occurs in nature is obscure, but experimentally the disease can be reproduced by inoculating the organism in a variety of ways. Route of infection may have some bearing on the clinical signs seen.

Diagnosis

Typically, in cattle, sheep, and goats, the disease causes an encephalitis. The animal may stand off by itself looking rather dull and depressed or may wander aimlessly. If it comes to a fence or wall, it just stands there pushing against it. The animal may stand with its head and neck turned to one side; if you turn the animal's head the other way, it returns to the original position when released. A high percentage of, but not all, affected animals when they walk will move in a tight circle, always in the same direction, hence the common name, *circling disease*. Facial paralysis on one side with drooping of the ear, eyelid, and lip on the same side is typical of listeriosis. Commonly, animals with this sign will stand with some hay or feed in the mouth, making no effort to chew or swallow. Frequently, not all of these signs will be seen in the same animal, especially in sheep and goats, in whom the disease is more acute, causing death in 24 to 48 hours. Cattle tend to be more resistant, and the disease may run a course of 7 to 10 days. Once the first case is recognized, checking temperatures of other animals in the herd may distinguish those in the early stages of the disease, as fever is a consistent early finding.

Encephalitis, however, is not the only form of the disease. In monogastric animals, such as the pig, and occasionally in young calves, lambs, and foals, the disease will become generalized, involving the liver and other viscera. Affected animals show all the signs of acute septicemia: fever, lack of appetite, increased pulse and respiration, diarrhea, and early death. It can also infect the uterus, causing abortion and retained placenta with no other clinical signs. All three forms (encephalitic, septicemic, uterine) can occur in humans, although the encephalitic manifestation may be more frequent. Aborted fetuses and placenta and vaginal discharges are highly infective, and extreme caution should be taken when handling such material.

Strangely, herd outbreaks that may involve up to 10 percent of animals usually consist of all encephalitic or all septicemic cases. Abortions may occur without any other clinical signs of disease. Except when the unilaterial facial paralysis and circling are evident, diagnosis is sometimes difficult. The septicemic form looks like any other septicemia and the encephalitic form can be confused with other diseases causing brain disorders, such as thromboembolic meningoencephalitis, tumors, rabies, pregnancy toxemia in sheep, and the nervous form of ketosis in cattle. Blood tests are of little value because many normal animals have a strong antibody titer against *L. monocytogenes*. Culture of the organism in the laboratory from body tissues, coupled with the clinical signs, is most diagnostic but special techniques may be required. Listeriosis in cattle can be confused with bovine spongiform encephalopathy, rabies, polioencephalomalacia, and lead poisoning, among other things. The unilateral facial paralysis helps distinguish it. Because of the public health implications, animals with neurological signs should be seen by your veterinarian.

Treatment

Treatment of the septicemic form in all species and the encephalitic form in sheep and goats is worth trying but usually disappointing. By the time it is noticed, the disease is too far advanced and the sick animals die too soon. Because it runs a longer course in cattle, treatment may be more rewarding, but some recovered animals may show evidence of permanent brain damage. Without treatment, mortality approaches 100 percent. In any case, prompt treatment is essential, and at the first indication that the disease is present, temperatures should be checked on all animals in the herd or flock. Any with above-normal temperatures should be treated immediately, using broad-spectrum antibiotics or other drugs recommended by your veterinarian. If corn silage is a part of the diet, especially for feedlot lambs, it should be removed.

Because the organism is widespread and its mode of infection is unclear, specific control measures are hard to define. Thus far, satisfactory bacterins have not been developed. Because of the apparent circumstantial relationship, the best present recommendation, particularly for sheep and goats, is to introduce silage to the diet gradually and to avoid feeding spoiled silage entirely.

Lyme Disease

This disease, named for Lyme, Connecticut, where it was first diagnosed, is caused by a spirochete, *Borrelia burgdorferi*. It is transmitted by ticks and primarily affects humans and dogs, but has been occasionally reported in horses and cattle. The principal host for the immature tick larvae is the white-footed mouse, and for adults the white-tailed deer. The disease has been reported in most of the continental United States, and infections occur most frequently in summer and early fall, when tick activity is at its peak.

Symptoms

In horses and cattle, the primary signs are fever and lameness caused by arthritis, particularly involving the joints of the foreleg. The affected joints feel hot and swollen and are painful. The arthritis may be transitory or it may become chronic. The clinical signs are not sufficiently definitive to provide a positive diagnosis. A tentative diagnosis can be confirmed by an ELISA test of blood serum.

Prevention

As with all disease, prevention is preferable to treatment; however, the disease does respond to early treatment with antibiotics such as ampicillin, penicillin, and tetracycline. Prevention consists of those measures that keep animals and ticks separated. Fence off brush areas, or cut the brush where ticks reside and keep pastures clipped. During the high-risk season, examine animals daily and remove any ticks found. Frequent use of acaricidal dips or tick repellents is helpful.

Lymphadenitis, Caseous

This disease, most important in sheep and goats, is caused by *Corynebacterium pseudotuberculosis*. In these species, caseous lymphadenitis is characterized by chronic abscesses of the superficial lymph nodes. It rarely infects cattle, but in the horse may cause an ulcerative lymphangitis, with enlargement and nodule formation in the subcutaneous lymphatics of the lower leg. In the horse, it's important that the disease be distinguished from a much more significant equine disease, *glanders*. The latter has been eradicated from the United Sates but could reappear.

Caseous lymphadenitis in sheep and goats is primarily a wound infection. The organism gains entrance through an abrasion, especially following shearing, and is carried to the lymph nodes, where it colonizes to develop abscesses that may not be apparent until several months after the actual infection occurred. Although the disease causes pain and fever in the horse, it is relatively innocuous for sheep and goats except in the rare instance when abscesses develop in vital organs such as the liver and kidneys.

The disease is important economically in sheep, however, because affected carcasses or parts thereof are condemned at slaughter. In goats the disease is unsightly, and particularly troublesome to exhibitors of purebred animals. While wool hides the lymph node enlargement in sheep, the enlarged nodes are readily apparent in goats, particularly where they rupture to drain a caseous greenish pus and then heal, leaving an unsightly scar.

Prevention

Once it appears in a herd or flock, prevention of further cases is difficult. Vaccines may reduce the incidence of new infections, but will not prevent all new infections and will not cure those animals already infected. Draining abscesses discharge the organism onto the ground, thereby contaminating the premises and increasing the possibility of further infections. The organism can survive for months on the ground, on shearing equipment, in feeders, and so on. An important control procedure for the goat herd is to isolate any animals with draining abscesses, preferably in an area with an impervious floor that can be readily disinfected. The same advice is valid but usually impractical for the sheep flock, as detection of infected sheep is so difficult. Serologic testing for the disease has no value, and severely affected animals should be culled. The best procedures for the sheep flock are to use the shears carefully and to disinfect them frequently. Cuts or abrasions should be treated with a topical disinfectant such as iodine. Shorn sheep should not be held in a corral, where the concentration of the organism is likely to be high, but should be turned out to pasture immediately to take advantage of the natural dilution factor.

If detected early, before abscesses form, the infection responds well to penicillin. The drug, however, will not reach bacteria inside an abscess. In goats, the ripe abscesses may be surgically drained and medicated as an open wound to promote healing with minimal scarring.

Mastitis

Without doubt, mastitis is the most prevalent disease afflicting dairy cattle, but its prevalence is not limited to them alone. It is a common problem in sows and dairy goats; occurs sporadically in beef cattle and sheep; and, rarely, occurs in the mare. It may occur as a chronic, even inapparent infection, or as an acute febrile disease, causing generalized illness in addition to local pain and swelling. The acute form, especially in sheep and goats, may be complicated by gangrene. This condition, commonly called *blue-bag,* is life-threatening, and at the very least usually results in sloughing of the infected gland.

There are a number of bacteria that have the potential to cause mastitis, including *Streptococcus agalactiae, Streptococcus dysgalactiae, Streptococcus uberis, E. coli,* and several species of *Staphylococcus.* Infections due to *Pseudomonas aeruginosa, Arcanobacter (Corynebacterium) pyogenes, Enterobacter (Aerobacter) aerogenes, Klebsiella* species, and *Mycoplasma* are less common. Although *Mycoplasma* mastitis is not common, it is highly contagious and incurable.

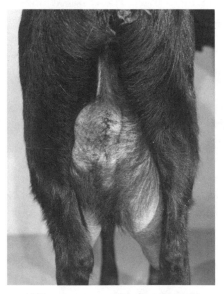

Udder abscess occasionally occurs with the chronic form of mastitis.

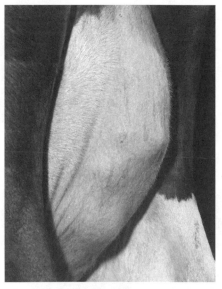

Hard intramammary nodules result from tissue destruction during the acute phase of mastitis.

There are regional and species differences in the prevalence of these organisms as udder pathogens. *E. coli* is the predominant cause of mastitis in the sow and is often incriminated as a part of the metritis, mastitis, agalactia (MMA) syndrome. *Staphylococcus, Streptococcus,* and *E. coli* are the most common causes in the cow, ewe, doe, and mare.

Clinical Signs

Diagnosis of acute mastitis is not difficult. Clinical signs of acute mastitis include abnormal milk; a hot, swollen udder that is often painful; fever; lack of appetite; and greatly reduced milk flow. The latter has serious implications for the offspring of animals that are nursing their young. Agalactia in sows is a prominent cause of death loss of piglets due to starvation.

Acute mastitis, as a result of treatment and occasionally spontaneously, may subside into a chronic form with a latent infection that subsequently flares up again, particularly when udder resistance is lowered. Localized abscesses are not uncommon as a sequel, nor is scar tissue, which develops from tissue destruction during the acute phase. This results in unbalanced udders with "slack" quarters. Abscesses and lumpy scar tissue are palpable if not actually visible, and animals with such evidence of past severe infection are not good prospects for herd replacements.

Diagnosis of the Chronic Form

Chronic mastitis is not as easy to diagnose. Characteristically, *S. agalactiae* produces a low-grade chronic infection that causes a gradual attrition of secretory tissue and loss of production. This unobserved infection accounts for production losses as high as 20 percent in some dairy herds, and lost production is the most costly part of chronic mastitis.

Daily use of the black plate strip pan will help to identify cows with chronic mastitis. A few squirts of milk on the plate prior to milking will reveal milk that is watery or contains clots and flakes. As a matter of routine, it takes only a few seconds, and as a fringe benefit it helps to stimulate letdown, thereby facilitating milking.

An indirect but more sensitive and objective method of detecting abnormal milk is the use of a leukocyte screening test, such as the California mastitis test (CMT), Wisconsin mastitis test (WMT), or modified Whiteside test (MWT). Of these, the CMT is the easiest to do at the side of the cow. These tests provide an estimate of numbers of somatic cells in milk. Because the leading cause of high numbers or cells in milk is mastitis, it follows that test results will give a reasonably good indication of udder health.

CMT test kits are available from most dairy farm supply dealers. The kit consists of a four-compartment plastic paddle and a bottle of reagent. The reagent is a liquid detergent to which has been added a pH-sensitive dye, usually brom-cresol purple. Milk from each quarter is squirted into separate compart-ments of the paddle, and an equal amount of reagent is added. The mixture is then gently swirled for 10 to 15 seconds and the reaction noted. An increase in viscosity and depth of color indicates the presence of somatic cells. The more cells that are present, the greater the viscosity will be. Results are recorded as negative, 1, 2, and 3, with 3 indicating the most cells. Quarters indicating 2 or 3 almost certainly have serious levels of infection.

Treatment of mastitis, however, should not be based solely on CMT results, because cows recently fresh and those drying off will give high test results in the absence of any infection. Udder injury from improper milking machine operation will also raise cell counts, but such injury also leads to mas-titis very quickly.

The U.S. Public Health Service has adopted the somatic cell count as a measure of milk quality, and all milk from commercial dairy herds is periodi-cally screened. The federal standard is set at 750,000 cells/mL of grade A milk, although many states and milkshed districts have adopted stricter standards. Because the screening is done on a pooled sample representing all cows in the herd, the dairy farmer who consistently meets the federal standard should not feel complacent about the mastitis status of his herd. When the somatic cell count of a pooled sample exceeds 200,000 cells/mL, it is virtually certain that there are cows with subclinical mastitis in the herd. The higher the count, the more mastitic cows there are.

Nor should the farmer be lulled into complacency by few observed acute or clinical cases. A British study in 1971 of 1,344 cows in thirty-one herds demonstrated that for every quarter showing evidence of clinical infection, there are thirty-two subclinically infected quarters. Similar results have been obtained in other studies in the United States. While obvious clinical cases are bad enough, it's the unobserved subclinical cases that cause the serious produc-tion loss due to this disease.

Prevention

Most of the staggering loss from mastitis can be prevented by application of inexpensive control methods if one understands the pathogenesis of the disease. First, a distinction must be made between udder infection and mastitis. It is possible, even common, for many potential pathogens to infect the mammary gland and not cause disease. Mastitis results when these pathogens are present in overwhelming numbers and resistance of the udder tissue is lowered.

Infection of the gland in all species occurs when pathogens enter the teat canal. For practical purposes, this is the only route of infection. It follows, then, that if pathogens are kept away from the teat end, infection will not result. The closer you can come to keeping the teat end sterile, the less the risk will be. Obviously it's impossible under farm conditions to keep teat ends sterile, but many simple procedures will help. The first is to keep the animal in as clean and sanitary surroundings as possible, to keep environmental pathogens down to a reasonable level. The use of inorganic material such as sand, rubber mats, or mattresses in the stall/bed further reduces the risk of environmental contamination. The animal that has no alternative but to lie down in mud and manure is more likely to get an infected udder than is one lying on clean dry ground or a well-bedded stall.

An exception should be noted. Although not common, mastitis in cows due to *Klebsiella* species is a serious disease that has been linked to use of contaminated sawdust, wood chips, or shavings as bedding. *Klebsiella* species is a common saprophyte on tree bark; therefore, the use of green sawdust is not recommended. Sawdust or shavings from kiln-dried lumber would be less hazardous.

There are other simple methods of reducing exposure. Milk known infected cows last so that infection will not be carried to others on your hands or the milking machine. Avoid the bad habit of stripping a little milk on the floor before attaching the milking machine. The highest concentration of bacteria is usually in the foremilk, and stripping the milk on the floor only increases the level of environmental contamination. Keep animals out of situations likely to lead to high infection rates. For example, serious outbreaks of coliform mastitis have resulted when cows were allowed to wade in contaminated ponds.

Use of Germicide. The single most effective procedure for preventing new infections due to contagious pathogens has proved to be spraying or dipping the teat ends with a residual germicide immediately after each milking. A number of approved teat dip products are available for the purpose. The teat is most vulnerable to bacterial invasion immediately after milking. The teat sphincter muscle is then relaxed, and it's not unusual to find a drop of milk on the teat end when milking is completed. This is an excellent medium for bacterial growth and subsequent invasion of the teat canal itself. Dipping the entire teat in a sanitizer prevents this from happening.

Germicides are also available for predipping. When used properly, they can be effective in preventing mastitis due to environmental pathogens.

Use of Antibiotics. As a control procedure, it has also been proved advantageous to infuse long-acting antibiotics into each quarter via the teat canal *after* the last milking before the dry period. This is the most practical time to treat the chronically infected cow, because milk doesn't have to be discarded and the antibiotic has a longer time to work. Over a period of time, by following good sanitary practices, dipping teats after each milking, and treating all quarters of all dry cows, a number of herds have become free of infection with *S. agalactiae* and some have even become free of *Staphylococcus.* Once *S. agalactiae* is eradicated from a herd, it will not reappear unless the infection is introduced via an infected cow added to the herd, because for all practical purposes, the organism lives only in the udder. In the badly infected herd, eradication of *S. agalactiae* can increase milk production by 20 percent or more.

While an assiduously followed program of teat dipping and dry cow treatment will greatly reduce udder infection as all the herd goes through the treatment cycle, it may sometimes be desirable to reduce the infection level much faster. With the aid of your veterinarian and a diagnostic laboratory, this can be done by collecting milk samples from each quarter and culturing them to identify the bacteria present. Once they are identified, and particularly if the organisms are checked for antibiotic sensitivity, the most effective antibiotic can be used to treat the infected quarters. This procedure is most effective for *S. agalactiae* eradication, as this organism is an obligate udder parasite. The procedure usually has to be repeated several times to eliminate the last vestiges of infection. Eradication of *Staphylococcus* species infection in a herd can be enhanced by combining vaccination with antibiotic therapy. Use of antibiotics alone for staphylococcal infections is usually disappointing.

Although the level of infection with other pathogens can be reduced in this manner, total eradication is difficult because reinfection occurs through environmental contamination. That's why sanitation and avoidance of teat and udder injury are so important in control of mastitis. Because infected cows are the main source of environmental contamination, judicious culling of chronically infected animals should be part of any control program. Treatment alone will never do the job!

Maintaining Milking Machines. The leading cause of teat and udder injury for the dairy cow is an improperly used or malfunctioning milking machine. While a detailed discussion of machine function is beyond the scope of this book, a few suggestions may be helpful. First, a great deal of research has gone into milking machine development, and it's safe to say that all new milking equipment, properly installed and maintained, will do an adequate job. Trouble arises when dairy farmers forget that the milking machine operates more hours than any other machine on the farm and therefore requires periodic maintenance. All too often it is forgotten until it quits.

The milking system should be checked by a factory-trained serviceman every 6 months. He will check such things as airflow, vacuum level at the pump, and stall cock and teat end, as well as pulsation rate and interval. On some types, the pulsators must be dismantled and cleaned and worn parts replaced. The rubber teat cup liners must be properly cared for and replaced frequently. The life of teat cup liners containing natural rubber can be extended by boiling them weekly in lye solution to remove butterfat accumulation. This is not recommended for liners made of synthetic materials, however, which should simply be replaced when signs of wear, such as loss of elasticity, become apparent. The vacuum pipeline should be flushed periodically to remove accumulated debris that restricts airflow. If you don't know how to do this, your serviceman can show you.

Milking machine problems seem to be more frequent in the small expanding herd. Too many people, as they add more cows, simply add more milker units until they unwittingly exceed the capacity of the vacuum pump and line. The effect is insidious because although the pump may be overloaded, the machines will usually still pulsate and milk cows. But because of inadequate vacuum, milking time will be increased, which means greater irritation for the udder. Be sure you don't exceed the rated capacity of your equipment.

Proper Milking Procedures. Even a properly functioning machine can cause udder problems if it is not used correctly. The longer the machine is attached to the cow, the greater the opportunity for organisms to enter the gland, resulting in infection. The vast majority of properly prepared cows will milk out in 5 minutes or less, and the machine should be removed as soon as milking is complete. Some of the new machines are designed to detach automatically when milk flow stops.

To reduce time spent on machine, letdown of milk must first be stimulated. Milk secretion occurs as a result of hormonal influence. The udder is not a bagful of loose milk, as some people think. It is a gland whose cells secrete milk in response to oxytocin, a hormone released by the pituitary gland under certain stimuli. One stimulus is washing the udder with warm water, which has the added benefit of removing any accumulated dirt. Individual paper towels are recommended for this purpose, to avoid spreading infection from one cow to another and to wipe excess water from the teats and udder.

In the milking parlor, a warm-water spray accomplishes the same goal with less risk of contamination. After washing the udder and wiping it dry, use the strip pan, as explained earlier (see page 181), and then attach the machine. The stimulative effect of udder massage is lost in a few minutes if the machine is not promptly attached. Addition of a sanitizer to the wash water has some germicidal effect, but only if the water is changed frequently, because most sanitizers are rapidly inactivated by organic debris.

Proper milking requires undivided attention, and it's a rare individual who can do a good job in a stanchion barn handling more than two milker units. As soon as milking is complete, turn off the unit, break the vacuum by pressing the base of one teat against the side of the teat cup to admit air, and remove it. Remember that the teat cups are held on by a vacuum, and that the vacuum remains for a time after the unit is shut off. Pulling off the teat cups without first breaking the vacuum contributes to everted teat ends, which provide better avenues for infection.

Milking is by far the most important of all the work done on the dairy farm. As such, it requires attention to detail and the best of well-maintained equipment. After all, it is the only procedure that actually produces the milk that supports the entire operation. Yet it is surprising how many dairymen really don't like to milk cows. They are the ones whose herds are more likely to have serious mastitis problems.

Handling "Slow" Milkers. Some cows congenitally or as a result of injury have unusually tight teat sphincters and as a result are "slow" or "hard" milkers. The condition can usually be corrected surgically, but hard milkers should be milked last so they don't impede progress in milking the rest of the herd. The use of teat dilators is a necessary evil in management of some cases of teat injury, but they should not be used routinely for hard-milking cows. Anything introduced into the teat end carries with it a risk of introducing infection, despite the most sanitary technique, including first wiping the teat end with 70 percent alcohol. Routine use of teat dilators sooner or later results in mastitis and so should be avoided.

Vaccines. Although considerable research is in progress, results thus far in attempts to find a vaccine capable of preventing mastitis have been mixed. The J5 bacterins are highly effective in reducing the severity of mastitis due to *E. coli. Staphylococcus* bacterins and toxoids are commercially available, but reported results from their use are inconsistent. Many different strains of *Staphylococcus* species, each antigenically a little different, are capable of producing mastitis. If the mastitis in your herd is due to a strain incorporated in these products, they may be helpful. If not, they will be useless.

In herds with severe problems due to *Staphylococcus* species, some relief may be obtained by using an autogenous bacterin prepared from organisms isolated from the herd. Recent research indicates that *Staphylococcus* bacterins are more effective when used concurrently with intramammary infusion of antibiotics. Your veterinarian can advise you in this regard.

Minimizing Problems

Methods have been suggested to minimize problems with mastitis. *S. agalactiae,* the most prevalent and insidious pathogen, can and should be eradicated from every dairy herd for economic reasons, if nothing else. But despite your best efforts, there will be occasional cases of mastitis in all species, and these will generally be acute in nature, recognizable by heat, swelling, and abnormal milk. If the problem is limited to the udder, these may usually be handled by infusion of antibiotics into the affected gland in the cow, doe, ewe, or mare via the teat canals. The mammary glands of the sow are anatomically quite different, and parenteral medication routes must be used.

Your veterinarian may ask you to infuse follow-up medication using commercial preparations he provides or prescribes. You may even feel confident in doing this without veterinary advice. In any case, strip out all the milk you can and then wipe the teat end carefully, using a cotton swab and 70 percent rubbing alcohol. If this precaution is not observed, when introducing the tube or syringe cannula, you may push bacteria into the teat, making the problem worse. Simply because the gland is already infected doesn't mean it can't be infected concurrently with other organisms. Many serious yeast and mold infections occur this way. Use reliable products from reputable manufacturers, and don't buy on the basis of price alone. When an expensive animal is at stake, a few cents on a drug is a poor place to economize. Your veterinarian can advise you what to use when the need arises.

Complications

Acute mastitis is often complicated by generalized, septicemic infection in all species. In addition to the clinical signs involving the udder, there will be high fever, lack of appetite, and often dehydration. The animal will appear dull and depressed. Milk flow may cease entirely, especially in the sow, and the onset is usually rather sudden. The first observed sign in the ewe may be an unusual rear leg gait because of udder soreness. Pulse and respiratory rate are usually high early in the disease, declining as the temperature falls prior to death. Acute septic mastitis is a serious disease, calling for prompt vigorous treatment to save the animal's life.

Although *E. coli* and *Staphylococcus aureus* are common causes of septicemic mastitis, it is not possible to determine the causative organism with any degree of accuracy on the basis of clinical signs alone. A number of organisms identifiable only by culture can cause similar signs. Although culture results are useful as a guide for management of similar future cases in the herd, treatment must be initiated on the basis of clinical signs and good judgment, without waiting for a laboratory report.

Withdrawal Time

Before leaving the subject of mastitis, a precaution for those selling milk should be mentioned. Antibiotics given via any route for any purpose will appear at some level in milk. Concentration will be much higher when the antibiotic is infused into the udder. Every antibiotic approved for use in lactating animals has a milk-withdrawal time on the label, and the time varies with the product. Withdrawal time is the interval that must elapse between last treatment and sale of the milk. Typically it will be 72 to 96 hours. A withdrawal time is also given for use of meat from a treated animal. Read the label and observe the withdrawal time. Residues of antibiotics in animal products may result in penalties for the producers. Worse, in the long run, repeated violation will result in even greater restriction of the drugs that may be used in food-producing animals.

To reduce the risk of accidentally putting milk from treated cows in the bulk tank, put a marker on them when treated. A crayon mark on the flank or udder or a tag on the ankle or tail is a help. Commercial cow-side tests to detect antibiotics in milk help determine when the milk is safe to use.

Meningoencephalitis, Thromboembolic

This disease, commonly called *TEME* for convenience, is an acute, infectious, highly fatal disease limited almost entirely to feedlot cattle. It occurs rarely in cattle at pasture or in dairy cattle. Generally fewer than 10 percent of the cattle in the group are affected, but mortality of 95 percent is common.

Onset is sudden with high fever, stiffness, and reluctance to move. This is followed rapidly by normal or subnormal temperature, staggering, prostration, coma, and death. Death usually occurs anywhere from 1 to 48 hours after clinical signs are first observed. The disease seems to be occurring with increased frequency in recent years.

The organism thought to be responsible is *Haemophilus somnus,* but little is known about its mode of transmission. The primary lesions produced are in the brain, but it produces extensive damage to blood vessels and causes thrombi in other organs as well. Diagnosis based on clinical signs can be confirmed by isolation of the organism from affected tissue.

Prevention

Because the mode of transmission is unclear, it is difficult to make definitive recommendations for prevention. Vaccinating with *H. somnus* bacterin, decreasing concentrate intake, and increasing roughage may help. The disease affects cattle near the end of the finishing period in the 800- to 1000-pound range, raising the possibility of minimizing losses by marketing cattle early when an outbreak occurs. Early treatment with antibiotics is effective, with *early* being the operative word. Just a few hours can make the difference between survival and death. In the event of an outbreak, addition of tetracycline or chlortetracycline to the feed or water may reduce the number of new cases.

Navel Ill

The common name given to this septicemic infection of the newborn of all species implies that the route of infection is always via the navel. This is not necessarily so. Infection can also occur by ingestion of bacteria with subsequent invasion through the digestive tract. The navel is frequently the site of infection and invasion by a variety of bacteria that produce a septicemia that is especially serious and common in animals that have not received colostrum.

Symptoms

Depending on the organism and the animal species involved, a variety of symptoms can result, but the disease is perhaps most dramatic in the foal. Lethargy and diminished strength are frequent symptoms. If the organism invades the central nervous system, convulsions may be seen and death may occur in as few as 12 hours. In animals that live longer, arthritis, pneumonia, peritonitis, and diarrhea may be seen. A specific bacterium encountered in navel ill of foals, *Actinobacillus equuli,* is responsible for the condition known as *sleepy foal disease.* It commonly causes kidney disease and uremia.

Arthritis is a common sequel to navel infection in calves, pigs, lambs, and kids, but other clinical signs vary according to the organs affected by the particular invading organism. Umbilical abscess is a frequent complication in calves. Because umbilical hernia is also common in this species, don't attempt to open an umbilical abscess yourself unless you are certain of the diagnosis and know what you are doing. I had a client one time who did just that and found himself with a handful of intestines.

The variety of possible symptoms makes the diagnosis, especially of the causative organism, difficult at times. Where the disease is occurring as a

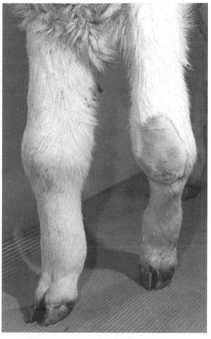

Suppurative arthritis is a common sequel infection.

herd problem, isolation of the organism from infected tissues and an antibiotic sensitivity test are helpful guides for treatment of future cases.

Treatment

A variety of antibiotics have been used successfully to treat early cases of navel ill. Treatment of long-standing cases is much less productive. Choice of antibiotic depends on the organism involved, but a broad-spectrum antibiotic such as oxytetracycline is a good starting point. Other symptomatic treatment is helpful. For example, if diarrhea is present, electrolytes administered intravenously and orally are indicated. Where the value of the animal warrants, blood transfusion is extremely effective.

Prevention

Because navel ill is both common and serious, measures to prevent it are most important. First, be sure that the area where the animal is to be born is clean and as sanitary as possible. Then *dip* the navel in tincture of iodine as soon as the umbilical cord separates; simply swabbing iodine on the navel is not sufficient. The best approach is to fill a widemouthed jar halfway with tincture of iodine, hold the jar firmly against the body wall with the stump of the navel in it, and slosh it around. This method ensures adequate penetration of the iodine solution, which kills all bacteria present. The alcohol in the tincture of iodine also has an astringent effect that helps to seal the umbilical blood vessels. Next, be sure the animal gets a meal of colostrum within the first hour after birth. If it won't or can't nurse, bottle-feed colostrum. Strict adherence to these suggestions will make navel ill a rare occurrence.

Ophthalmia, Periodic

This eye disease of horses and mules was much more prevalent at one time than it is now. The common name, *moon blindness,* was given to it many years ago because of its characteristic of recurrent acute attacks, which some people believed coincided with the phases of the moon. Periodic recurrences are typical, each causing additional damage, eventually resulting in total blindness, but the moon has nothing to do with it.

Symptoms

Onset of the disease is sudden, with profuse lacrimation and the eyelids held closed to protect the eyes from light. Slight swelling of the orbital area due to conjunctivitis is common. Typically, only one eye is affected at a time, but both can be involved. Some degree of corneal opacity may be present, and contraction of the pupil is a rather consistent finding. Toward the end of an acute attack, a yellowish exudate can often be seen at the bottom of the anterior chamber. The acute attack generally subsides in a few days, only to recur at intervals ranging from a few weeks to a year. Tags of fibrin and exudate, which can be detected between acute attacks with the aid of an ophthalmoscope, remain in the aqueous and vitreous humor of the eyeball. Examination for soundness of a horse should always include a careful ophthalmoscopic examination, but one should be aware that clinical signs may not appear until some months after infection.

Prevention

The cause of periodic ophthalmia is still debatable. It has been produced experimentally by infecting horses with *Leptospira interrogans* v. *pomona,* and vaccination with *L. pomona* bacterin may be a helpful preventative. But the disease is encountered more frequently in horses when the diet is marginal and the standard of husbandry poor. Supplementing the diet with riboflavin also gives a good degree of protection. Some researchers feel the disease is not a specific infection but a localized allergic reaction to another infection or toxemia.

Regardless of the cause, the disease has serious implications for the future eyesight of the horse and requires prompt veterinary attention. Antibiotics and corticosteroids relieve the acute signs, minimizing damage to the eye at the time of attack. Your veterinarian can suggest ways to reduce the possibility of future attacks.

Paratuberculosis

This chronic disease of cattle, sheep, and goats caused by *Mycobacterium paratuberculosis* is endemic on some farms, where its principal effect is unthriftiness and decreased production. The organism is related to *M. bovis,* and infection with either may give a positive intradermal test reaction. The common name of the infection is *Johne's disease,* and it is seen more frequently in cattle than in other species.

The incubation period is extremely long, with most cattle probably becoming infected as calves but not showing clinical signs until 2 years of age or older. Persistent diarrhea that occasionally subsides and then recurs, coupled with weight loss and decreased milk production, is the only clinical sign. Generally, there is no fever and appetite remains normal. Symptomatically, Johne's disease resembles Crohn's disease, a serious ulcerative bowel disease in humans. As yet, no direct link has been established between the two, but it is a cause for concern.

Diagnosis

Diagnosis and control of paratuberculosis are difficult because not only are the clinical signs minimal but also many infected animals show no clinical signs, yet they shed the organism in manure and thus are a hazard to others. The *intradermal test,* an allergy test utilizing avian tuberculin or *johnin,* a specific diagnostic agent, is often inconclusive. It is most reliably used on animals prior to development of clinical signs, but animals late in the disease may give a negative result. The *complement fixation test,* utilizing blood serum, is useful later in the disease. The ELISA test has proved more sensitive and is commercially available. Fecal culture, which may take a month or more, is good evidence of infection if culture results are positive, but the organism is both slow and difficult to grow, so a single negative culture may be meaningless.

Finding typical lesions at necropsy along with microscopic examination of tissues from the colon and adjacent lymph nodes is the most reliable. *M. paratuberculosis* localizes in the lower digestive tract, causing a thickening and corrugated appearance of the intestinal wall — particularly the lower small intestine, cecum, and colon. This thickening interferes with absorption of nutrients and especially fluids, so loose manure is common.

Control

If these tests and examinations are positive, the existence of the infection in the herd is confirmed, and it can be concluded that other animals are infected that may or may not show clinical signs later. Control of the disease is difficult at best. There is some indication that animals on a diet deficient in calcium will show clinical signs of infection more often, but this has not yet been proved. The organism is shed in manure and can survive under favorable temperature and moisture conditions for a year or more. It is resistant to many disinfectants, but doesn't survive long in direct sunlight.

Infection occurs when the animal eats feed or drinks water contaminated with manure containing the organism. Providing feed and water free of contamination is an essential part of control. This is relatively easy, of course, by using feed bunks and water troughs, but that doesn't solve the problem of pasture contamination. Nevertheless, sanitation is important. The risk of infection from contaminated pasture can be reduced by limiting the number of animals per acre, taking advantage of the dilution factor, and pasture rotation, provided the pasture at rest is clipped and manure is scattered with a drag to provide maximum exposure to sunlight. But these measures, though they will reduce the rate of new infections, will not entirely prevent the disease from spreading.

Separating calves from their dams at birth and raising them away from adult cattle, coupled with rigorous culling of mature cattle, are important components of a control program.

Utilizing the ELISA test and fecal culture, several states offer voluntary Johne's disease certification programs to assist farmers and ranchers who want to establish infection-free herds. Several types of vaccines have been used successfully in sheep and cattle in Europe, but they are not approved for use here except in a few states by permit. Vaccination interferes with the test for tuberculosis, which is considered a more important disease because of its economic and public health significance. Because of the economic loss it causes, the possibility of human infection, and the need to protect our livestock export market, it is probable that, in the near future, a national Johne's disease control program will be implemented. That program, if and when it comes about, will need and deserve the wholehearted support of livestock owners.

Pneumonia

Although the symptoms are rather clear-cut, pneumonia is a highly complex disease, with several different predisposing or contributing factors. Because of its complexity, pneumonia is often described by various terms. For example, pathologists will speak of *bronchopneumonia,* in which the infection involves primarily the bronchi and bronchioles and the alveolar tissue, or pneumonia may be described as *interstitial,* in which the lung connective tissue is the primary site of infection. We also speak of *inhalation pneumonia,* which results from inhalation of liquids, usually because of improperly administered medications, or *verminous pneumonia,* in which the underlying cause is parasites, particularly lungworms.

Several viruses can cause pneumonia, particularly in swine and calves. The myxovirus, parainfluenza-3, SF_4, or bovine respiratory syncytial virus, working in concert with *P. multocida* or *P. haemolytica,* causes a very serious form of pneumonia in cattle and sometimes in sheep. *Rhodococcus (Corynebacterium) equi*, which produces serious generalized disease in foals on some farms, commonly causes pneumonia as one of its principal signs. A very serious disease when pigs are brought together in large numbers, formerly called virus pig pneumonia, now is known to be due primarily to *Mycoplasma hyopneumoniae*. This disease and shipping fever, or pasteurellosis, in cattle are highly contagious and devastating when they appear in a herd. Regardless of the cause, the most serious effects of pneumonia are generally caused by bacteria, either as primary or as secondary invaders.

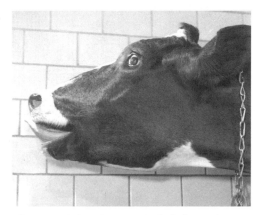

Onset

Management plays an important role in the onset of pneumonia. Most of the organisms that cause the disease can be found in apparently normal and healthy animals. Only under adverse conditions when the animals' resistance is lowered does the disease

Open-mouth breathing is typical of advanced severe pneumonia. Note the sunken eye, indicating prolonged illness and dehydration.

appear. Unsanitary conditions, overcrowding, poor ventilation, drafts, and other stress are known to be predisposing factors. Pneumonia can occur in all species but is most commonly seen in cattle and pigs, perhaps because these are the species most likely to be kept under crowded circumstances.

Symptoms

The clinical signs of pneumonia are generally not difficult to recognize. There is fever, coughing that is more pronounced on exertion, and labored breathing to varying degrees. Usually the respiratory rate will be fast, but the depth of respiration may be shallow, probably because of pain. In most cases of pneumonia, there is some inflammatory involvement of the pleura, the membrane lining of the chest cavity and covering the lungs, which causes considerable discomfort when the chest is expanded during inspiration.

Pneumonia is an inflammation of the lungs, and with the inflammation there is an accumulation of mucus and debris in the smaller air passages as well as some swelling of the lung tissue itself. This results in an interference with airflow and absorption of oxygen, which is necessary to convert carboxyhemoglobin in red blood cells back to hemoglobin.

When the inflammation is severe, oxygen deficiency results in varying degrees of cyanosis, with labored breathing to the point where the head and neck are outstretched and the tongue is protruding. Needless to say, this is a very grave sign, and points out the need for early effective treatment. In human medicine, administration of oxygen helps alleviate the condition. But oxygen is difficult to administer to animals because of the restraint problem. The exudate in the lungs, when air passes through or around it, will give rather typical abnormal lung sounds if one listens over the chest cavity with a stethoscope. If a portion of the lung becomes so congested that no air passes through, no sounds will be heard, which is just as significant if not more so than the abnormal sound.

Pneumonia of Pigs

A contagious pneumonia of pigs, sometimes called *enzootic pneumonia,* more commonly called *Mycoplasma pneumonia* and formerly called *virus pig pneumonia,* is probably the most important disease encountered in the swine industry from an economic standpoint. It is caused by *M. hyopneumoniae,* which, while not classified as a bacterium, causes a chronic disease that is made much more acute in the presence of a secondary bacterial invasion. The severity of the lung lesions that it causes is also increased in the presence of migrating ascarid larvae or lungworms.

The disease is more prevalent in swine herds, where replacements are frequently added from random sources. It differs from the usual concept of pneumonia in that typically it does not produce a serious febrile reaction, nor do the pigs go off feed. But it does cause lung lesions and a chronic cough, a combination that leads to decreased rate of gain and therefore increased cost of pork production. It is widespread, and its principal effect is economic. When complicated by secondary bacterial infection, the clinical signs more nearly approximate those of the types of pneumonia we have discussed thus far.

The disease is more prevalent and more persistent in younger swine beginning at about age 3 weeks and older. Unlike bacterial pneumonia, mycoplasma pneumonia will appear at any time of the year, with no increased prevalence noted during fall and winter. The organism persists for months in infected pigs, and transmission to susceptible pigs is by direct contact or aerosol inhalation.

Mortality Low. Generally, a high percentage of the younger pigs in the herd will be infected, but if the disease is not complicated by other factors, mortality will be rather low. Coughing aggravated by exercise and unthriftiness are the principal and often the only clinical signs. But diagnosis can be confirmed by serological tests or postmortem by typical lesions found in the lungs. By special cultural techniques in the laboratory, the organism can be isolated from infected pigs, which confirms the diagnosis.

Attempts to control the disease and treatment have generally been unsuccessful. Antibiotics and sulfa drugs are ineffective against *M. hyopneumoniae,* but they do have value in controlling secondary bacterial infection that may occur, thereby reducing pig mortality. Control of ascarids and lungworms through the use of good sanitary practice and anthelmintics when indicated also helps to reduce losses from mycoplasma pneumonia.

Methods of Control. Control of the disease in some herds has been accomplished by rather radical changes in swine herd management. Where the infection rate is severe, perhaps the best solution is depopulation of the entire herd and replacement of breeding stock with pigs purchased directly from specific pathogen-free (SPF) herds. Once this step is taken, however, to maintain an infection-free herd one must buy all subsequent herd replacements from herds of equal or better disease-free status. This may limit the options and choice of breeding stock and usually increases the cost of those replaced. The improved performance of the pigs in the herd, however, may well justify the added cost.

A second, moderately successful, method used where physical facilities permit is to attempt to provide a degree of isolation within the herd between infected and noninfected pigs. With this method, sows are farrowed in isolation to help ensure that there is no cross-infection between litters. The litters are then observed for clinical signs of infection, and those that appear to be free of infection, at least on observation or even necropsy of one of the piglets, can be grouped together and segregated from all other pigs on the farm. If the infected and noninfected groups can be kept separate, the infected group can be gradually eliminated, leaving only the noninfected breeding stock. While both of these methods present obvious problems, the economic effect of this disease is so great that any control attempt is worthwhile. *M. hyopneumoniae* apparently stimulates some immunity, as older swine are less frequently found to be infected than the younger groups.

Mycoplasma bacterins are available that will mitigate the symptoms somewhat when used in conjunction with improvements in ventilation. Because the disease is chronic and the carrier state exists, however, the most effective management technique remains the "all-in/all-out" system

With the exception of contagious pasteurellosis in cattle and mycoplasma pneumonia in swine, most cases of pneumonia in livestock, as in people, are isolated and sporadic. Each must be managed on the basis of clinical signs observed and then be treated accordingly.

Pododermatitis

Pododermatitis, commonly called *foot rot,* is a disease of cattle, sheep, and, to a lesser extent, goats. In cattle, the disease is caused by a soilborne organism, *Fusobacterium necrophorum,* that gains entry via minute cracks or abrasions. In sheep, *F. necrophorum,* working in concert with another pathogen, *Dichelobacter (Fusiformis) nodosus,* appears to be responsible. The latter organism seems capable of penetrating unbroken skin, causing severe foot lesions that may affect entire flocks, particularly during warm, wet weather. Foot rot in cattle is more sporadic, rarely affecting more than 10 percent of the herd at one time.

The first clinical sign noted is generally lameness, which gets progressively worse. In cattle, usually only one foot at a time is affected, whereas in sheep infection of all four feet is not uncommon. In cattle, the infection commonly starts at the bulb of the heel and extends up to the fetlock and into the interdigital space, causing swelling and tissue necrosis. This dead and dying tissue has a characteristic odor that gave the disease its early name *fouls*. As the disease progresses and swelling extends, cracks open that permit infection with a variety of secondary invaders. Left untreated, the infection may extend into the coffin joint, causing permanent lameness. The lameness and acute pain, of course, lead to rapid weight loss and, in the dairy cow, decline in milk production. Foot rot is a troublesome and costly disease on some farms, and any effort expended to control it is well worthwhile.

Although foot rot is common, relatively little research has been done on it. As a result, there is confusion in terminology and even etiology. It may involve the sole, the heel, the interdigital space, or the skin on the posterior aspect of the pastern, and be named according to the anatomical site of the initial lesion. *Thrush,* which involves the frog of the horse's hoof, is a form of foot rot attributable to poor foot hygiene.

The organisms causing foot rot thrive in a warm, moist, anaerobic environment. Underrun soles and cracks in the feet provide an ideal environment for them. A good foot rot control program, therefore, includes regular periodic examination and trimming of the feet.

Regardless of the name or the multiple etiology, the measures outlined here will do much to control the disease.

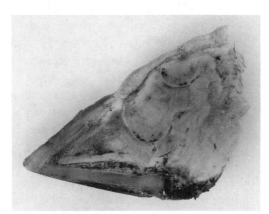

This sagittal section through one claw of the bovine foot shows infection extending into the coffin joint, which causes severe lameness.

Early Treatment

As with all diseases, treatment is most effective if started early. The first essential step is to examine the foot and carefully pare away all dead and underrun sole tissue. Foot rot is not the only cause of foot swelling and lameness. On more than one occasion I have seen cases that didn't respond to intramuscular injection of antibiotics because there was a nail in the foot or a stone lodged between the claws. *Always* examine the foot. When only a few animals are

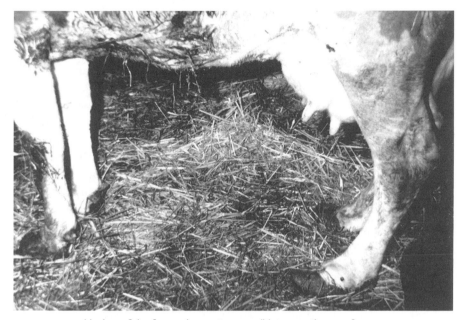

Neglect of the feet and unsanitary conditions contribute to foot rot.

involved, it's practical and advantageous to treat the infection locally and to bandage the foot. This is more comfortable for the animal and promotes more rapid healing. Rubber boots are available to provide extra protection to the foot.

Once the infected area has been debrided and cleaned, several different medications can be used. Among these are 20 percent icthammol ointment, copper naphthenate solution, 5 percent formalin solution, and sulfanilamide powder to which has been added copper sulfate powder at the rate of 5 percent. Any of these will be beneficial when coupled with parenteral administration of penicillin or one of the approved sulfonamides. Some other antibiotics and sulfa drugs work equally well; the choice is largely one of preference and economics and, in the case of food-producing animals, legality. Aside from helping the animal, bandaging the foot has value as a control procedure. An open, discharging foot rot lesion sheds millions of organisms onto the ground to serve as a source of new infections. For this reason, infected animals should be segregated from the rest of the herd or flock. Occasionally infection will actually invade the joint of one or both claws. This is a severe sequel that doesn't respond well to medical therapy. However, when one claw is involved, it can be amputated surgically by your veterinarian. The results are usually good and the cow can complete her lactation. The alternative is culling, which is a substantial loss, especially when antibiotic residues from prior treatment are present.

Footbath

When too many animals are involved to make bandaging practical, and as a general control procedure, a foot bath of 5 percent copper sulfate through which the animals must walk at least daily is helpful. The trough containing the solution should be about 4 inches deep and wide enough that the animals can't jump over it. In freezing weather or when solutions are objectionable, the same thing can be accomplished with a shallow box filled with a mixture of 5 pounds of copper sulfate powder to 100 pounds of hydrated lime. This, of course, must be placed in an area protected from rain or snow. The use of ethylenediaminetetraiodide (EDDI) as a feed additive or in salt blocks has been recommended as a control procedure, but results have been inconsistent.

F. necrophorum can survive in the soil for long periods, so once infection appears in a cattle herd, new cases will appear sporadically thereafter. Rotating pastures and reducing the concentration of cattle in the pasture lessens the rate of ground contamination, but won't prevent it entirely. Prevalence is greatly reduced when cattle are kept in a paved drylot that is regularly cleaned.

Pododermatitis in Sheep

F. nodosus, a component of the disease in sheep, is an obligate parasite that probably doesn't survive outside the sheep for more than a week. This makes it possible to eradicate the disease, and many flock owners have done so. Eradication involves some effort but is worth doing. It requires examination of the feet of each individual sheep and separation of infected and noninfected animals. The noninfected sheep are then given a dose of antibiotic, usually penicillin, and put into a pasture that has not held any sheep for at least 2 weeks. It also helps to walk them through a footbath as described above as they enter the clean pasture. As individuals in the infected group recover, they are given additional antibiotic and added to the clean flock in the same manner. The clean flock should be carefully observed every day for a week or two for any sign of lameness. Lame sheep should immediately be put back with the

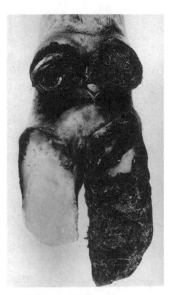

The sole of the left claw of this neglected foot has been trimmed for comparison.

infected flock. Once the entire flock is free of infection, special measures must be taken to keep it that way.

If possible, replacement sheep should be purchased directly from flocks known to be free of infection. Where the history is unknown, they, and your own animals returning from a show, should be considered infected, treated with antibiotics on arrival, and kept separate from the main flock for 2 weeks. At the end of that time, if no problems develop, they can join the clean group.

A word of caution should be added. Don't forget that you can carry *F. nodosus* on your shoes or boots from the infected to the clean flocks. As long as any vestige of infection remains, *always* disinfect your boots when moving from one flock to the other.

A vaccine for prevention of foot rot in sheep appears to be a useful aid, but does not supplant the need for the control measures outlined above.

Polyserositis

It has been estimated that about 2 percent of the swine in the United States suffer some degree of polyserositis manifested primarily as an arthritis. At least two distinct organisms, *Haemophilus parasuis* and *Mycoplasma hyorhinis*, are capable of producing the disease. Both are common inhabitants of the upper respiratory tract, where they normally do little harm. But under conditions of stress, they may produce generalized infection with localization in the joints.

Polyserositis in weanling pigs due to *H. parasuis* tends to be more acute, with fever ranging to 107°F, a high percentage of the herd infected, and death losses up to 10 percent or more. Hot, swollen, painful joints are a common part of the syndrome regardless of the cause. Infection caused by *M. hyorhinis* tends to be less acute, with an incubation period of 4 to 5 days and recovery in about a month.

Mycoplasma hyosynoviae has also been shown to be capable of producing arthritis in older pigs. It is difficult, if not impossible, however, to determine the causative organism on the basis of clinical signs alone. Isolation of the organism from joint fluid is the only sure way, although serologic testing may also be helpful.

A retrospective diagnosis can sometimes be made based on response to therapy. Infection caused by *H. parasuis* responds fairly well to treatment with a variety of sulfonamides and antibiotics. Infection due to *Mycoplasma* species, on the other hand, responds better to tylosin, lincomycin, or erythromycin.

Polyserositis is a complex disease with no specific control measures available. Older swine act as unaffected carriers and are a constant source of infection. Any degree of isolation between age groups that can be achieved will be helpful, as will avoiding stress situations such as rough handling, shipping, and abrupt changes in diet. Where the problem is severe, depopulation and establishment of a specific pathogen-free herd may be the best answer. This is obviously expensive, but the economic loss from reduced weight gain of infected pigs in severely infected herds is equally costly.

Pyelonephritis

This is a serious but fortunately sporadic infection of the urinary tract, most commonly encountered in mature cattle and more often in cows than bulls. The causative organism, *Corynebacterium renale,* can also infect horses and sheep, but such infections are rare.

Pyelonephritis is generally referred to as an ascending urinary tract infection — that is, infection enters the tract via the urethra and proceeds upward to the bladder, then via the ureters to the kidneys. The probable source of infection is vulvar contact with contaminated bedding, or tail switching and spreading contaminated urine droplets from one cow to another. The use of unsterilized urinary catheters is an excellent way to spread the infection. The disease is seen most often in cows during advanced pregnancy or under the stress of inclement weather.

The organism thrives in urine and causes inflammation of the walls of the urethra, bladder, and ureter. In the kidney it causes destruction of functional tissue and small abscesses, eventually destroying so much kidney tissue that the animal dies from uremia. This occurs over a period of weeks or months.

Symptoms

The typical history is a gradual loss of appetite and weight with no fever. The animal may have intermittent periods of colicky abdominal pain due to restricted urine flow, evidenced by kicking at the belly, frequent urination, and straining. The urine usually has flakes of pus and clots of blood in it, which makes the diagnosis at that point relatively easy. The entire urinary tract and kidneys will be greatly enlarged, and detection of this enlargement by rectal palpation helps to confirm the diagnosis. The organism is quite easy to culture from urine samples.

Other than good sanitary practices and isolating infected cows, there are no specific preventive measures to be taken.

Treatment

If the damage already done is not too great, the infection responds well to treatment with penicillin. Relapses following apparent recovery are common, however, so overall the prognosis is guarded. It's well known that once infection appears in a herd, occasional additional cases are likely to occur. For that reason, it seems prudent to remove the first case from the herd as soon as possible in hopes of preventing further cases from occurring.

Pyelonephritis in Pigs

A closely related organism, *Actinomyces (Corynebacterium) suis,* causes pyelonephritis and cystitis in sows. The disease in pigs is a bit different in that clinical signs are not so pronounced. Apparent sudden death may be the only clinical sign — if that can be called a sign. Necropsy of infected sows will show an enlarged thickened bladder and ureter containing pus and blood. There is another difference in the swine disease, too. It occurs most commonly 3 to 4 weeks after breeding, leading to the possibility that it is a venereally transmitted disease in pigs.

Because there is a strong possibility of venereal transmission, boars that have been used on sows that developed pyelonephritis should not be used again until cultures of preputial swabs and semen are negative for *A. suis*. Fortunately, the disease is not common in pigs or cattle and is of relatively little economic significance except in the few herds where it is endemic.

Pyoderma

This is a nonspecific and noncontagious disease occasionally seen in all species but most commonly in the horse as a sequel to saddle sores. By definition, the name means "pus in the skin," and it is usually due to one or more species of *Staphylococcus*. The infection starts initially in the hair follicles to cause swelling and extreme sensitivity. It may remain superficial or go into the deeper layers of skin to cause abscessation and fistulous tracts. Involvement to this degree may cause fever and other signs, such as lack of appetite, depression, and enlargement of regional lymph nodes.

Treatment

The superficial infection responds well to local treatment with antiseptics. Scabs and crusts should first be softened with wet packs or ointments and gently removed before applying the antiseptic. Deeper infection with fistulous tracts underlying the skin is much more difficult to treat, and surgical drainage may be required in addition to local and systemic treatment.

Cleanliness and frequent careful grooming will do much to prevent this condition from occurring.

Rhinitis, Atrophic

This chronic debilitating disease of swine causes considerable economic loss on some farms each year. The most obvious change when it occurs is lateral deviation or shortening of the snout due to atrophy of the nasal turbinate bones. This does not occur in all infected pigs, however, and its incidence seems to depend on the age at which infection occurs. The younger the pig when first infected, the more likely the characteristic "twisted" snout is to occur. Older pigs may show little, if any, change following infection.

The disease has been recognized since the early 1800s in Europe and since the early 1940s in the United States. As might be expected, over the years many agents, ranging from bacteria, viruses, and protozoa to nutritional deficiencies, have been suggested as the cause. The gross pathological changes in the nasal turbinates can be produced experimentally by feeding diets deficient in calcium and phosphorus, or an imbalance of the two. More recent evidence indicates that a specific organism, *Bordetella bronchiseptica,* is the primary cause. Concurrent infection with *B. bronchiseptica* and toxigenic *P. multocida* results in a more serious form of the disease. Nevertheless, elimination of *B. bronchiseptica* carriers from the herd effectively prevents occurrence of atrophic rhinitis. Overcrowding and inadequate ventilation contribute to the spread of the disease, which often appears following introduction of new animals to the herd.

Diagnosis

The earliest sign in young pigs is excessive sneezing and snuffling, occasionally with discharge of mucopurulent material from the nose and eyes. In some severe cases, mild to profuse nosebleed occurs. Temperatures are usually normal, and the pigs continue to eat. This is not sufficient evidence on which to base a diagnosis, however; many other conditions produce similar signs. On most farms, the majority recover from these mild symptoms, although some become carriers. Especially if concurrent infection with organisms such as *P. multocida* is present, some of those infected pigs go on to develop the turbinate atrophy and snout deviation typical of the disease. Once it occurs, this deviation is irreversible and may result in reduced rate of gain and, hence, economic loss. The disease usually is not fatal but may be complicated by secondary pneumonia.

In the absence of obvious snout deviation, a positive clinical diagnosis cannot be made. Often, however, even though no external signs can be seen, turbinate changes can be detected when the snout is sectioned with a band saw at necropsy. This doesn't do much for the pig being examined, but it can establish the presence of the infection in the herd. A more useful technique is laboratory culture of nasal swabs taken from representative pigs in the herd. Your veterinarian can provide this service for you to determine the presence of *B. bronchiseptica.*

Treatment

Treatment of the infection is possible on some farms using sulfamethazine in the feed or sulfathiazole in the drinking water for several weeks. It is not always successful because some strains of the organism are resistant. Treatment of the young animals is less satisfactory than treatment of older stock. Because treatment results vary, several other means have been developed to control the prevalence of astrophic rhinitis. Because spread is primarily via aerosol transmission from one generation to the next and turbinate atrophy is more likely to occur when infection occurs early in life, a good degree of control can be obtained by removing piglets from the sow as soon as they have nursed colostrum. They are then kept separate from other mature swine and reared by hand. A modification of this is to confine the sow in such a manner that piglets are kept away from her head and have access only to her udder at feeding time. A third method is the same as that used to establish a specific pathogen-free herd. This is to take the piglets by caesarean section or by collecting them in clean plastic bags as they are born and then rearing them in isolation from all other swine. All of these methods present obvious management problems.

Identifying Carriers

The advent of a reliable, economical culture technique makes it possible to identify carrier animals, so the herd can be divided into clean and infected groups. The infected group can then be treated or sold for slaughter as circumstances indicate. They must be kept separate, however, and the clean group should have two additional cultures taken to be sure that, in fact, no infected animals are part of it. It should also be protected from access by dogs, cats, and rodents because these species may carry *B. bronchiseptica.*

All of these techniques as well as periodic herd depopulation have been successfully employed to control atrophic rhinitis. But the most promising technique may prove to be the routine use of intranasal *B. bronchiseptica* bacterin and/or *P. multocida* bacterin/toxoid in sows and gilts prior to farrowing.

Salmonellosis

This disease, affecting all species including humans, is caused by species of the genus *Salmonella* and is sometimes called *paratyphoid.* Several hundred species and subspecies are widely distributed in nature, but fortunately only a few are highly pathogenic. *Salmonella typhimurium* and *Salmonella dublin* commonly affect livestock. *Salmonella abortus equi* was once commonly incriminated as a cause of abortion in horses but seems to have virtually disappeared from the United States. *Salmonella cholerasuis* is limited primarily to pigs.

Diagnosis

Positive diagnosis of salmonellosis in the living animal is difficult because of varying clinical signs and resemblance to many other diseases. A positive fecal culture, coupled with history and clinical signs, is helpful, but recovery of the organism is sometimes difficult, and several samples taken at different times may be necessary for a positive result. Infected but asymptomatic animals shed the organism intermittently, so by itself a positive fecal culture may not mean much. Recovery of the organism from tissues at necropsy is more diagnostic.

Prevention of the infection also presents some problems and depends primarily on scrupulous sanitation. Commercially prepared salmonella bacterins may help if they contain antigen for the particular species causing the trouble. Autogenous bacterins prepared from isolates from the farm would be more helpful, but sanitation is still the most important component.

Salmonellosis is likely to be more of a problem in intensive rearing operations common to the veal and pork industries. For these, the "all-in/all-out" method allows time for adequate cleaning and disinfection of the barn before the next group of animals is brought in. Avoiding rodent contamination of feedstuffs, removing leftover feed, and thorough cleaning of feed utensils following each use are all important parts of a control program. Continuous low-level feeding of antibiotics may help to keep the *Salmonella* species population in check, but that procedure, too, is not looked on favorably by the FDA because of the risk of inducing antibiotic-resistant strains of the organism. Producers of meat products, especially beef, veal, and poultry, need to be cognizant of the effect of *Salmonella* species contamination of their products. Outbreaks of human salmonellosis due to food contamination are not unusual, but they draw widespread adverse publicity. This in turn causes great economic loss to the producer and processor. Reduction of *Salmonella* species contamination begins at the farm.

Forms

Three distinct forms of salmonellosis are recognized: peracute, acute, and chronic. The peracute form occurs primarily in young animals, especially those such as calves and pigs maintained under concentrated husbandry methods. It is a septicemic (that is, generalized), rapidly fatal disease that in calves is indistinguishable from the septicemic forms of colibacillosis, although it is inclined to occur sometimes in calves a week or so older. It causes high fever, dullness, depression and death in 24 to 48 hours. Foals, piglets, and lambs show similar signs. The peracute form generally occurs in animals under 4 months of age. Calves infected with *S. dublin* may also develop staggering and incoordination. In piglets where the infection is due to *S. cholerasuis,* a red to purple discoloration of the skin of the ears and abdomen occurs, along with weakness, paralysis, and convulsions prior to death.

In adult animals and humans, salmonellosis usually takes the form of an acute enteritis, or intestinal disorder. Onset is sudden with fever, abdominal cramps, and watery diarrhea. As the disease progresses, the fever disappears but blood clots may appear in the feces. The diarrhea is accompanied by straining, and often mucus and mucous casts of the intestinal lining may appear. To the inexperienced, these mucous casts may look like the intestinal lining itself. Lack of appetite is usually complete, and affected animals dehydrate rapidly and show extreme thirst. Horses will show violent colicky symptoms, and pigs, in addition to the above, may show signs of central nervous system disturbance. Abortion is a common sequel in all species.

S. dublin is reported to cause abortion in cows and ewes without any other clinical signs. The acute form of the disease in the majority of animals terminates fatally in 2 to 5 days. Those that survive are debilitated for long periods of time. In horses, onset of acute enteric salmonellosis often follows the stress of transportation.

Chronic Salmonellosis

In pigs and sometimes in cattle following the initial acute attack, the disease will become chronic with persistent diarrhea, emaciation, and occasional episodes of fever and blood clots in the feces. Chronically infected animals should be culled from the herd.

Salmonella is ubiquitous, and many animals become infected without showing signs of disease. Development of clinical signs is dependent on the size of the infecting dose, pathogenicity of the particular organism, and resistance of the animal. The organism colonizes in the bile ducts and gallbladder and is intermittently shed in feces. Recovered and subclinically infected animals remain carriers, and fecal contamination from them is the primary source of infection. Under favorable conditions of moisture and temperature, the organism can survive for long periods of time outside the body.

Rats and mice are common carriers of *S. typhimurium,* and contamination of feedstuffs by them is a common source of herd outbreaks. Salmonellae multiply rapidly in liquid or moist feeds. Milk replacer and pig feed in slurry form, if mixed in batches and allowed to stand at room temperature, will rapidly become a thriving salmonella culture if the organism is present. For the same reason, to prevent human infections, it's important to keep cold foods, especially those containing poultry products, refrigerated until served.

Treatment

Treatment of salmonellosis in food-producing animals sometimes presents a dilemma. The organism develops antibiotic resistance quite rapidly, and a limited number of antibiotics are effective against it. Ampicillin, oxytetracycline, and ceftiofur are among the drugs used to treat the septicemic form of the disease. Supportive therapy such as intravenous fluids and corticosteroids to combat shock is often indicated. In view of these and other complications, including the difficulty of making a positive diagnosis, treatment of this disease is best left to your veterinarian.

Strangles

Prior to the advent of antibiotics, and when horses were congregated in large numbers in stables, remount depots, and so on, this disease caused by *Streptococcus equi* was rampant. Its occurrence now is limited primarily to occasions when groups of horses are assembled for summer camps, rodeos, and shows. The disease is often referred to as *distemper* or sometimes *shipping fever,* the latter because it often occurs 3 to 4 days after a group of horses are brought together. It is possible that the stress of trucking predisposes to infection if an animal in the group is carrying the infection. Strangles bears no relationship to shipping fever in cattle, however, and does not cause pneumonia.

Disease Progression

Onset of the disease is sudden, with the first signs being lack of appetite and fever as high as 106°F. These are followed by a clear nasal discharge that soon becomes purulent. A mild conjunctivitis, or eye inflammation, sometimes occurs concurrently. The disease causes a severe pharyngitis, sufficiently painful that affected horses are reluctant to swallow and sometimes hold the neck outstretched to relieve the pain. Within a few days, abscesses develop in the lymph nodes of the throat region, and accumulation of pus in the guttural pouches is common. Many of these abscesses break and drain to the outside, yielding a thick creamy yellow pus from which pure cultures of S. equi can be obtained.

The disease affects younger animals primarily, but those over 5 years old who have had no prior exposure to it are also susceptible. In the individual it runs a course of about 2 weeks, but in a band of horses it may be several months from the time of the first case until the last one recovers. Mortality from strangles averages less than 2 percent, but once it appears, all horses in the group generally will be affected.

Occasionally abscesses will get large enough to interfere with breathing, and a tracheostomy will have to be done to save the animal's life. The possibility always exists, too, that a few organisms will be carried in the bloodstream to other organs, especially liver, kidney, and brain, to form abscesses in these locations as well. Such cases usually are fatal.

Purpura hemorrhagica, a disease thought to be due to circulating bacterial protein, is a not uncommon sequel to strangles, occurring about 2 weeks after the initial infection. Damage to the lining of blood vessels results in swelling, especially of the head and legs, with varying degrees of subcutaneous hemorrhage and anemia. This is a serious complication that is fatal about 50 percent of the time.

S. equi is a more resistant organism than the majority of streptococci and can survive, for example, in a contaminated stall for up to a month. The route of infection is primarily by inhalation or ingestion. Therefore, an infected animal should be isolated from all others and the stall where it was kept thoroughly cleaned and disinfected. Infected animals may continue to shed the organism for a month or more following apparent recovery.

Although the disease is not as prevalent as it once was, it still exists and every precaution should be taken to avoid it. By all means, if you are taking a horse to a show, take along your own feed and water utensils. The use of community feed troughs or water buckets is an ideal way to spread the infection. Try to keep your horse isolated from others at the show as much as reasonably possible. These measures may help to prevent other infections as well.

Treatment

Treatment of strangles is quite effective if started early in the course of the disease. The organism is sensitive to penicillin, tetracycline, and the sulfonamides, but relapses are common unless treatment is continued for 4 to 5 days after the initial signs disappear. Antibiotic therapy after abscesses have formed is much less valuable, and some people feel it actually prolongs the course of the disease. Surgical drainage of mature abscesses may hasten recovery, but if breathing becomes labored due to obstruction, tracheostomy may be required.

A bacterin from *S. equi* is available for immunization against strangles, but its use is not without complications. It is given in two or three doses 2 weeks apart, and a few horses after the second dose may develop an allergic reaction. Also, local irritation at the site of the injection is common enough to cause concern. An avirulent strain of *S. equi* used as an intranasal bacterin may prove to be more effective. Follow the advice of your veterinarian on whether to vaccinate, depending on local circumstances.

Tetanus

Humans, horses, and sheep are the most susceptible to tetanus, or *lockjaw*, as it is commonly called, but the disease occasionally occurs in cattle, goats, and pigs as well. The clinical signs are caused by a neurotoxin produced by *Clostridium tetani*. Tetanus is a wound infection disease most common with deep penetrating wounds, when tissue damage is extensive. The organism requires anaerobic conditions for growth and will not thrive in a surface laceration where the blood supply is good. The interval between infection and clinical signs may range from 4 days to several weeks, and it's not unusual for a puncture wound of the foot to be completely healed on the surface when symptoms of tetanus develop. The disease is usually individual and sporadic, although serious outbreaks have been reported following castration, shearing, and docking of pigs and lambs. The use of elastic bands for castration and docking is conducive to conditions favoring growth of *C. tetani*.

As infection proceeds, neurotoxin travels along nerve pathways, increasing irritability of the motor nerve end plates, so the effect is an overreaction to external stimuli. This may be seen first as muscle stiffness, particularly in the legs, muscles of the jaw, and around the wound itself. This progresses rapidly to a point where muscle rigidity increases. Difficulty in chewing or swallowing is responsible for the common name, lockjaw. One of the early diagnostic signs in the horse is a "flash" of the third eyelid in response to a loud noise or sudden movement. Temperature is usually normal at the outset, but the exertion of constant muscle contraction may cause sweating and temperature rise a few hours before death. Affected animals move with great difficulty if at all. Extensive rigidity of leg muscles may cause a "sawhorse" stance, and if the horse should happen to fall, fractures are a distinct possibility.

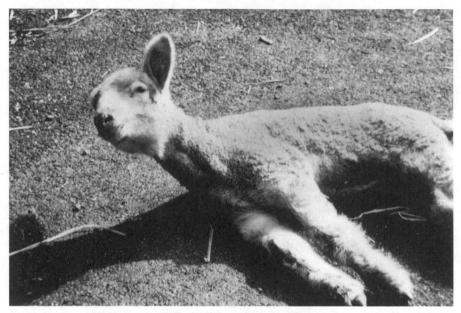

Severe muscle rigidity characterizes the latter stages of tetanus.

Prevention

Prevention of tetanus is far more rewarding than treatment. Mortality is high in horses and sheep, less so in other species. Treatment with massive doses of penicillin and antitoxin is helpful, but the excitement of treatment itself may stimulate a fatal spasm. Use of sedatives, tranquilizers, and anesthetics may be helpful. Good nursing care is essential.

Prevention is far more satisfactory. Proper sterilization of surgical instruments between animals when castrating or docking will help to prevent infection, as will careful cleaning and debridement of wounds. *C. tetani* spores are commonly found in soil and in the digestive tracts of animals, especially horses. It's safest to assume that any penetrating wound is contaminated, so give tetanus antitoxin along with the usual wound treatment. Horses can be permanently immunized with two doses of tetanus toxoid given a month apart, followed by an annual booster dose.

Tuberculosis

Through the ages, tuberculosis has been a major scourge of humans and animals, and in many parts of the world it still is. It is caused by members of the genus *Mycobacterium,* and several distinct strains — human, bovine, and avian — are recognized. Of these, the human type tends to be the most host specific, rarely being found in species other than humans, although occasionally dogs contract the infection from their owners. A classic example of this occurred in New York City many years ago. A child was found to have tuberculosis, but other members of the family were negative and the source of the infection was obscure. Epidemiologic investigation subsequently revealed a dog that was a neighborhood pet that customarily played with all the children living nearby. The dog was tested and found positive, and its owner was found to be infected as well. The infection apparently passed from owner to dog to child.

The bovine type is least host specific and infects not only cattle but also humans, swine, goats, horses, and sheep, in about that order of frequency. The avian type is commonly found in older birds and readily infects swine and, to a lesser extent, cattle and sheep. The human type readily infects cattle as well.

Tuberculosis is best described as a chronic wasting disease, typically without overt clinical signs early in the disease. Except with the avian type in birds and swine, the initial lesions usually develop in the lung and thoracic lymph nodes. The organism slowly develops tumorlike masses called *tubercles*. These may be few or numerous and may become quite large. The center of the tubercles degenerates into a caseous or cheesy mass that may undergo calcification in long-standing cases. Although the primary lesions are usually in the chest cavity, generalized or miliary tuberculosis does occur, and the organism can thrive anywhere in the body. Bovine tuberculosis in humans, for example, commonly locates in the spine to cause serious spinal deformities. One of the outstanding contributions of veterinary medicine to human health has been control of tuberculosis. The precipitate decline in the disease in humans during the last 60 years exactly parallels the rate of eradication in cattle.

The tubercle bacilli are shed in saliva, feces, and milk from infected cows. Infection may occur by inhalation or ingestion. Because of this, the disease is more likely to occur in stabled animals than in range cattle. Signs of the disease are variable depending on location. With lung involvement, a persistent cough and intermittent low-grade fever may be seen as the disease progresses. Gradual weight loss to the point of emaciation is the usual sequel, despite adequate food intake. The avian type in swine occurs primarily in the digestive tract, as it does in birds, and may not cause any visible signs. The principal loss in swine is through condemnation of carcasses or parts of infected carcasses at slaughter.

Diagnosis

Diagnosis of tuberculosis in animals, because of the absence of clinical signs early in the disease, is sometimes difficult. In cattle, the intradermal tuberculin test is routinely used as a part of the official tuberculosis eradication program. Tuberculin is prepared from a culture of *M. bovis* and is basically a standardized culture filtrate. A small amount injected intradermally in the tail fold of a cow sensitized by exposure to the organism will cause a swelling at the injection site in 48 to 72 hours. Those with no prior exposure do not get any reaction. The test is really an allergy-type test, and, unfortunately, exposure to other related organisms will give a similar response. The comparative cervical test, wherein both avian and mammalian tuberculin are used and the responses measured, is more sensitive. Despite this shortcoming, the tuberculin test has been an effective tool in reducing the level of infection in cattle in the United States to a small fraction of 1 percent. By the end of 1999, every state except zones within Texas and Michigan was eligible for Accredited Tuberculosis Free Status for cattle, bison, and goats. Nevertheless, isolated sporadic cases may occur, and it is imperative that the source of these be found.

Although it's frustrating to owner and veterinarian alike to see a good cow slaughtered because of a positive test and have a postmortem report come back marked "No visible lesions," the test should not be condemned. A percentage of those may be in the early stages of infection with lesions too small to be seen. Loss of an occasional cow is a small price to pay for healthier cattle and human populations. A greater deficiency is its failure to identify cattle with advanced tuberculosis because they have lost their sensitivity.

Control

Test and slaughter is the proven, effective control method for bovine tuberculosis. The disease rarely occurs in sheep and goats unless they are exposed to infected cattle, but the same test technique applies. In poultry, the disease can be kept under control by marketing all birds at the end of their first laying period, as the disease is more of a problem in old birds. Swine can be protected by keeping poultry away from them and by keeping wild birds out of the farrowing and finishing houses.

Before leaving tuberculosis, a word of caution is in order. Nonhuman primates (such as monkeys and chimpanzees) are highly susceptible to and notorious carriers of tuberculosis. If you have any inclination to keep one as a pet, try to resist it because they are nothing but trouble. But if you can't resist, by all means have the animal tested for tuberculosis before you bring it home.

Diseases Caused by Viruses and Chlamydia

VIRUSES, AS PATHOGENS, DIFFER in many respects from bacteria. Physically, virus particles are much smaller than bacteria, and cannot be seen with the ordinary optical microscope. With the magnification afforded by the electron microscope, virus particles can be seen as symmetrical geometric shapes without a nucleus or cell wall. The lack of a cell wall assumes importance in their response to antibiotics, because many antibiotics exert their effect by disrupting the integrity of the bacterial cell wall. Consequently, these drugs have no effect whatsoever on viruses, and at the present time, we have very few drugs available that will substantially influence the course of a viral infection. Treatment of viral diseases, therefore, depends on symptomatic therapy, prevention of secondary bacterial infection, and immunologic techniques, such as administration of antiserum or gamma globulin from previously immunized animals.

Although most viral infections follow a recognizable pattern of symptoms, confirmation of the diagnosis by culture of the pathogen is not as easy or reliable as it is with bacterial infection. In general, viruses will not survive long outside the animal, except under special conditions such as freezing, and attempts to isolate viruses from sick or dead animals frequently fail. Laboratory diagnosis of viral infections, therefore, depends heavily on serologic technique, such as a rise in serum antibody titer concurrent with clinical signs or specialized tests such as fluorescent antibody (FA) and agar gel immunodiffusion (AGID). Because of the special techniques required, some of which are quite time-consuming, laboratory diagnosis of viral diseases tends to be more expensive than other diagnostic testing procedures.

Although there are exceptions that will be pointed out, most viral diseases tend to spread with great rapidity through the herd, with all susceptible animals quickly becoming infected. With some viral diseases, the carrier state is quite common. As a general rule, viral infections are characterized by sudden onset, fever, depressed white blood cell count (leukopenia), absence of pus formation, and lack of specific response to drug therapy. For these and other reasons, some viral infections assume great importance in animal and human medicine.

Abortion, "Foothill" (Epizootic Bovine Abortion)

This abortion disease of cattle confined thus far to the western United States, especially California, Oregon, and Nevada, is caused by one of several viral pathogens carried by an insect vector, the soft-shelled tick. *Chlamydia* species is the most likely cause, although there is still some question about this. Abortion is the only clinical sign, and the disease gets its name from the frequency of occurrence in cattle pastured in the foothills. The mode of transmission is not known, but its restriction to a particular terrain and isolation of the organism from ticks and rodents suggests that it is a vector-borne disease. Also, that abortion typically occurs only during the first pregnancy or in cattle newly introduced to the area indicates that infection confers some degree of immunity. Abortion rates as high as 75 percent in susceptible cattle have been reported. Abortion usually occurs about the middle of gestation, and retention of the placenta is a common sequel.

The disease produces characteristic lesions in the fetus that are useful in making a diagnosis. One method of control to reduce abortions is to pasture heifers in endemic areas prior to breeding. This exposes them to the organism at a time when it does no harm but produces immunity to prevent abortion.

Enzootic Abortion of Ewes

A similar, if not identical, disease called enzootic abortion of ewes (EAE) occurs in sheep. In sheep, it is believed, infection occurs at lambing time through ingestion of the organism present in aborted fetal membranes or contaminated forage and remains latent until conception occurs. Isolation of aborting ewes and proper disposal of aborted fetuses, therefore, are important control procedures. Interestingly enough, it's not unusual for only one lamb of a set of twins to be affected. In some cases, the lambs are not aborted and become mummified. Ewes carrying mummy lambs, from whatever cause, often show signs of systemic illness such as rapid weight loss. As in cows, however, abortion is generally the only clinical sign. The disease has not been reported to be a problem in goats. That it occurs in both cattle and sheep, however, leads one to believe that it could occur in goats as well, and it should be considered as a possible cause of unexplained abortion in goats in the endemic areas.

At the moment, isolation of aborting animals until all vaginal discharge ceases and disposal of aborted fetuses by deep burying or burning are probably the most practical controls. Broad-spectrum antibiotics such as tetracycline in rather high doses will control the disease, but administration under range conditions is difficult. Inactivated vaccine given prior to breeding is helpful in controlling this disease in sheep, but does not provide absolute protection.

Anemia, Equine Infectious (Swamp Fever)

In terms of the number of animals affected, equine infectious anemia (EIA) is not the most important viral disease of horses and other members of the horse family, although the consequences for the infected individuals are generally serious. It is a disease marked by confusion and misunderstanding on the part of some horse owners and occasionally by heated emotion when state regulatory programs become a factor.

Spread

Equine infectious anemia is spread from horse to horse by transfer of a droplet of blood from an infected horse to one that is susceptible. For all practical purposes, this is the only means of spread, although intrauterine infection of foals from infected dams has been reported and the possibility does exist of virus transfer during copulation if there is any bleeding. In nature, the virus is transferred from one horse to another by biting insects, especially the horsefly. Transfer of infection depends on the level of virus in the blood and the volume of blood transferred. Because volume is a factor, the biting flies are of more concern than mosquitoes. Horseflies are the principal natural vector and rarely range more than a few hundred yards, so the spread of the disease is slow. It has been recognized for more than one hundred years, yet just a small percentage of the horse population is infected.

Spread of the disease is more rapid and dramatic in stables where contaminated hypodermic needles or surgical instruments, even dental floats, have been used successively without sterilization between horses. Needles and dental floats should be sterilized between uses; disposable needles should be used and then properly discarded.

Symptoms

Symptomatically, three forms of the infection are recognized: inapparent, acute, and chronic. Equine infectious anemia attacks red blood cells, and the acutely affected horse will have a fever, marked anemia, signs of jaundice, and occasionally edema or swelling of the lower part of the abdomen and the legs. The pulse rate and the respiratory rate will be high due to the reduced oxygen-carrying capacity of the blood. The acutely affected horse will be weak, depressed, and may die in a day or two or apparently recover.

Those that recover from the initial attack remain infected for life, and usually suffer periodic recurrences during the stress of heavy work or other illness. The majority of horses chronically infected with EIA virus lack the stamina for racing and other competitive events. Sooner or later (which may be years), most of them die from the effects of the disease. A few horses become infected and never show any clinical signs of disease. Nevertheless, they do harbor the virus and can serve as a source of infection for others. All evidence to date indicates that every infected horse carries the infection for life, although the level of viremia varies from time to time, being highest at the time of the acute attack.

Periodically, EIA has had devastating effects where large numbers of horses were congregated, such as at racetracks, with disastrous economic effects. Recognizing this, the Standardbred industry and the State of New York supported research at Cornell University by Dr. Leroy Coggins that led to the adaptation of the agar gel immunodiffusion test (AGID) for the diagnosis of EIA. This was a major breakthrough in control of the disease, and after several years of extensive testing, the AGID, or Coggins test, was adopted by the state governments and the U.S. Department of Agriculture as the official test for EIA. In capable hands this has proved to be the most accurate serologic test ever devised for any disease. Prior to the AGID test, the only reliable diagnostic tool for EIA was inoculation of test ponies or horses with suspect blood, a very time-consuming and expensive procedure. The enzyme-linked immunosorbent assay (ELISA) for EIA will provide more rapid response, but positive results should and, for regulatory purposes, *must* be confirmed by Coggins test.

Control

The advent of a reliable diagnostic test has made control of the disease a practical possibility, and many states now have official regulatory programs in effect. In general, these programs provide for a test when the animal is to be moved off the home premises. If the initial test is positive, it is confirmed by a second test. If both are positive, the animal is identified by a permanent freeze brand and quarantined to the farm.

Such programs have aroused strong emotions in some people, which is not difficult to understand. Horses are livestock, but for many people they are pets as well and part of the family. How do you explain to the tearful girl that although her horse appears normal it carries EIA virus, is a danger to other horses, and therefore must be quarantined to the farm or destroyed? It isn't easy. Yet EIA is a disease that could be totally eradicated in a relatively short time if the decision were made to devote sufficient resources to the effort. Only a small portion, probably not more than 2 percent of the total population, is infected; the disease spreads very slowly; and a good economical diagnostic test is available. In New York State, for example, where 50,000 to 60,000 horses were tested annually between 1973 and 1978, the rate of positives dropped from over 3 percent to 0.6 percent. Although the federal government now requires a negative test before horses can be moved interstate, relatively few states require a negative test for movement within their borders. Those states are primarily in the Northeast, perhaps following the lead of New York, which was the first to adopt a program aimed at eventual eradication of EIA. As a result, of 179,000 samples collected in the northeastern states and tested in 1998, only three were found to be positive.

Treatment

There is no specific treatment for EIA, and there is no vaccine available despite intensive research. It behooves the prudent horse owner to do everything possible to prevent infection. Those with a single horse that never gets near other horses have little to worry about. The greatest risk is in commercial stables, at racetracks, and at shows where there is considerable traffic in horses. Requiring that every horse brought in have evidence of a negative Coggins test will go a long way to protect the others. Beyond that, a good fly-control program and careful cleaning and scrubbing of curry combs, brushes, and other paraphernalia between successive uses will help. Perhaps most important is sterilization of hypodermic needles and surgical instruments, including dental floats and hoof knives. Disposable needles should be used and properly discarded.

Arteritis, Equine Viral

This specific viral disease of horses can be readily confused with influenza and equine viral rhinopneumonitis (EVR). It is caused by a herpesvirus and produces an illness characterized by rapid onset, acute upper respiratory distress, and abortion in pregnant mares. Unlike EVR, however, with equine viral arteritis abortions occur concurrently with clinical signs, whereas with EVR, the abortions occur several weeks or months after infection takes place. The disease tends to be more severe than either influenza or EVR and laboratory confirmation is generally required to make a definitive diagnosis. Viral arteritis is more commonly encountered when large numbers of horses are brought together, such as at racetracks and shows.

The incubation period ranges from 1 to 6 days, and although the clinical signs of the disease may be quite severe, recovery usually begins in about a week. Fever is the first sign, followed rather quickly by a clear nasal discharge that may become purulent. Conjunctivitis and congestion of the nasal mucous membranes are common. Coughing and labored breathing due to pulmonary edema may occur. A few individuals may develop a severe diarrhea.

One of the lesions that distinguishes this from other equine viral infections is damage to the lining of the smaller arteries and arterioles. The resulting interference with blood circulation in some cases causes edema or swelling of the legs, especially in horses that are stabled. Edema of the prepuce and sheath of stallions and geldings is common. Infected stallions tend to remain carriers and shed the virus in their semen. Venereal transmission is a significant part of the epidemiology of the disease.

Despite the vascular damage that can occur, mortality from this disease is not high, provided the sick horse is given complete rest and good nursing care. No specific treatment is indicated, but antibiotics are usually given as a precautionary measure to prevent secondary infection. Spread of the disease is generally thought to be via direct contact, so it's important that sick horses be completely isolated from all others, especially during the acute phase of the disease. A modified live-virus vaccine is available, but because of the hazard of reversion to virulence, its use is carefully regulated.

Bluetongue

This is an important disease of sheep, cattle, and goats that, thus far, is limited primarily to the southern and western United States. The disease is seasonal in occurrence, a reflection of the fact that it is spread by biting insects, especially midges, and is seen concurrently with peak populations of these insects. Because a specific midge, *Culicoides varipennis,* is the primary vector, the disease in the United States is limited principally to the western and southern states where the midge is found. Many different serologic types have been identified worldwide, and five types have been found in the United States. Each is antigenically distinct, and vaccination against one type will not protect against the others.

Symptoms

Of all ruminant species, sheep appear to be the most susceptible. After an incubation period of about a week, they develop fever, labored breathing, loss of appetite, and depression. Ulcers and erosions of the lips, tongue, and dental pad are commonly seen, and in advanced cases, the tongue becomes swollen and cyanotic, hence the name *bluetongue.* The saliva may be blood-tinged and frothy due to the mouth lesions. A secondary pneumonia is not uncommon, and mortality may range up to 30 percent of a flock. Swelling and cracks at the coronary band, in the interdigital space, and at the bulb of the heel causing severe lameness are not unusual. The principal effect of bluetongue virus is exerted on capillaries, resulting in loss of blood supply to the area served by the affected blood vessel. The result is tissue necrosis in that area. This is most dramatic in cattle, where patches of skin may die and slough. The same thing may happen to one or more digits on the feet, with the horny part actually sloughing off. Animals thus affected lose weight rapidly because the pain of moving about to graze is more than they can tolerate.

Abortion is a common sequel to bluetongue infection and this, coupled with severe weight loss, damage to the fleece, and death loss, makes bluetongue a serious economic matter when many animals in the flock are affected. Because of its economic importance, countries that do not now have the disease, such as Australia, prohibit importation of sheep from countries where the disease is present. Canada has imposed a negative bluetongue test requirement on cattle from the United States prior to importation.

Treatment

Treatment of the disease, other than good nursing care, is of little value. Affected animals should be housed and fed good-quality hay if they will eat. Isolation of infected animals is of little or no value, as the disease is not directly transmissible. Recovery confers a solid immunity, and lambs born of immune ewes will have a passive immunity lasting about 6 months.

Insect control will help reduce the spread of bluetongue, but vaccination is the most satisfactory control procedure. Annual vaccination of sheep in the age range of 6 months to 3 years is commonly practiced in the endemic areas. Older sheep are generally

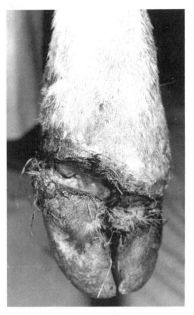

Sloughing digits can be caused by ergot poisoning and bluetongue, among other things.

immune. The vaccine should be used cautiously in pregnant ewes during the first 6 weeks of gestation because abortions and deformed lambs have been reported following vaccination. Unfortunately, the vaccine currently available is not wholly effective, as it protects against only one serotype of virus and is not approved for use in cattle or goats. Therefore, the virus serotype in the area must first be determined and then the appropriate vaccine used. Because the vaccines used are modified live virus, it is preferable to use them during seasons of the year when midges are not active to prevent dissemination of vaccine virus. A polyvalent vaccine has been reported highly successful in South Africa, but a similar vaccine has not yet been licensed in the United States.

Bluetongue is a serious disease. It you have reason to suspect it in your flock or herd, call your veterinarian immediately.

Cholera, Hog

At one time hog cholera was, by any measure, the most costly disease of swine in the United States, with annual losses running into millions of dollars. In addition to the direct losses, many foreign countries, free of the disease, refused to import U.S. pork products because of the risk of introducing infection. The hog cholera virus can survive several months in pickled pork and for years in frozen pork. Thanks to an intensive state-federal eradication campaign and the cooperation of swine producers, the disease appears to have been eradicated. No cases have been reported in the Untied States since the summer of 1976. This should not be cause for complacency, however, because prior to that episode, the disease had not been seen for almost 2 years.

Symptoms

Hog cholera is an acute, highly contagious disease of swine, causing high fever, lack of appetite, constipation followed by diarrhea, incoordination especially in the young, prostration, coma, and death in a high percentage of cases. With an incubation period sometimes as short as 2 days and extremely rapid spread, it was not uncommon to hear of a producer's herd being wiped out overnight. Mature swine tend to be more resistant, with an incubation period sometimes as long as 30 days and recovery more common. Even then the economic loss through reduced rate of gain and abortion was highly significant.

Vaccination

With such a devastating disease, it's not surprising that vaccination played an important role in its control. The earliest attempt, which was used at great cost for many years, was the simultaneous administration of live virus and antiserum at two different sites. The theory, which worked most of the time, was that the live virus would stimulate immunity but the antiserum would control its replication so disease would not result. Breaks were not unusual,

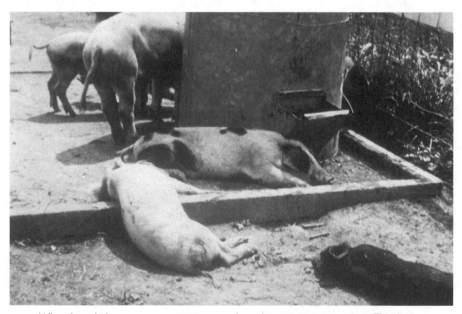

When hog cholera was rampant, scenes such as this were not uncommon. The disease advanced to death in a high percentage of cases.

however, due to improper administration or antiserum of inadequate potency. Use of live virus in any immunization program guarantees perpetuation of the disease.

The next development, never totally satisfactory, was the use of live virus inactivated with crystal violet. Unfortunately, the inactivation was occasionally incomplete and vaccine breaks occurred. With improved knowledge of virology techniques, attenuated or modified live-virus vaccine became available and was widely used until the early 1970s. Despite occasional vaccine breaks, it helped to reduce the prevalence of hog cholera to a manageable level. When it became feasible to eradicate the disease, all vaccination was stopped by law because at that time most of the cholera being seen was due to vaccine failures, and, in fact, the last outbreak in New England was traced to illegal use of vaccine. A stockpile of vaccine is maintained under federal control in case of emergency.

It's interesting that the hog cholera virus and the virus causing bovine virus diarrhea (BVD) in cattle are antigenically related. In the laboratory, pigs vaccinated with BVD vaccine withstood challenge by hog cholera virus. However, as a control procedure, use of BVD vaccine never found much favor.

Caution

Hog cholera can be diagnosed on the basis of clinical signs, FA test, and virus isolation. The disease is so important, although it appears to be eradicated, that anyone with a pig having a fever as part of the clinical picture should isolate the pig and call a veterinarian immediately. Although most veterinarians today have never seen a case of cholera, they do know the clinical signs and have access to epidemiologists and laboratories to aid in the diagnosis. There is always the possibility that, if not hog cholera, the disease could be African swine fever, an equally devastating foreign animal disease that resembles cholera.

Diarrhea, Bovine Virus (Musocal Disease)

Based on serologic testing surveys, bovine virus diarrhea (BVD) may well be the most prevalent viral infection of cattle. Positive antibody titers indicate that upward of 75 percent of our adult cattle have encountered the virus and become immune. Fortunately, only a small percentage of these ever show clinical signs of the disease.

Two distinct forms of the disease are recognized, which at one time led to the belief that BVD and mucosal disease were separate entities. The term *mucosal disease* was given to a disease that affects many cattle, but with low mortality. It occurs primarily in feedlot cattle. The other form sporadically affects few cattle, primarily yearlings, but with high mortality and is seen more often in dairy cattle. Further research has established that the two diseases are caused by the same virus. The difference in clinical signs may be a reflection of stress at the time of infection, immune status of the animal, or viral mutation. Two biotypes of BVD virus are recognized, cytopathic and noncytopathic, both capable of producing disease and both antigenically related to hog cholera virus.

Spread

Widespread distribution of the virus makes it apparent that it can be carried from farm to farm by many routes, probably including carrier animals and contaminated clothing and vehicles, as well as by other animals and perhaps birds. Experimentally, infection can be produced by administering virus orally, intranasally, or by injection. Most naturally occurring cases probably result from ingestion of virus. Cattle infected as fetuses may become persistently infected (PI) after birth and are a major source of virus.

Symptoms

The earliest clinical sign is high fever and loss of appetite occurring 4 to 7 days following infection. The virus has an affinity for epithelial and lymphoid tissue, and typical lesions are small erosions on the lips, dental pad, tongue, and palate. At necropsy, the same lesions may be seen throughout the digestive tract. The erosions may coalesce to form a larger lesion in some areas, but they tend to heal quickly. When present, they help greatly to confirm the diagnosis but, unfortunately or fortunately, depending on one's point of view, they do not occur in all cases. Concurrent with onset of fever, a profuse watery diarrhea develops, sometimes accompanied by violent straining. Extreme dehydration and rapid weight loss accompany the diarrhea. In cases of a few days' duration, the diarrhea subsides to be followed by periodic expulsion of small amounts of black, tarry stool. Lacrimation and an ocular discharge sometimes occur, and the muzzle is frequently crusty, with the nostrils partially plugged with sticky mucus. Lameness due to laminitis is not uncommon, and on some animals the skin in the neck region will get scruffy and wrinkled.

Those that recover generally show improvement in 4 to 5 days, but apparent recovery followed by periodic bouts of diarrhea and unthriftiness lasting a period of several months is not unusual. Mortality is high, however, and death may occur anywhere from 3 days to a month or more after the onset of clinical signs. In recent years, the disease has been seen more frequently in yearling cattle and is generally limited to those in the group that are unthrifty for unrelated reasons. Although the preceding description may seem perfectly straightforward, the actuality is somewhat different. These symptoms will typically be seen in different animals in the herd but usually not all in the same animal. The clinical signs observed in infected animals range from none to death, depending on the pathogenicity of the particular virus, age of the animals, stage of pregnancy, and immune status.

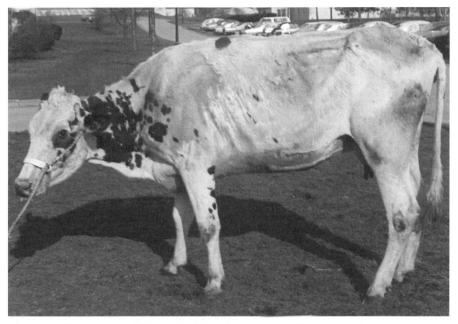

Emaciation and dehydration such as the is typical of bovine virus diarrhea.

Abortion

While the clinical signs of the disease occur infrequently, they may only be the tip of the iceberg as far as the economic importance of BVD is concerned. The virus can cause abortion at any stage of gestation, and when the fetus becomes infected during the first 3 to 6 weeks of gestation, cerebellar development is arrested. Many of the calves that survive to term are born with physical incoordination due to cerebellar hypoplasia. If they can stand at all, they stand with legs outspread to keep from falling and move with a peculiar jerking gait. Cataracts of one or both eyes often accompany this condition. It's entirely possible that many of the unexplained early embryonic deaths and abortions that occur in cattle each year are the result of inapparent BVD virus infection.

Diagnosis

Better diagnostic tools would help to resolve this question. Clinical signs and lesions at necropsy usually define the cause of death without difficulty. It is not so easy in those with minimal lesions that survive. In these cases, diagnosis must be based on a rise in antibody titer that occurs between the time of initial infection and 3 weeks later. This diagnosis requires two separate blood samples and is retrospective — by the time a laboratory report is received, the animal is either dead or better. Its chief value is to establish the presence of the virus in the herd. This can serve as a guide for future vaccination programs.

Vaccine

An effective modified live-virus vaccine is available singly or in combination with other antigens for the prevention of BVD. When given to animals at least 6 months of age, it provides immunity of long duration. It can be given earlier but, if so, should be repeated later because of possible interference from maternal antibody. The vaccine does have drawbacks, however. If given during pregnancy, some cows may abort. Also, it is a live virus and there is an element of risk in using it on animals that are under stress, because a few may develop serious illness.

This presents a difficult choice for the feedlot operator. At the time they enter the feedlot, cattle are under the stress of shipment, change in diet, and new surroundings. These factors combine to make them good candidates for a variety of infections and poor candidates for vaccination at that time. In consultation with their veterinarians, many operators will weigh the odds and accept a few vaccine-induced illnesses in preference to the possibility of a larger number of natural infections. A killed-virus vaccine is available for BVD and produces adequate immunity with less risk, but generally two doses are required.

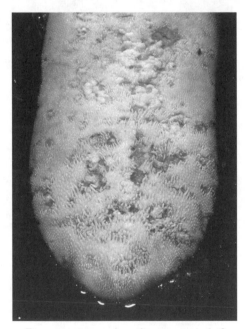

Treatment is of little value, and control, aside from vaccination, is difficult. Because the disease is so widespread, a high percentage of cattle will show a positive blood test, but testing of herd additions has some value. Viral isolation from blood or nasal swabs is more useful as an indicator of persistent infection. It is especially important that breeding bulls be free of persistent infection because bull semen can contain high levels of virus. Embryo donors and recipients should also be free of BVD virus.

Tongue erosions such as these are typical of bovine virus diarrhea.

Diarrhea, Viral, of Calves

Viruses belonging to the two groups, rotavirus and coronavirus, have been identified as the cause of a contagious diarrhea seen in some herds. The original virus isolations were from herds in Nebraska.

Rotavirus infection affects calves primarily in the 1- to 3-day age bracket, whereas coronavirus is more common in those a few days older. Much is yet to be learned about the significance of these viruses as they relate to the calf diarrhea complex. Both are apparently capable of causing pathological changes in the intestinal epithelium that result in rapid fluid loss, dehydration, and death of some calves, with or without concurrent bacterial infection. It's possible, however, that the most severely affected calves are those with concurrent infection due to other pathogens such as *Escherichia coli.*

Transmission as far as is known is by direct contact, and the calf hutch or elevated tie stall system of housing helps control the spread of disease.

Vaccine

A vaccine for the calf rotavirus and coronavirus is commercially available, but mixed reports follow its use. To be effective, it must be given immediately after birth. When used this way, some herd owners report a marked decline in calf diarrhea problems; others report no detectable difference. From this it must be concluded that the vaccine may be useful in those herds where calf diarrhea due to rotavirus is endemic, but the vaccine is not the answer to the entire calf scours complex. Because the specific etiologic agent is rarely identified early in outbreaks of calf diarrhea, ensuring that calves get colostrum immediately after birth is still the most effective recommendation to be made.

Dysentery, Winter

This baffling disease occurs primarily in stabled dairy cattle during the winter months and is more prevalent in the northeastern United States than elsewhere. Although beef cattle can be affected, it is seen mostly in the dairy breeds and rarely in young stock. It appears suddenly, rapidly affects the majority of the herd, and disappears as quickly as it came. Older texts state unequivocally that it is caused by *Campylobacter (Vibrio) jejuni,* but attempts to reproduce the disease with the organism have been unsuccessful, and its rapid spread indicates that other agents must be involved. A bovine coronavirus has been shown to produce the disease.

Recovery seems to confer some immunity, because once it appears in a herd, a recurrence is not likely the following year. Where the infectious agent stays between outbreaks is unclear; the precipitating factors are not well understood. *C. jejuni* is known to be a cause of severe diarrhea in humans, and it is not unusual for an episode of diarrhea to appear in the household concurrent with that in the barn.

Symptoms

Abdominal discomfort, uneasiness, and slightly depressed appetite are the earliest clinical signs. These are followed in a few hours by a profuse, watery, explosive diarrhea having a fetid odor. The diarrhea is so profuse and forceful that it behooves one to be very alert when walking behind cows with the disease. An effective range of 10 feet is not unusual! Temperatures are usually in the normal range, and in some cases the diarrhea becomes quite bloody. Dehydration caused by the fluid loss may be severe, and a milk production decline of 50 percent is not uncommon. Mortality is low if there are no complications. In a very few cases, intestinal hemorrhage accompanying the diarrhea may necessitate blood transfusion. When the disease is unduly prolonged, acidosis may contribute to death.

Treatment

A great variety of intestinal astringents and protectives have been used to treat the disease, but their value is difficult to assess. It has been said that the uncomplicated case of winter dysentery recovers in 72 hours with treatment; otherwise it takes 3 days. There is little doubt that oral medication with any of the currently available drugs recommended, coupled with electrolytes given orally and intravenously, will help to minimize the effects of the disease, particularly on milk production. But with half or more of the herd to be treated at one time, the labor requirement to do so may not be justified. This does not apply, of course, to the few individuals whose symptoms are so severe that vigorous treatment is necessary to save their lives. The normal course of the disease in the individual is about 3 days, and on a herd basis the whole unpleasant episode usually passes in 2 to 3 weeks. For the dairyman and his cows, however, those weeks are messy, unpleasant, and costly in terms of milk production.

Prevention

Because the causative agent and mode of transmission are not well defined, specific preventive measures are elusive. Circumstantially, it appears that the agent can be carried from farm to farm on boots, clothing, and vehicles. Many instances have been observed where the disease appeared in herds successively down the road about 2 days after a visit by an inseminator, drug and feed sales representative, cattle dealer — or veterinarian. Purchase of replacement animals during the season when winter dysentery is likely to occur is an obvious risk. Thus, at present, the best recommendations that can be made are to avoid overcrowding, keep the barn well ventilated, keep the barn as clean as possible, and, perhaps most important, keep new animals and new people out.

Ecthyma, Contagious (Sore Mouth)

The virus causing contagious ecthyma has an affinity for the lips of lambs and kids. Mature animals rarely show lesions with the exception of ewes nursing infected lambs, which, unless solidly immune, may develop lesions on the teats and udder. The disease occurs worldwide, and most outbreaks in the northern hemisphere occur in late summer, fall, and early winter.

The infection spreads primarily through contact with the lesions. However, the virus is highly resistant to drying, among other influences. Dried scabs falling to the ground may remain infective for years, so once the disease appears on a premise, additional cases can and should be expected in subsequent years.

Symptoms

Small reddened papules on the lips are the first clinical sign. These soon become vesicles that rupture, becoming pustular prior to scab formation. Adjacent vesicles may coalesce to become rather extensive lesions involving the entire lip. Occasionally, similar lesions occur inside the mouth. With extensive involvement, the lips and mouth become quite sore. Some affected lambs are reluctant to nurse and, as a consequence, lose weight and become weak. A few may actually die from starvation. The problem is compounded if the disease is transmitted to the ewe when the affected lamb tries to nurse. The lesions on her teats may be so sore that she won't allow the lamb to nurse. Sometimes, lesions develop on the feet, causing lameness.

Contagious ecthyma can readily be confused with a much less common viral disease of sheep called *ulcerative dermatosis*. The latter, however, causes actual ulcers on the lip, muzzle, feet, and, unlike sore mouth, also on the prepuce and occasionally the penis of rams. Both diseases can be complicated by secondary bacterial infection and screwworm infestation.

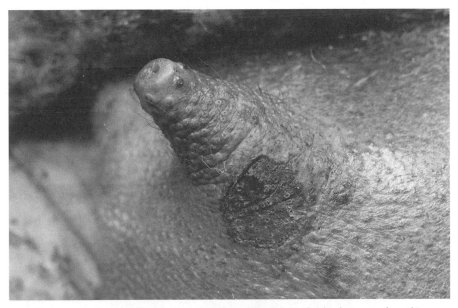

Ewes nursing lambs infected with contagious ecthyma may develop lesions such as this on the teats and udder.

Vaccine

Contagious ecthyma is preventable by vaccination; however, vaccination against this disease is actually planned infection using a suspension of live virus. Therefore, the vaccine should not be used on farms where the disease has not appeared before. The usual procedure is to apply virus suspension to a lightly scarified area on the inside of the thighs of lambs when they are about a month old. Repeating the procedure several months later provides a more solid immunity. Recovered animals are solidly immune.

Treatment of the disease is of questionable value. Antibiotic ointments or antiseptic solutions may prevent secondary infection and promote earlier healing, but the labor requirement in a commercial flock may be more than the effort is worth. In the majority of cases, the lesions are completely healed in a month or less.

Caution

A word of caution is in order when handling infected animals or vaccine. The disease is transmissible to humans, causing lesions on the hand and face not unlike those in sheep. In humans the disease is referred to as *orf.* Because contact is the mode of transmission to humans as well as animals, it's prudent to wear rubber gloves when handling lesions or vaccine and to scrub thoroughly with soap and water when through.

Encephalomyelitis, Equine (Sleeping Sickness)

Several viruses are capable of causing encephalitis in horses. These are classified as *arboviruses* because the virus is transmitted by arthropod insects, such as mosquitoes, which are the principal vectors, or carriers, of equine encephalomyelitis. Although the clinical signs produced by the several viruses are similar, the viruses are antigenically slightly different. Also, their distribution, with some exceptions, is generally limited to specific geographic areas, and from this they are variously designated as California, eastern, St. Louis, Venezuelan, western encephalitis, West Nile virus. At the present time, only eastern and western types are of major significance in the United States.

Diagnosis

Occurrence of the disease is sporadic and seasonal. In areas where the disease is endemic, outbreaks can be anticipated a week or two following the peak mosquito population. In the northern areas, this is generally late August and September. The seasonality of the disease is an aid to diagnosis, although occasional cases may occur earlier or later. In the horse the disease is characterized by fever, lack of appetite, drowsiness, partial or complete blindness, aimless wandering, incoordination, staggering, paralysis, and death. With eastern encephalitis, mortality ranges up to 90 percent; mortality is a bit less with the western type.

There is no specific treatment for viral encephalitis, but supportive therapy and good nursing care help to reduce mortality. Serologic testing has limited value in diagnosis because many horses die before antibody develops. Isolation of virus from brain tissue confirms the presumptive diagnosis and provides a logical basis for vaccinating other horses in the area and all horses in subsequent years. A vaccine incorporating antigen for eastern, western, and Venezuelan types, singly or in combination, is available. This is given in two doses initially, with a booster in spring every year thereafter. The vaccine is relatively safe and gives a good immunity. Anyone who cares about his horses should have them immunized.

From a professional standpoint, eastern equine encephalomyelitis is an interesting disease. Birds are the principal reservoir of the virus but are rarely affected themselves. Eastern encephalitis has, however, caused serious losses in flocks of pheasants raised in captivity. Mosquitoes are the vector by which the virus is transmitted from birds to horses — and to humans. Horses are actually a dead-end host for the virus because most of them die and the virus dies with them. In that sense, the term *equine encephalomyelitis* is really a misnomer. It is really a disease of birds causing inapparent infection that accidentally gets transmitted to horses by mosquitoes. Whether or not horses get the disease is a matter of chance. First, there must be birds in the area carrying the virus. Second, there must be mosquitoes available to bite the bird. Then sufficient time must elapse for the virus to replicate in the mosquito salivary gland to reach an infective dose level, and then the mosquito must bite a susceptible horse. When all these factors come together in the right sequence, the disease appears. Remove any one of them and disease will not occur. Mosquito population control and vaccination of horses, therefore, are valuable tools in preventing this disease.

Venezuelan Encephalitis

Although, symptomatically, Venezuelan encephalitis is similar to eastern and western encephalitis, it differs in two important respects. Mammals in addition to birds can be unaffected carriers, and there is evidence that the virus can be transmitted by aerosol transmission between horses in addition to transfer by mosquitoes. This disease has appeared sporadically for years in the northwestern countries of South America, but during 1969 and 1970, it progressed northward though Central America and across Mexico, and was reported in Texas in June 1971. An intensive and expensive control program kept it confined to that state, but several thousand horses died from it. No new cases have been reported in the United States since December 1971, and the virus has apparently disappeared from this country.

All three types of equine encephalitis virus are capable of infecting humans, and the disease must be considered a public health hazard. During the Texas outbreak, a number of human cases developed and the symptoms were reported to be similar to influenza. The eastern and western types, however, cause an encephalitis in humans similar to that produced in horses — with equally serious implications. In humans, as in horses, mosquitoes are the vector.

Control

Because of its fatal potential for horses and people, every effort should be made to control equine encephalomyelitis. The most logical approach is through vaccination of members of the horse family about a month before the mosquito season starts and again 4 months later. Where mosquitoes are active year-round, annual vaccination is indicated. When outbreaks occur, area spraying for mosquito control may be helpful, but spraying is of less value on individual premises. Stabling horses at night when mosquitoes are active is more useful.

Fever, Malignant Catarrhal (Malignant Head Catarrh)

Malignant catarrhal fever (MCF) is an infectious, sporadically occurring disease of cattle that is usually fatal. Generally, only a small percentage of cows in the herd are affected, but in some herds the disease may persist to cause significant losses over a period of time. Sheep and goats are apparently unaffected carriers of the virus, and the majority of cases occur in herds where the cattle are kept in close proximity to sheep. The virus of MCF can cause overt disease in farmed deer and is a concern of zoological parks because it also can infect several species of antelope and wildebeest.

Symptoms

The signs of MCF are variable, but typically onset is accompanied by high fever, lack of appetite, and a clear discharge from the eyes and nose. The nasal discharge soon becomes mucopurulent and dark with encrustation of the nostrils. Conjunctivitis, inflammation of the eyelid, is commonly seen, and breathing may become labored. Dehydration is a consistent complication contributing to the high (90 percent) mortality. Encephalitis and blindness may occur. On the basis of clinical signs alone in the individual cow, MCF can easily be confused with BVD, acute shipping fever, or rinderpest, a foreign animal disease.

A few cases develop a profuse diarrhea with severe straining that, when accompanied by signs of encephalitis, may be suggestive of rabies. The incubation period may range from several days to several months, and in all its most acute forms the disease is usually fatal in 10 days or less. Occasionally affected cows live longer, but recovery, if it occurs at all, is a slow process.

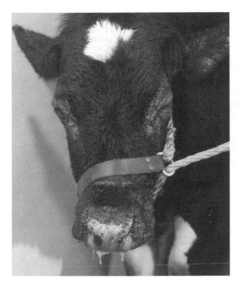
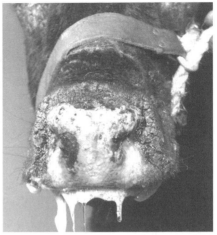

*Drooling, crusty muzzle, and facial dermatitis
are typical of malignant catarrhal fever.*

Vaccine

No vaccine is available to prevent the disease, and considering the relative infrequency of its occurrence, it's doubtful that the potential market would justify the cost of vaccine development and licensing. Similarly, presently available drugs do little to influence the course of the disease. Past experience indicates that destroying the animal may be the most humane course to take, except in the case of valuable purebred animals, where the cost of vigorous therapy, including intravenous fluids, blood transfusion, and antibiotics, can be justified.

Keeping sheep and cattle completely separated is the best method of preventing the disease, and, of course, isolating any infected cattle from the herd.

Fever, West Nile

The virus causing West Nile fever, considered a foreign animal disease for many years, appeared in the New York City area in 1999. Dead birds from which the virus was isolated confirmed the presence of the disease.

The clinical signs in animals and humans are those of encephalitis, and several people in the New York City area, as well as nine horses on Long Island, died. The virus seems to be endemic now in wild birds, especially crows, as it was found in Massachusetts and Connecticut birds during summer 2000 and again in summer 2001.

As yet, there is no vaccine available to protect against the disease, but a diagnostic test has been developed that readily helps to distinguish the disease from others, such as rabies, causing signs of encephalitis. The virus is transmitted from birds to humans and to horses by mosquitoes. Serological evidence indicates that horses can be infected without showing clinical signs.

In the absence of a vaccine, the most effective control method used is to reduce the concentration of mosquitoes. Area spraying with insecticide seems to have been effective in the New York City region but would be impractical over wide areas. For the individual owner in the endemic area, it would be wise to confine horses in a screened stable at night when mosquitoes are most active. Using insect repellents will help, as well as draining areas where mosquitoes breed. Simple things such as emptying cans or bottles and pails that have stagnant water in them will also help. Reducing the mosquito population will keep you more comfortable in the evening, too.

Gastroenteritis, Transmissible

Transmissible gastroenteritis (TGE) is a major disease of swine, most prevalent in the swine-producing areas of the Midwest during winter and early spring. Although swine of all ages can be affected, its effect on piglets under 2 weeks of age can be devastating.

Profuse, watery diarrhea, preceded sometimes by vomiting and rapid dehydration, is the principal sign in very young pigs. The incubation period may be only a matter of hours in some outbreaks, and rapid spread through adjacent litters in the farrowing house is a common characteristic. Mortality in young pigs can range up to 100 percent after an illness of 1 to 5 days. Less severe diarrhea without the early vomiting characterizes the disease in older swine. After several days' illness, older swine generally recover, but they may continue to shed virus in the feces for a couple of months after all clinical signs have disappeared. These virus shedders are a source of infection for susceptible new pigs added to the herd, and if sold into other herds carry the virus with them.

Transmissible gastroenteritis should be suspected whenever a rapidly spreading diarrhea affecting all ages but fatal only to the very young occurs. The virus causes a physical change in the intestinal lining that results in rapid fluid loss. This in turn produces an extreme dehydration that even very young pigs try to counteract by drinking copious amounts of water. The diagnosis can be confirmed in the laboratory by fluorescent antibody techniques or by virus isolation.

Treatment and Prevention

Treatment is of very limited value because of the peracute nature of the disease. Antibiotics generally don't have much effect on the outcome. Antidiarrheal drugs such as carbadox and oral electrolytes by drench or added to the drinking water may save a few pigs that would otherwise succumb.

Prevention is generally more rewarding than treatment. A number of techniques have proved helpful. Avoiding introduction of the virus to a clean herd is highly desirable. The feces of infected pigs are thoroughly contaminated with virus, and the virus can be mechanically carried from one farm to another on equipment and dirty footwear and by dogs, rodents, and wild birds. The first step, then, is to keep all unnecessary traffic — human, avian, animal, and vehicular — away from the pigs and particularly away from the farrowing house. To further isolate the most susceptible population, separate cleaning and feeding equipment, boots, and coveralls should be kept and used only in the farrowing house. And, of course, new breeding stock should be kept isolated from the remainder of the herd until danger of disease transmission has passed. These measures will help to prevent other contagious diseases as well.

While these measures are ideal, under some husbandry conditions they may not be practical, and other measures must be taken to cope with TGE. When the disease has occurred on the farm or the risk of infection is high, immunization can be useful. Immunization through planned infection was used prior to the advent of a vaccine and is still widely practiced. Deliberately exposing sows to virus in dead pigs during early pregnancy will stimulate antibody transferable in milk to piglets when they are born. This will protect many, but small losses may still occur. Vaccination of sows increases antibody in colostrum to protect newborn pigs.

Influenza

This is among the most interesting of viral diseases for the number of species it affects, including humans, and for the variability and adaptability of the viruses that cause it.

Equine Influenza

Among livestock, equine influenza is the most economically significant. Two myxoviruses, designated A/equi-1 and A/equi-2, are responsible for most cases in horses in the United States, although the A/equi-2 type has not been seen in recent years. Symptomatically, in the horse the disease closely resembles human influenza. The incubation period is short, usually 1 to 3 days, and the onset is sudden with high fever, coughing, weakness, and lack of appetite. Duration of the acute signs is generally only several days, but the cough and weakness, aggravated by exercise, may last much longer. The disease spreads rapidly through the herd, and rapid spread is one of the characteristics that helps distinguish influenza from other equine respiratory ailments. Severity of the clinical signs is influenced by degree of immunity, age, debility, and stress.

Spread of the disease is by aerosol dispersion or by contact with horses in the early stages of the disease. Therefore, as with rhinopneumonitis, the risk of infection is greatest in situations where large numbers of unrelated horses are brought together. Influenza in the horse is a serious disease readily complicated by secondary bacterial infection. Absolute rest, good ventilation in the stable, and a nourishing diet help to speed recovery. Antibiotics, although routinely used to prevent secondary infection, such as strangles, have no effect on the influenza virus. It is sometimes necessary to control persistent high fever with aspirin or other antipyretics. This, coupled with rest and good nursing care, is usually all that can be done or is necessary once the disease occurs.

A vaccine is available for prevention of influenza in horses and should be used routinely to immunize horses at risk. It is usually given in two doses, with the second 3 to 8 weeks after the first and a booster dose 6 months later. The duration of immunity is relatively short, and horses at risk should receive a dose of vaccine every 3 to 6 months.

Swine Influenza

While the myxovirus causing equine influenza is host specific, the cause in swine influenza is not. In fact, there is evidence to indicate that the swine influenza virus, belonging to influenza virus type A, originated with humans during the great influenza pandemic of 1918–19. While this particular strain of virus has since disappeared from the human population, it has stayed with pigs. An exception was a few cases of influenza at Fort Dix in New Jersey identified as swine type A virus during early 1976. This aroused some medical and great political concern that a repeat of the 1918 epidemic was in the making for 1976–77. This concern culminated in a federally financed mass-immunization campaign that proved to be a fiasco. It did serve at least two purposes, however: (1) it alerted millions of people to the interrelationship between animal and human disease, and (2) it helped demonstrate, once again, that medicine and politics don't mix.

Swine influenza is most prevalent in the Midwest, where swine are concentrated. It is a disease that occurs primarily during the inclement weather of fall and winter, indicating that stress is a factor in the appearance of the clinical signs of fever, lack of appetite, coughing, muscular weakness, depression, and death of 1 to 2 percent of affected pigs. The disease spreads rapidly through a herd, with sudden onset involving most of the herd and disappearance of the more conspicuous signs in 3 or 4 days. The principal loss is economic through stunting and reduced weight gain.

The mystery in swine influenza is where the virus survives between outbreaks. Because these occur primarily in fall and winter, and the life of a pig from birth to slaughter is only about 6 months, the usual concept that a virus particle requires living cells to survive wouldn't hold true. Of course, there is no problem with that theory where breeding stock are kept over from one year to the next. The question arises on farms where swine influenza is endemic but only feeder pigs are kept.

Part of the answer lies in intermediate hosts. At the time of acute attacks, the virus infects the swine lungworm. Lungworm eggs containing virus are passed out in pig feces and in turn are ingested by earthworms. The earthworm population thus becomes infected and months later, when new pigs out on pasture eat infected earthworms, they also get a dose of virus. The virus in the pig then remains more or less dormant until the pig's resistance is lowered by the stress of chilling and especially by concurrent infection with *Haemophilus suis.* This accounts for the characteristic rapid spread of the disease in the herd. It is as much simultaneous activation of latent infection as it is spread from one pig to the next. Recovered animals have been shown to harbor the virus for up to 3 months after all clinical signs have passed.

Fortunately, swine influenza is not a major problem in pigs because prevention is difficult due to the mode of transmission. As with prevention of any disease, good management, including clean, dry, draft-free quarters, and avoidance of stress are important. For the commercial hog grower, vaccination is useful but doesn't provide total protection for the herd. Buying only specific pathogen-free (SPF) breeding stock or feeder pigs and keeping them in paved feedlots would help, but it is not practical in all situations. Antibiotics in feed or drinking water and reduction of stress to minimize weight loss during an outbreak are usually the best bet.

Leukosis, Bovine (Bovine Lymposarcoma, Bovine Leukemia)

Bovine leukosis is undergoing intensive study as a model for further understanding of the pathogenesis of leukemia in humans. Bovine lymphosarcoma is a viral-induced neoplastic disease of cattle that in adults is slow in onset and eventually fatal. There is evidence to indicate infection occurs *in utero* or via colostrum and becomes manifest months or years later. Also, familial predisposition is a factor. The disease is more prevalent in dairy cattle than in beef cattle, and it has been produced experimentally in sheep and in goats.

Diagnosis

A consistent finding of elevated white blood cell count, principally lymphocytes with many immature forms, is typical of the disease. This leukocytosis may precede clinical signs by months or years. The most readily recognized clinical sign in adult cattle is enlargement of the superficial lymph nodes. Enlargement of the thoracic or abdominal lymph nodes may cause clinical signs that mimic other diseases such as respiratory distress and digestive dysfunction. Diagnosis in these cases is usually an accidental finding during rectal palpation or exploratory surgery.

Although the primary lymphosarcoma is to be found in lymph nodes, metastatic tumors may develop in a variety of locations, including liver, kidney, spinal cord, and brain, in which case clinical signs are those to be expected due to pathological change in the organ involved. Otherwise, unexplained decline in milk production and weight loss are reasons to suspect lymphomatosis. Occasionally, lymph nodes in back of the eyeball will enlarge, forcing the eye outward to give the cow a pop-eyed appearance. Once tumors appear, the condition of the animal deteriorates over a span of weeks or occasionally months with fatal termination. A similar disease sometimes occurs in young calves causing generalized lymph node enlargement, lymphocytic infiltration of bone marrow, and anemia prior to death. Some investigators believe the causative agent to be an aberrant host cellular protein, designated a *prion,* which can bring about formation of additional abnormal protein. Much more research needs to be done and is, in fact, under way with regard to bovine spongiform encephalopathy.

Better understanding of the disease, including its viral etiology, has led to development of a specific serological test. Interpretation of test results requires some discretion, however. A positive test indicates only that the animal has encountered the virus at some time and has circulating antibody, not that it has lymphosarcoma. Several surveys based on serologic testing indicate that 20 percent or more of our dairy cattle have been exposed, but prevalence of the clinical disease is probably less than 1 percent. There is no present evidence of any relationship between enzootic bovine leukosis and leukemia in humans.

Prevention

Several northern European countries have initiated test-and-slaughter programs based on high leukocyte counts in an attempt to eradicate the disease, with moderate success. For the individual dairy farmer, prevention is difficult

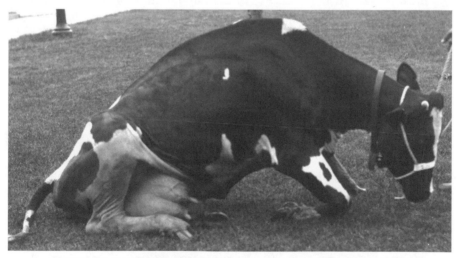

Metastatic tumors resulting from lymphosarcoma may compress the spinal cord, causing posterior paralysis.

at best. Certainly any clinically affected animals should be removed immediately from the herd. Where the disease is a herd problem, it is possible that a combination of a positive blood test and a high leukocyte count could be used to identify incipient disease and provide a logical basis for removing these animals from the herd. The same criteria could be applied to prospective herd replacements to keep the disease out of the herd.

Mammillitis, Bovine

Fortunately, this disease is rare in the United States, because it can cause considerable grief for the dairy cow and the person who has to milk her.

Lesions are confined to the teats and udder, starting as reddened, thickened areas that soon develop into vesicles or blisters. These slough, leaving denuded areas, ranging in size from a dime to larger sections involving the whole side of the teat or the teat end. These heal rapidly in the dry cow, but in the lactating cow, healing is delayed due to the constant irritation of milking. The raw areas left after the skin sloughs are painful, and the response of affected cows when milking is attempted is, as one might expect, a swift kick.

The virus causing mammillitis is a member of the herpes group and in other countries causes thickened lumps on the skin of the neck and back as well as the lesions described on the teats and udder. It could easily be confused with lumpy skin disease, a serious cattle disease we don't have in the United States, and when the lesions are confined to the teats and udder, it resembles a severe case of pseudocowpox.

The source of the virus in the few domestic outbreaks is unknown, as is the mode of transmission. There may be a mild febrile reaction early in the disease, but generally the skin lesions are the only clinical sign noted. The skin lesion, coupled with a rising serum neutralization antibody titer, is diagnostic. The disease is more common in first-calf heifers, particularly when the udder is edematous.

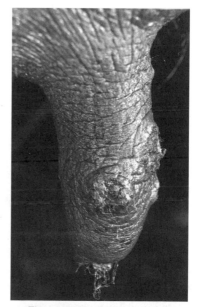

These teat lesions are typical of herpes mammillitis.

Management of the disease is largely symptomatic. Affected cows should be isolated from the rest of the herd or at least milked last. Antibiotic ointment applied to the teats helps to reduce secondary infection and to keep the scabs soft. Where the teat end is involved, infusion of antibiotics into the quarter will help prevent mastitis as a secondary complication.

Papillomatosis

This impressive-sounding name is the medical term for the common skin condition seen in most species called *warts.* The most dramatic of these are the large cauliflower-like lesions seen most frequently on the skin of the head and neck of cattle. These may occur singly and reach the size of a softball, or they may be smaller and quite numerous. Warts of this type, although they are unsightly, do not seriously impair the health of the animal. However, they do bleed easily and profusely if torn at the base and do provide a good site for screwworm infestation in areas where the screwworm is endemic.

Smaller warts occur on the teats of cattle and often interfere with milking. These may be broad-based or rather long and pedunculated. Warts are rare in sheep but do occur in goats and particularly around the muzzle of young horses. A particular type of wart, fibropapilloma, occurs occasionally on the penis of young bulls and in the vagina of heifers. These are particularly troublesome because they often bleed during coitus, and even a small amount of blood is lethal to sperm cells.

Wart tissue is an overgrowth of epithelial basal cells that enlarges and erupts through the epidermis. This overgrowth is stimulated by papillomatosis virus, and virus is present in wart tissue. Fibropapillomas occasionally occur in the mouth, pharynx, and even the esophagus of cattle. Warts in the esophagus, although rarely reported, may interfere with swallowing. There is some indication these may be due to papular stomatitis rather than wart virus.

Wart virus is quite hardy and readily spread by hypodermic needles, tattoo instruments, and tagging pliers. In nature, spread is probably via direct contact or indirectly by rubbing against a post or wall where infected cattle have recently rubbed themselves.

Warts are most common in young animals and may disappear spontaneously as they get older. This is especially true of the large proliferative type seen on the skin. It's a common observation, too, that surgical removal of one or two hastens disappearance of the others. Commercially available wart vaccine given in repeated doses at monthly intervals is an aid to removal of warts in cattle. Wart virus, however, is host specific and the cattle vaccine has little if any value when used on other species. When warts are a herd problem, an autogenous vaccine prepared from wart tissue taken from an animal in the herd may be more effective than commercial vaccines. Your veterinarian can arrange to have an autogenous vaccine made for you.

The small "seed warts" commonly found on the teats are less responsive to vaccine. If the base is broad, surgical removal is probably the best bet. Those with a narrow stalk or pedicle can frequently be twisted off or snipped off with sharp scissors.

Since antiquity, a variety of concoctions for topical application have been recommended for removal of warts. With the possible exception of silver nitrate or caustic potash carefully applied to small warts, these have little value. Vaccine or surgery is the best approach.

While prevention of warts through vaccination is possible, it is usually not feasible because of the need for repeated doses, short duration of immunity, and cost, as well as the minimal effect of warts on animal health.

Parainfluenza

The significance of this disease of cattle due to a myxovirus, parainfluenza-3 (PI$_3$), is not clearly understood. The virus is widely distributed in the cattle population, where by itself it causes little if any clinical disease. However, in conjunction with *Pasteurella multocida,* under conditions of stress, it is a factor leading to the contagious pneumonia called shipping fever.

Shipping fever is a major disease, and in an effort to provide the best vaccines possible to control it, several vaccine manufacturers now market vaccine containing killed or attenuated PI$_3$ virus. There is mixed opinion among virologists on how effective the PI$_3$ component is, but it apparently does no harm, and anything that may help to prevent shipping fever is all to the good.

Parvovirus, Porcine

This virus is widespread in the swine population. It is a very small and resistant virus that tolerates wide ranges of pH and temperature. Although it is capable of infecting any body cell, it exhibits a preference for embryonal and fetal tissue.

Serological studies indicate that up to 80 percent of sows have antibody to the virus, indicating prior infection, but the percentage of exposed gilts is not as high. The virus has been isolated from boar semen. Considering its adaptability to a variety of tissues and its wide distribution in the swine population, it is probable that the route of infection is oral or nasal and perhaps venereal.

The only outward sign of parvovirus infection in swine is reproductive failure. Infected animals appear to be healthy. The significance of the infection is its effect on the embryo or fetus and the resulting infertility it produces.

Infection of the embryos at about 12 to 20 days after conception results in embryonal death and a delayed return to heat. Infection at 21 to 35 days when the fetus is larger results in fetal resorption and pseudopregnancy. Typically, a sow may be diagnosed as pregnant but fail to farrow. Later infection, at 35 to 55 days, produces a high percentage of mummified fetuses. If the entire litter is infected, abortion may occur. Infection occurring at 55 to 80 days may produce mummies and stillborn pigs, although a few in the litter may survive. Infection after the 80th day of gestation does not seem to be as much of a problem.

The economic implications of parvovirus infection, which is a part of the SMEDI (stillbirth, mummification, embryonic death, infertility) complex, are obvious. Reproductive failure can be a disaster for the swine producer.

Although vaccination of gilts is recommended, management for prevention is of paramount importance. Maintaining a closed herd is most desirable. The alternative is planned infection at a time when litters will not be affected. This means exposing new boars and gilts to older sows that may be carriers at least 2 weeks prior to breeding. This allows time for them to develop antibodies and become immune without endangering subsequent litters.

There is no treatment for parvovirus infection, and it should be suspected whenever reproductive failure occurs in a swine herd. Diagnosis can be confirmed by laboratory examination of fresh mummified fetuses or placenta. A positive antibody titer in blood samples from sows in the herd will confirm presence of the virus but will not establish parvovirus as the cause of the problem.

Polyarthritis, Chlamydial (Serositis)

Distribution of chlamydial polyarthritis, caused by a large-particle-size virus of the genus *Chlamydia,* thus far seems limited to the upper Midwest and western United States. The disease, occurring in lambs, calves, and swine, causes primarily an arthritis. The organism can be found in joint fluid and also in urine, feces, and eye discharges. The disease does not occur commonly, but herd or flock outbreaks can involve half or more of the young animals.

Lambs show varying degrees of lameness, and if checked, some of them will have a moderate fever. This helps to distinguish the disease from other conditions causing stiffness or lameness such as white muscle disease.

Calves, in addition to fever and lameness, frequently develop diarrhea. Swelling of the joints is usually more noticeable in calves than in lambs and is quite noticeable in pigs. The disease in pigs is often complicated by nasal congestion, sneezing, labored breathing, and conjunctivitis.

History, clinical signs, and joint lesions seen at necropsy all must be considered in arriving at a diagnosis, but laboratory confirmation may be required. The principal effect of the disease is economic, through reduced rate of gain or outright starvation; lame animals are so reluctant to move that they won't nurse.

Although little work has been reported on the pathogenesis of the disease, it's reasonable to assume that carrier animals perpetuate the infection from one season to the next and introduce it to new herds. Broad-spectrum antibiotics are useful in treating it, and daily low-level antibiotic feeding in the feedlots helps to control it. This practice, however, is under scrutiny by the U.S. Food and Drug Administration and may be banned.

Pox Diseases

Almost every species, from human being to mouse, is subject to infection by pox viruses. The viruses tend to be host specific, with some exceptions, although — except for sheep and goat pox — they are clearly related. Sheep pox causes a very severe, frequently fatal disease, transmissible by inhalation, much like smallpox in humans. Fortunately, sheep and goat pox do not exist in the United States. Horse pox, although it may exist, is rare. Pox infections of cattle and swine are the most commonly encountered.

Symptoms

In cattle and swine, the disease is spread by contact, appearing first as a small raised red area on the teats and udder of cattle and on the belly of swine. These are variable in size and soon develop into vesicles that rupture, leaving a craterlike lesion that generally scabs over and heals uneventfully. The disease tends to be localized with no general effects. However, secondary bacterial infection may occur, which delays healing. Lesions on the teats and udder, of course, interfere with milking of dairy cows.

Cowpox and Pseudocowpox

Immunologically, there is an interesting historical note to cowpox. It is transmissible to humans, causing a disease referred to as *milker's nodule*. Many years ago, when smallpox was ravaging Europe, it was noted that those who had had cowpox, or milker's nodule, were immune to smallpox. This discovery became the basis for the smallpox immunization. People were infected with cowpox (vaccinia) by placing a suspension of virus on a lightly scarified area. This immunized them against smallpox (variola) and cowpox. Because of the presence of live vaccinia virus, people recently vaccinated against smallpox would not go near cows until the vaccination site had healed because they could infect cows. With the eradication of smallpox from the United States and the rest of the world, routine vaccination against smallpox during childhood is no longer done.

Although true cowpox does not occur any longer in the United States, a disease very similar in appearance to cowpox, called *pseudocowpox* and caused by a parapox virus, is a common occurrence in dairy cattle.

Control

Control efforts for the disease in cattle are aimed at reducing further spread by segregating infected cows and milking them last. The virus is readily transmitted on milking equipment and the milker's hands. Treatment is generally not necessary, although antiseptics applied to the lesions may hasten healing. Ointments applied after each milking help to soften the larger scabs, making the milking process less traumatic for the cow.

Pseudorabies

Swine are the natural host of this viral disease, which is endemic in the major swine-producing states. Adult swine may be unaffected carriers, and clinical signs are generally limited to suckling pigs. Since 1976, the disease has been reported much more frequently in the upper Midwest.

The disease spreads via contact with nasal and oral secretion from carrier animals, and the clinical picture in piglets is one of fever, paralysis, coma, and death in as little as 24 hours. The virus is a member of the herpes group, and typical of this group, latent infection may be activated in adults to cause abortions or stillborn pigs.

Most other animal species are susceptible, and in these the symptoms are much more dramatic and consistently fatal. While encephalitis occasionally occurs in pigs, it is common in species such as cattle, sheep, goats, and dogs. The clinical presentation in these animals is primarily intense itching, so much so that infected animals literally rub or lick themselves raw prior to death. This behavior gives the disease its common name, *mad itch.*

At necropsy, typical lesions can be seen microscopically. Diagnosis can further be confirmed by virus isolation and serologic testing. Serologic tests can be used to identify carrier swine, and many states now require a negative test as a prerequisite to importation.

Outbreaks in species other than swine can be prevented by keeping them away from swine. In the swine herd itself, serologic testing and removal of reactors from the herd may be necessary. Herd replacements should be from herds known to be free of the disease or should be negative on serologic testing. A vaccine is now available for use in states where the disease is endemic. Vaccination with either attenuated or inactivated vaccine will prevent clinical signs of the disease but will not prevent infection, and infected vaccinates may intermittently shed the virus to infect others. Vaccination may confuse the issue when serologic testing is done as part of an attempt to build a negative herd or to meet shipping requirements. This interference with test results can be avoided by using vaccine from which certain genes have been removed to prevent virus replication. A regular vaccination program gives good control of the infection in swine herds.

It should be noted that pseudorabies is a legally reportable disease, and states free of the disease generally do not permit vaccination.

Rabies

In terms of death losses, animal or human, in the United States this disease is almost inconsequential at present. Because of the anxiety and worry it causes and the actual discomfort thousands of people undergo each year from antirabies therapy, however, it must be considered an important disease.

The rabies virus is capable of infecting all animals, and the virus is transmitted in saliva via bite wounds. At one time this was thought to be the only route of infection. However, there is good evidence now of transmission in bat colonies via aerosol dispersion. This probably has significance, however, only for bats and for spelunkers who explore caves where bats reside. Rabies is a reportable disease that is almost invariably fatal, and all of the state health departments and the federal government maintain records of prevalence of the disease. Skunks, foxes, raccoons, and bats are statistically the most important wildlife reservoirs of the virus, but the infected dog or cat, because of its close association with humans, is the greatest threat to humans. All states require that dogs be vaccinated for rabies and a few require cat vaccination as well.

Disease Progression

Rabies is a neurotropic virus that follows the nerves from the point of virus inoculation (bite wound) to the brain and then via peripheral nerves to the salivary glands. The incubation period of the disease varies from days to months, with the interval between infection and onset of clinical signs being determined in part by the proximity of the bite wound to the brain and the species of animal under consideration.

Skunks and bats can remain asymptomatic carriers for many months, unlike other species, in which the disease is consistently and rapidly fatal. Incubation periods up to 6 months have been reported in humans, but this is exceptional. Immune status of the individual, the size and location of the infective dose, and individual resistance also play a role in determining the length of the incubation period. Although the disease is invariably fatal for domestic animals and must generally be considered so for humans, there is a record of a human case in which the individual survived. The odds against survival are so great, however, that rabies must be considered a public health hazard with serious potential.

Rabies in livestock occurs in the United States as a result of a bite by an infected animal — usually a dog, fox, coyote, raccoon, or skunk. In Central America, vampire bats are important vectors of the disease. Furthermore, its occurrence is generally limited to those areas where the disease is known to be endemic in wildlife. Thus, geographic distribution is a help in distinguishing rabies from other neurological disorders. However, when the clinical signs indicate, rabies should always be considered.

Symptoms

The earliest sign of rabies common to all species is a change in normal behavior. Usually there is loss of appetite and a pattern of obscure clinical signs easily confused with such things as indigestion, inability to swallow, and foreign objects in the mouth. Early in the disease, normally sociable animals may seek solitude and wander off by themselves, whereas others, normally shy, will become unduly friendly. Reports of rabid foxes, raccoons, and skunks walking into a barn or even a house are not unusual.

Within about 48 hours, either an excitatory or a paralytic stage begins to develop. The mention of rabies usually conjures up in most people's minds the image of a dog frothing at the mouth, running down the street biting anything that moves. This does occur, and it occurs in livestock species as well. Cattle with the excitatory stage of rabies will urinate frequently, strain, and run aimlessly in the pasture, bellowing as they go, with their tails in the air. While the ruminants — cattle, sheep, and goats — are less prone to bite, rabid horses and pigs will, and one should exercise extreme caution in their presence.

The paralytic form of the disease follows the premonitory directly in some individuals, while in others the excitatory stage may precede it by a few hours to a day or two. The earliest indication of the paralytic stage is an inability to swallow. The drooling that results gives rise to the expression "frothing at the mouth." This pharyngeal paralysis is easily confused with the signs produced by a foreign object caught in the mouth or throat. The first inclination is to open the animal's mouth and reach in to see if anything is there. Where the possibility of rabies exists, don't do it! The promising career of a good friend and colleague came to an early end some years ago indirectly as a result of failure to heed this admonition. The paralytic stage proceeds rapidly to total collapse, coma, and death.

Treatment

There is no economically feasible or effective treatment for rabies in livestock, and because of frequency of failures, the temptation to try postexposure immunization should be avoided. Animals bitten by a known rabid animal should be destroyed immediately. In case of bites by an animal not known to be rabid, the bitten animal should be confined and carefully observed for a minimum of 14 days.

If an animal shows signs of rabies, call your veterinarian immediately. He will advise you what to do and will notify the appropriate health authorities. Generally, infected animals should be allowed to die or be humanely destroyed without damaging the brain. Brain tissue is necessary for laboratory diagnosis to confirm the disease.

Prevention

Rabies is best prevented by area control procedures, including mass immunization of dogs and control of susceptible wildlife populations, especially foxes. With few exceptions, immunization of livestock is usually not necessary. An exception would be when the prevalence of rabies in an area is high, with proportionate risk of infection.

Vaccines

All rabies vaccines currently marketed in the United States for use in livestock are inactivated and thus incapable of producing the disease. Duration of immunity ranges from 1 to 3 years. A few countries permit the use of modified live-virus vaccine. Every year, the National Association of State Public Health

Veterinarians updates the protocol for rabies control and lists the vaccines currently licensed by the U.S. Department of Agriculture (USDA). Because of the seriousness of the disease, for anything to do with rabies — diagnosis or vaccination — call your veterinarian.

Respiratory Syncytial Virus, Bovine

Like PI_3 virus, the significance of this virus as a component of the respiratory disease complex in cattle, sheep, and goats is uncertain. Serologic testing indicates that a high percentage of the cattle population has been exposed to it. It can produce mild or acute respiratory disease, but present indications are that stress factors coupled with secondary bacterial infection are necessary for acute disease to result. The virus primarily affects younger dairy and beef cattle, with all the signs commonly associated with respiratory tract infection: fever, coughing, runny eyes, lack of appetite, and, in many cases, secondary pneumonia.

Pulmonary edema is a complicating factor in respiratory disease where this virus has been incriminated. Bovine respiratory syncytial virus (BRSV) antigen is included in some vaccines for prevention of respiratory disease in cattle.

Rhinopneumonitis, Equine (Equine Virus Abortion)

Equine rhinopneumonitis is a common upper respiratory infection of young horses caused by equine herpesvirus (EHV) type 1 or 4. It is a major problem where large numbers of horses are brought together. Although the upper respiratory infection is bad enough, its major economic significance is that it causes abortion in mares pregnant in late gestation, usually without producing any signs of illness in the mare.

The upper respiratory infection in young horses is characterized by fever, clear discharge from the eyes and nose, coughing, pharyngitis, and lack of appetite. Secondary bacterial infection is common and may cause the nasal discharge to become mucopurulent. The clinical disease runs a course of about 10 days, although the cough may persist longer. Mortality is low, but infection of yearlings generally disrupts training schedules. On breeding farms or at training stables, the entire episode may span several months from the time of the first case to the complete recovery of the last. Treatment will not alter the course of the viral disease, but it may help prevent secondary complications. There is evidence that some recovered horses will harbor the virus in a latent state for months or even years. It must be considered, therefore, that most horses are infected with the EHV-1 and/or the EHV-4 type of the virus.

Equine herpesvirus 1 (EHV-1) is but one of several that contribute to what is often referred to as the equine respiratory disease complex. Influenza, parainfluenza, and occasionally arteritis may all produce similar respiratory signs. Several other viruses are known to produce respiratory disease in horses but the extent to which they are a factor is unknown at present. In each case, the primary mode of transmission is probably by aerosol dispersion.

Where the upper respiratory tract involvement is the only sign noted, a definitive diagnosis must be based on serological tests. However, if abortions in otherwise normal mares follow an episode of respiratory infection in young horses on the same premises by anywhere from 1 to 4 months, you can be reasonably sure you are dealing with EHV-1. Characteristic lesions, especially in the liver of the aborted fetus, help to confirm the diagnosis. A variety of laboratory tests can make it unequivocal. In some outbreaks a few horses may develop neurological signs, ranging from mild incoordination to paralysis.

Vaccination

The disease can be prevented or its effects at least minimized by vaccination. The necessity for vaccination depends somewhat on circumstances. On the one hand, the pet horse kept in the backyard and rarely in contact with other horses will probably never encounter the virus, and vaccination would be a needless expense. On the other hand, horses on the show circuit or at the racetracks will almost certainly be exposed. Those under 3 years old should routinely be immunized with modified live-virus vaccine. Those in the older age brackets tend to be resistant through prior exposure and are less likely to show clinical signs. The resistance of the pregnant mare, however, may not be sufficient to protect her foal; mares, depending on exposure risk, should be vaccinated using inactivated vaccine. On breeding farms, particularly when outside mares are brought in for service, all horses on the premises should be vaccinated annually.

Occasional adverse reactions to the vaccine have been reported, but these have not been sufficiently frequent or severe to preclude its use when necessary. Vaccination coupled with good isolation and quarantine procedures for new arrivals is the best available means for controlling the disease at present. It should be emphasized that efforts to control this disease by vaccination alone will be disappointing. A vaccination program must be accompanied by sound management practices.

Rhinotracheitis, Infectious Bovine (Rednose)

Infectious bovine rhinotracheitis (IBR) is a common upper respiratory infection of cattle that is most prevalent in fall and winter. Symptomatically, the typical case is not unlike a severe head cold in humans, with fever, coughing, eye and nasal discharge, and depressed appetite.

The first indication of the disease is usually a dry, hacking cough involving just a few animals. This cough is accompanied by fever, lack of appetite, and a clear nasal discharge, which later in the disease becomes mucupurulent. The disease affects cattle of all ages and is occasionally fatal for young calves. Unless complicated by secondary pneumonia, IBR is rarely fatal for adult cattle, and its principal economic effect is lost production during the acute attack. Like BVD virus, however, it will cause abortions, usually beginning about 3 weeks after the episode passes. In the individual animal, recovery takes place in about 4 to 7 days. The virus spreads rapidly through the herd by aerosol dispersion, however, and it may be 2 months before all signs of disease disappear from the herd.

Eye Involvement

While the foregoing symptoms may be considered a description of typical IBR, the effect of the virus can be quite variable. Concurrent with an acute attack, a few individuals may develop a corneal opacity easily confused with pink eye. With pink eye, the opacity spreads *outward* from a central ulcer of the cornea, whereas with IBR, in most cases the opacity spreads *inward* from the periphery and there is no ulceration. With eye involvement the sclera, or white part of the eye, becomes reddened. The term *rednose* developed from the appearance of the white nose of Hereford cattle in the feedlots. Just as we get a reddened sore nose when we have a bad head cold, so do cattle, and this is most striking in cattle with a white muzzle. In a herd outbreak, a few animals may develop raised, whitish plaques on the lining of the nostrils and vagina. These lesions, if present, are good evidence that IBR is the problem.

Occasionally, a more severe genital infection called *infectious pustular vulvovaginitis* occurs in cattle. It is caused by the same IBR virus and is spread primarily during breeding. Whether the virus affects the respiratory system or the genitalia seems to be determined by the route of infection.

IBR virus can be very insidious. It may pass through a herd without any observable clinical signs, but a month or two later a rash of unexplained abortions may occur. Careful necropsy of an aborted fetus may reveal lesions suggestive of IBR. If the tissue is fresh, the fluorescent antibody test can be used to confirm the diagnosis. Testing the dam's blood serum for antibody has limited value. If it is negative, then the abortion was probably not due to IBR. If the sample is positive, it means only that sometime in the past the cow was exposed to IBR. That exposure may be entirely unrelated to the abortion.

Transmission

Once infected with this member of the herpesvirus group, some cattle will harbor the virus for indefinite periods and shed virus particles intermittently, especially during periods of stress. This shedding serves as a source of infection for new animals added to the herd and for contact animals at fairs and shows. It is also a concern of bull stud managers because it has been shown that the virus can be transmitted in semen, although such transmission is uncommon. Nevertheless, bulls in the reputable studs are routinely tested for IBR, and many stud managers will not buy bulls that have been IBR vaccinated because the vaccine virus–antibody titer confuses test results.

Treatment

Like all virus diseases, there is no effective treatment for IBR. Antibiotics are routinely used, however, to prevent secondary infection. The best way to handle the disease is by protection through vaccination. Both killed and modified live-virus vaccines are available and provide good immunity when properly used. The killed vaccine must be used annually, while the modified live virus will provide much longer immunity. Because of the risk of vaccine virus–induced abortion, the latter should not be used on pregnant cows. It is available singly or in combination with BVD vaccine. If given to all calves at 6 to 8 months of age, an immune herd can be maintained.

Infectious bovine rhinotracheitis is the first cattle disease for which a vaccine has been developed that is administered by spraying it into the nostrils (intranasal instillation). It must be repeated annually but has the advantage of producing rapid local immunity in the respiratory tract with few, if any, adverse side effects. The variety of vaccines available makes the choice difficult for an individual without the training and experience to make an intelligent decision. For that reason, an immunization program worked out with the advice of your veterinarian and designed for your herd circumstances is more likely to be successful. By all means, don't do what I have seen many farmers do — wait until a few cows start coughing before deciding to vaccinate. Vaccination when the infection is already present has little if any value and may actually make a bad situation worse. The time to vaccinate is *before* the need arises, while the cattle are still healthy.

Scrapie

Although uncommon in the United States, this disease of sheep and goats is an enigma in many respects. First, the causative agent was once theorized to be a virus, although virus has not been isolated from affected sheep. Some investigators believe the causative agent to be an aberrant host cellular protein, designated a *prion,* which can bring about formation of additional abnormal protein in genetically susceptible individuals. Much more research needs to be done and is, in fact, under way with regard to bovine spongiform encephalopathy. Nevertheless, the disease has been reproduced in test animals by inoculation of brain suspension from those showing clinical signs, indicating that it is a transmissible disease. Second, it appears in certain bloodlines of sheep more than others, especially in the Suffolk breed. Third, it doesn't appear until sheep are 2 years of age or older, and it is more likely to occur in the progeny of those who later develop the disease. The mode of transmission in nature is most commonly from ewe to newborn lambs via uterine fluid and placenta.

The earliest sign may be excitability, with almost imperceptible tremor of the head and neck. As the disease progresses, there may be a peculiar high-stepping gait or even convulsions in response to external stimuli. One of the more obvious clinical signs, reminiscent of pseudorabies, is intense itching sufficient to interfere with eating or sleeping. The wool may come out in patches where the animals rub themselves. The clinical signs intensify over weeks or months, eventually terminating in death.

Similar transmissible spongiform encephalopathies have been reported in mink, mule deer, elk, and cattle. In England in 1991–92, a major outbreak in cattle is thought to have resulted from feeding processed animal protein from sheep to dairy cattle. In cattle, the disease is called *bovine spongiform encephalopathy,* or more commonly *mad cow disease.*

At the moment, the disease is not prevalent, but the sheep grower should be aware of its existence and know the clinical signs. Scrapie is a legally reportable disease, and the established control program, once a diagnosis is made, is quarantine and slaughter of all affected and exposed animals. While this may seem radical, with a disease such as this with low prevalence, unknown epidemiology, and fatal consequences, it is the most logical approach.

Stomatitis, Vesicular

Cattle, horses, and swine as well as a number of wild animals are susceptible to this vesicular disease, and human cases have occasionally been reported. This is one of a group of viral diseases referred to as *vesicular* because of the blisterlike vesicles that the virus produces. Several serious foreign animal diseases, foot-and-mouth disease, swine vesicular disease, and vesicular exanthema produce identical lesions, so prompt and accurate diagnosis is important.

Symptoms

Vesicular stomatitis occurs sporadically in all parts of the United States, usually during the warmer months, and is recognizable by fever and development of vesicles on the lips and tongue, on the nostrils and muzzle of cattle, and frequently in the interdigital space and on the bulb of the heel in cattle and swine. In fact, lameness may be the first sign noted in swine. Excess salivation and drooling usually are a sequel to the mouth lesions. The incubation period is up to 5 days, and the disease may spread rapidly through the herd by direct contact, because the vesicular fluid is teeming with virus, and probably also via insect vectors. Appetite is depressed due to soreness when mouth lesions are present. The disease is self-limiting, usually with complete recovery in about 2 weeks. Recovered animals are immune to further infection for about a year. Dairy cows may develop vesicles on the teats and udder, and when the teat end is involved, secondary mastitis may occur.

The disease occurs sporadically with several years elapsing between outbreaks in a given area, and the natural reservoir of the virus is unknown. Because of the commonly long interval between outbreaks, the use of vaccine is indicated primarily to protect animals at risk when an outbreak occurs.

Treatment

No specific treatment is available, although topical application of antibiotic ointments may reduce the complication of secondary infection. The disease is generally not of sufficient importance or sufficiently common to warrant special precautions to prevent introduction to the herd other than the usual caveat, "Raise all your own replacements." Vaccine is used to control the disease in some South American countries.

The chief importance of vesicular stomatitis is its similarity to the much more serious foreign vesicular diseases. Diagnosis can be confirmed by serologic test or virus isolation, but animal susceptibility is the classic and perhaps most certain way of distinguishing between them. Table 8-1 shows the varying susceptibility of different animals to each disease.

TABLE 8-1	DISEASE SUSCEPTIBILITY		
	HORSE	COW	PIG
Vesicular stomatitis	+	+	+
Foot-and-mouth	–	+	+
Vesicular exanthema	–	–	+
Swine vesicular disease	–	–	+

+ = susceptible; – = resistant

Diseases Caused by Yeasts, Molds, and Fungi

WITH A FEW EXCEPTIONS, most organisms in this category are not pathogenic and cause disease only rarely as secondary invaders. The exceptions, however, deserve some discussion.

Abortion, Mycotic

Abortions due to mold infection of the fetus and placenta occur sporadically in all species but perhaps most commonly in the cow. Mold species of the genera *Aspergillus* and *Mucor* are generally responsible. In most cases the mold spores are probably introduced at the time of breeding, although some researchers believe occasional infections occur when spores are conveyed via the circulatory system to the placenta. Frequently, aborted fetuses will have skin lesions that look like ringworm, and the placenta is always greatly thickened, with evidence of necrosis, especially in the cotyledons.

Although mold infections are a minor cause of abortion, they contribute to the overall problems of reproduction, and effort to prevent them will help to improve breeding efficiency. For this and other reasons, moldy feed should be avoided insofar as possible.

The cleanest technique possible should be used when breeding by either artificial insemination or natural service. Scrub the vulva and surrounding area thoroughly with soap and water, and wipe it dry prior to inserting the insemination pipette. This helps reduce the risk of introducing other miscellaneous infections. The same procedure applied to the prepuce and sheath of the bull will help improve conception rates by natural service. Equine stud managers have learned by experience that cleanliness at breeding time is essential, and the same applies to other animal species.

Mycotoxicoses

This name is given to a group of disease conditions caused not directly by molds themselves but by the poisons they produce, mycotoxins.

A *mycotoxin* is a fungal metabolite that exerts a deleterious effect on a biological system. For example, most antibiotics are mycotoxins, which, at therapeutic levels, are more toxic for bacteria than they are for animals. Historically, ergot was the first known mycotoxin. Epidemics of dry gangrene and nervous derangement in humans, undoubtedly due to ergot, were recorded as early as the eleventh century. The source was contaminated rye used in bread. Interest in mycotoxins has paralleled the interest in antibiotics and has accelerated since 1940.

More than one hundred molds are known to produce toxic metabolites under certain conditions of temperature, moisture, oxygen tension, pH, and type of substrate. Of these, twenty-five to thirty have been associated with animal disease. They produce a wide variety of effects, some clinically dramatic and others clinically unrecognizable. Toxins may be produced by molds on the standing crop or in stored feeds. Mycotoxin, when present, may be in the mold itself or diffused into the substrate. It is visually unidentifiable.

There is considerable species variation in susceptibility to mycotoxins. Swine and poultry are quite susceptible, followed by horses, cattle, sheep, and goats. Humans and fish are near the top of the list. Similarly, some feedstuffs favor the growth of toxigenic fungi more than others. Aflatoxin, for example, is commonly found in peanuts, cottonseed, copra, corn, grain, sorghum, barley, and apple juice. Many mycotoxins are heat-stable and survive canning, pelleting, and other such processes.

Detection of mycotoxins in feeds is difficult. It is possible to have grossly moldy feed without any mycotoxin present. Conversely, feeds without obvious mold may contain mycotoxins. Distribution of mycotoxin in stored feeds is rarely uniform, and detection presents a problem. Black-light screening for mold fluorescence is a moderately good rough method, but it is effective only when the mold is living and does not indicate the presence of mycotoxin. Chemical analysis is the most satisfactory detection method. Unfortunately, few laboratories are equipped to do it, and those that will accept samples for analysis are generally set up to test for only a few of the known mycotoxins.

With a few exceptions, the clinical signs of mycotoxicoses in animals have not been well defined. Much of the available data are from experimental work with laboratory animals that has been extrapolated to livestock. Therefore, it is difficult to say with certainty that a particular syndrome is attributable to a specific mycotoxin.

Note: It is probable that some unexplained disease syndromes in livestock may be in fact due to a mycotoxicosis; however, we should avoid the temptation to attribute every obscure syndrome to mycotoxins. Fortunately, except for fatalities, the effects of most of the mycotoxicoses are reversible once the toxin is removed. The prudent course is to avoid the use of moldy feeds, but if moldy feeds must be used, they should be fed cautiously to a few animals to observe the effects rather than fed to the entire herd at the outset. Because the effect of mycotoxins is dose related, it may occasionally be possible to salvage moldy feed by diluting it with feed that is not moldy.

Aflatoxin

The best known of the mycotoxins in stored grain is aflatoxin from *Aspergillus flavus* and *Aspergillus parasiticus.* The aflatoxins are a group of toxic metabolites that vary in their toxic and carcinogenic potential. The susceptibility of different animal species to aflatoxins also appears to be variable. Acute aflatoxicosis causes hepatitis, hepatic cell necrosis, and prolonged clotting time. Affected animals often die with severe hemorrhages, and feeds containing as little as 1 ppm can cause acute poisoning in some animals. In *subacute poisoning,* the changes in the liver include cell destruction, regeneration, and repair, with areas of scar tissue formation and bile duct proliferation. Growth rate and protein formation are depressed, but the animal may or may not die. *Chronic poisoning,* in addition to retarding rate of growth, lowers resistance to disease, and in turkey poults has been shown to impair the immune response to vaccination. Chronic poisoning results in icterus and liver cirrhosis. Prolonged consumption of as little as 0.5 ppb is carcinogenic in some animals.

Ergot

Ergot poisoning is due to the alkaloids produced by the fungus *Claviceps purpurea.* There are two forms of ergotism commonly observed in domestic animals: a convulsive form and a gangrenous form. The *convulsive form* is characterized by vertigo and muscle spasms of the hind limbs, followed by temporary paralysis. The *gangrenous form* is characterized by lameness, which can be followed by loss of the limbs, tail, and ears. In cattle and sheep, in addition to lameness, the animals commonly have decreased rate of gain and increased body temperature and respiratory rate. In swine, although there are reports of decreased rates of gain and feed efficiency, the most common signs are agalactia and dead pigs at birth. There is some evidence that ergot interferes with reproduction.

Ochratoxin

Ochratoxin A, from *Aspergillus ochraceous,* causes hepatic and renal damage in rats. It also causes fetal resorption and abortion in pregnant rats. Similar signs have been seen in livestock fed moldy feeds, although in these cases ochratoxicosis has been diagnosed retrospectively.

Rubratoxin

Rubratoxins are potent hepatotoxic, hemorrhage-inducing metabolites of *Penicillium rubrum* and *Penicillium purpurogenum,* common soil fungi that frequently contaminate animal feeds. The role of these substances in naturally occurring disease is suspected, but has not been demonstrated definitively.

Slaframine

This mycotoxin from *Rhizoctonia leguminicola* found in red clover has been identified as the cause of excessive salivation and reduced milk production and body weight in dairy cattle. Salivation is the most consistent sign, followed by lacrimation, diarrhea, frequent urination, and anorexia.

Tremortina

This toxin from several species of *Penicillium* induces tremor, ataxia, and tonic, clonic convulsions when administered to animals. In experimental work, 2.5 mg/kg was sufficient to cause clinical signs. The first sign of toxicity in calves was a fine tremor that increased in severity with forced movement or excitement. With continued consumption, the tremors became more severe; the calves stood with legs stiff and spread apart and swayed rhythmically. When forced to move, their gait was stilted and they were ataxic. In the most severely affected, there was lateral recumbency with paddling, intermittent extensor rigidity, opisthotonos, and severe tremors.

T-2 Toxin

Fusarium tricinctum is consistently the most toxigenic fungus isolated from moldy corn. Its principal effect is necrosis of the skin, oral mucous membrane, intestine, and liver. Fatal doses can be absorbed through the skin, with large necrotic areas developing at the point of absorption. Sublethal doses produce a hemorrhagic syndrome similar to that of other mycotoxicoses. The death of seven out of thirty-five cows in a Wisconsin herd was attributed to T-2 toxin in 1971.

Fescue foot, a progressive lameness of cattle, with heat, swelling, pain, and later gangrene, has long been recognized as a hazard of grazing on pastures containing tall fescue. More recent evidence indicates that the condition is due not to the fescue itself but to a mycotoxin form mold growing on the fescue. The clinical signs strongly resemble those produced by *F. tricinctum* toxin.

Zearalenone

The effect of F2 or zearalenone, from *Fusarium roseum* and related species, on swine is well known. It is a potent estrogenic substance producing characteristic sexual changes, such as swelling of the vulva, enlargement of the mammary glands, and uterine hyperplasia. Stunting of male and female swine has also been observed following consumption of *F. roseum*–contaminated corn. Evidence exists that the fungus produces several interrelated substances that may affect animals synergistically, inasmuch as contaminated corn has a much greater effect on pigs than does an equivalent amount of purified F2 toxin. Other fungal metabolites associated with vomiting and feed refusal have been found in *F. roseum*–contaminated corn and cause significant economic effects.

Zearalenone is a not an uncommon cause of sow infertility.

Ringworm

In terms of frequency of occurrence, this is the most important fungal infection of livestock. Several species of the genus *Trichophyton* are responsible for most cases, and the disease is seen most frequently in cattle, horses, swine, goats, and sheep — in that order.

If you have studied biology, you may recall that fungi grow with many branching hyphae and reproduce by sporulation. Infection occurs within the surface layer of the skin, and hyphae extend down into the hair follicles and sometimes into the hairs, causing the hair to break off or fall out.

Symptoms

Ringworm in cattle is more common in calves and yearlings than in adults and is more prevalent during the winter months, although it can occur throughout the year. The face and neck are the most frequent sites of infection in cattle, and the early lesions appear as small, slightly raised areas with the hair roughened rather than smooth. This hair falls out, leaving grayish circumscribed areas

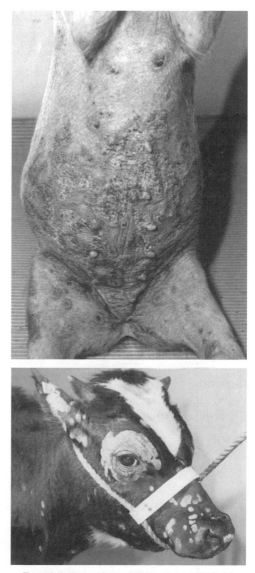

Typical ringworm lesions are seen in a pig (top) and a calf (bottom).

varying in size, from almost imperceptible to large patches at least 3 inches in diameter. It is not unusual to see a gray ring completely around the eyes of cattle.

The lesions in the horse are somewhat similar but are more inclined to be moist and weeping and located where parts of the harness rub. In swine the lesions appear more like ringworm in humans, starting as a reddened area that gradually enlarges, with the center healing as the disease progresses outward. This leads to lesions that appear as circles, which gave rise to the superstition years ago that the infection was caused by a "*ring* worm." Although the name stuck, we now know that the condition is caused not by a worm at all but by a fungus. Although it causes itching and discomfort, ringworm is not a serious disease and tends to be self-limiting, although it may persist for months. Nevertheless, it is unsightly and, more important, contagious to humans. Effort should be made, therefore, to control and treat it.

Prevention

Prevention of ringworm through the usual isolation and quarantine procedures applied to infectious diseases is not effective. Spores of *Trichophyton* species are ubiquitous, and most animals carry some spores on the skin all the time, with no evidence of infection. The disease is more likely to occur in the presence of filth, when nutrition is marginal, and when sunlight is lacking. Calves kept in dark, damp, filthy pens on a marginal diet almost invariably develop ringworm. Ultraviolet rays from the sun help to reduce development of ringworm spores, and particular attention should be paid to the content of vitamin A in the diet, as vitamin A plays an important role in maintaining the resistance of epithelium. Frequent grooming is helpful, especially for horses, using clean brushes and curry combs. These should be cleaned and disinfected after each use to help prevent spread of infection.

Diagnosis of ringworm is generally not difficult because of the characteristic nature of the lesions. However, if there is any question, microscopic examination of deep skin scrapings in the laboratory will generally reveal the typical hyphae of the organism. It can also be cultured on selective media, but this takes considerably longer.

Treatment

Treatment is not as easy as the diagnosis. The organism is susceptible to a variety of drugs if the drugs reach it. The single most important thing in treatment is to remove the scabs with soap, water, and a stiff brush, because the organism is in the skin. Simply painting the lesions with iodine or similar solution without this important first step usually gives disappointing results. Many different drugs are effective, including copper naphthenate, tincture of iodine, and even ordinary household bleach diluted in water (1 part bleach to

10 parts water). When the lesions are extensive, these simple remedies may not be practical. In these cases, high-pressure sprays using fungicides such as lime sulfur may be required. The latter is not cleared by the U.S. Food and Drug Administration (FDA) for use on food-producing animals, however. Before embarking on a heroic treatment plan such as spraying or dipping, the advice of your veterinarian would be a good investment.

Sporotrichosis

This disease, caused by a fungus, is seen primarily in horses and occasionally in goats. The condition takes the form of multiple small, painless nodules on the skin that discharge small amounts of pus. Initial infection probably occurs via wound contamination. The disease does not spread rapidly, and the lesions usually heal in 3 to 4 weeks. Occasionally, however, the infection may spread via the lymphatics to other areas and organs of the body, causing serious disease. Outbreaks are more likely to occur when horses are stabled, due to a higher concentration of mold spores in the environment.

The disease responds well to treatment and most cases can be prevented by careful disinfection of cuts and abrasions. It should be noted that sporotrichosis can be transmitted to humans, particularly those who may be immunocompromised.

Yeast Infections

Infections with organisms of this group, especially *Candida* species, often follow prolonged indiscriminate antibiotic therapy. Yeast mastitis in cattle and goats causes an acute inflammation, with fever, swelling of the udder, change in milk consistency to almost a creamy pus, and virtually total cessation of milk flow. Treatment other than symptomatic attention is of little use. In most cases, recovery occurs in about 2 weeks, but some cows never return to their former level of full production.

Almost invariably the infection is introduced during faulty udder infusion technique or via contaminated medication. Serious herd outbreaks have occurred when mastitic cows were treated with "homemade" antibiotic mixtures that became contaminated. Multiple-dose vials should *never* be used to treat cows for mastitis.

Prolonged use of oral antibiotics can also promote overgrowth of yeast in the intestinal tract, causing chronic enteritis in young animals. Yeasts are essentially microflora in the gut that can become pathogenic when people unwisely interfere.

Diseases 10 Caused by Protozoa and Rickettsia

ALTHOUGH, AS A GENERAL RULE, protozoan diseases are more of a problem in the Tropics than domestically, several species of pathogenic protozoa are economically significant in the United States. *Protozoa* are single-cell organisms, much larger than bacteria, and are widely distributed in nature. Those that are pathogenic tend to be host specific, and about half of them require the assistance of a vector to spread from one animal to the next.

Anaplasmosis

There is disagreement among taxonomists as to whether *Anaplasma marginale*, the organism responsible for this disease, is a protozoan or whether it more properly should be classed with the bacteria family Rickettsiaceae. For our purpose it makes little difference. Suffice to say that it is a blood-borne parasite causing anemia in cattle, sheep, and goats that is a major problem, especially in the Gulf and Pacific Coast states. Isolated cases have been identified in the north-central and northeastern United States, but the disease is not endemic in those areas.

The effect of anaplasmosis on the animal is variable, depending on age, resistance, and possibly the size of the infecting dose. Young animals are more resistant to anaplasmosis than are adults, which is atypical of most diseases. With most infectious diseases it is usually the other way around, with adults having sufficient immunity through prior exposure to be resistant.

Symptoms

The incubation period may be as long as 3 weeks, and onset of clinical signs is marked by persistent high fever, lack of appetite, and depression. The organism attacks red blood cells, causing anemia, which in turn results in rapid pulse and respiration, pale mucous membranes, dehydration, and weight loss. Exertion may result in collapse of the animal due to hypoxia. The disease may be peracute, with death in 1 or 2 days; acute, lasting 10 days to 2 weeks; or chronic. A few animals never recover completely and remain thin and unthrifty. In adult cattle, especially range cattle, where the disease may not be recognized and treated early, mortality up to 50 percent may occur.

In nature the organism, *A. marginale,* is spread from infected to susceptible cattle by biting insects, particularly ticks and biting flies. Of these, ticks are the more important vector, and the organism may survive in the tick for several months. In the United States, prevalence of the disease tends to parallel the natural distribution of the several ticks serving as vectors. Anaplasmosis is not transferable through direct contact but instead requires mechanical transfer of a droplet of infected blood. On occasion, humans have done this more effectively than insects. Serious herd outbreaks have occurred when animals were vaccinated with the same contaminated needle. In endemic areas it's especially important to sterilize surgical instruments, hypodermic needles, tattoo instruments, tagging pliers, and other implements after each use. Recovered animals commonly remain carriers for life. A few may relapse to clinical disease when subjected to stress from any source. In areas where the disease is endemic, exposure of young animals resistant to the disease helps to establish an immune population.

Treatment

When the disease is detected early, infected animals respond fairly well to treatment with broad-spectrum antibiotics such as chlortetracycline and oxytetracycline. Elimination of the carrier state requires therapy with these drugs for 30 to 60 days. Several different serologic tests are available to confirm the diagnosis, but during the acute illness, microscopic examination of a stained blood smear usually reveals the organism at the margin of red blood cells.

Prevention

Prevention of the disease depends on vector control through spraying or dipping with insecticides, careful disinfection of surgical instruments, and vaccination. A killed vaccine is available that does a reasonably good job of preventing new infections.

Babesiosis

Several species of *Babesia* infect horses, cattle, sheep, and swine in various parts of the world, but currently in the United States — specifically in Florida — only *Babesia caballi,* which causes infection in horses, is of importance. This was not always the case, and cattle babesiosis, also called *Texas fever* or *cattle tick fever,* at one time was a serious threat to the beef industry in the Southwest. Babesiosis is spread by ticks, and eradication of the specific tick responsible for Texas fever in the United States through quarantine and cattle dipping programs was a major milestone in the history of veterinary medicine.

Symptoms

Like anaplasmosis, *Babesia* species invade red blood cells, causing anemia and sometimes jaundice. They also cause red cells to swell, with a resulting sludging of cells in the capillaries. When this is sufficiently severe, circulatory impairment occurs, and symptoms associated with organ dysfunction such as hepatitis and nephritis result. Severity of signs is a function of the size of the infecting dose and resistance of the animal. In horses the disease is called *piroplasmosis,* and clinical signs include high fever, jaundice, anemia, subcutaneous edema, rapid pulse, and general weakness. Many infected horses develop petechial hemorrhages in the conjunctiva, and some show signs of colic. The disease may be acute, with death occurring within 48 hours; subacute, with apparent recovery in about 2 weeks; or chronic, in which case the animal fails to gain weight and lacks the stamina for hard work.

Prevention

At the moment, prevention is basically a matter of keeping infected ticks and susceptible horses apart by daily grooming and application of insecticides to the horse or, if prevalence warrants, area spraying. The latter is not widely used due to the adverse effect of insecticides on other insects. Similarly, some of the most effective insecticides cannot be used legally on animals because of their environmental persistence. Although it would be possible technically to eradicate this disease in Florida through vector eradication, as was done with Texas fever, it is highly unlikely that such a program will be undertaken because of possible adverse effects on other insects and wildlife. It should be remembered that, like anaplasmosis and other blood-borne diseases, equine piroplasmosis can be spread by contaminated surgical instruments.

Coccidiosis

This is the most common protozoan disease in the United States, affecting virtually all species of animals. Its effects are serious in cattle, sheep, and goats, occasionally in swine, and much less commonly in horses.

Symptoms

Coccidia have an interesting life cycle that has bearing on the characteristics of the disease they produce. The principal clinical sign in all species is profuse, often bloody, diarrhea. Clinical signs follow ingestion of infective oocysts, which have been passed out in the feces of other animals that may or may not have been clinically ill themselves. Infective oocysts contain sporozoites that escape from the oocyst and invade intestinal cells, where they develop into schizonts.

These divide asexually into merozoites, which invade additional cells to cause extensive intestinal inflammation. After several of these asexual cycles, a sexual generation occurs, with development of micro- and macrogametocytes, ultimately forming a zygote that becomes encapsulated as an oocyst and is passed out in the feces. At this point, the oocyst is not infective and must undergo further development outside the body. Under favorable moisture and temperature conditions, sporozoites form in the oocyst in about a week and they are then infective. Typically, an initial acute attack of coccidiosis will subside only to recur in 1 to 2 weeks. The apparent recovery occurs when the oocysts are forming and before reinfection with the sporulated oocysts occurs.

Eimeria and *Isospora* are the two most common pathogenic genera of coccidia, and there are many species within each genus. The species tend to be quite host specific. While infection of aberrant species may occur, it is usually transitory and inconsequential.

Coccidiosis is a disease primarily of young animals. Mature animals, although commonly infected, usually have developed sufficient immunity that clinical signs do not develop. They periodically shed oocysts, however, and are probably the source of infection for younger generations on the farm.

The effect of acute coccidiosis can be quite devastating, with diarrhea, rapid dehydration, and sufficient blood loss to require blood transfusion to save the animal's life. Some animals may be less severely affected and show only inappetence and reduced rate of gain. The history, clinical signs, and microscopic identification of the organism in the feces are sufficient to confirm the diagnosis. A single negative microscopic finding may be misleading, because in the early stages, oocysts may be present in the feces only in very small numbers. This goes back to the life cycle explained above, and a few days later overwhelming numbers of oocysts may be seen in a fecal sample.

Treatment

Left untreated, mortality of calves, lambs, and goats may range up to 10 percent or more, and those that recover from the acute attacks undergo a long recuperative period that reduces weight gain and growth rate. Furthermore, the debility caused by the disease often leads to complications such as pneumonia. Therefore, treatment early in the disease is important. Blood transfusion when indicated and sulfonamides orally or intravenously are the usual effective treatments. Individual treatment is most desirable, but in a flock or herd outbreak the labor requirement may make this impossible. In such cases, medicated feed or drinking water may be the only feasible route. Lasalocid, one of a group of drugs called *ionophores,* has been approved as a feed additive for prevention of coccidiosis in lambs. It also has the advantage of improving feed-conversion efficiency in beef cattle as well as in lambs. Other drugs such as monensin, amprolium, and decoquinate are used in the same manner.

Prevention

As with every other disease, prevention is far more rewarding than treatment. Because infection occurs by ingestion of oocysts, and these originate in manure of infected animals, it follows that overcrowding of animals in a given area will increase the concentration of oocysts on the ground. This is the reason coccidiosis is more of a problem in beef and lamb feedlots. The problem is obviously greater when animals are fed on the ground, where feed rapidly becomes contaminated. The same thing happens when the only source of drinking water is pools or streams. To reduce the risk of infection by coccidia and other internal parasites, don't overcrowd pastures, rotate pastures frequently, and in confinement such as feedlots, put feed in bunks or troughs protected from fecal contamination. In feedlots where coccidiosis has been a problem, some operators have found it advantageous to begin medication of animals when they arrive, as a prophylactic measure during the stress period, until they become adapted to the new surroundings and diet. On the dairy farm, rearing calves in individual hutches, as described earlier, will almost completely eliminate the problem.

Eperythrozoonosis

The significance of the disease caused by an *Eperythrozoon* species capable of infecting cattle, sheep, goats, and pigs is not clearly understood. It is a blood-borne parasite, found in pigs more often than in other species, that is transmitted by biting lice. In other species, transmission is primarily by ticks. The organism attacks red blood cells, producing clinical signs similar to those of anaplasmosis and babesiosis.

Early treatment with broad-spectrum antibiotics such as tetracycline is helpful. Prevention is best accomplished through control of insect vectors.

Neosporosis

This disease, caused by the protozoan *Neospora caninum,* has only recently been recognized as a major cause of abortion in cattle in the United States. Dogs are the natural reservoir of the organism, and in addition to cattle, it can infect sheep, goats, deer, and horses. Symptoms of the disease in cattle are not pathognomic and can easily be confused with the stillbirths and abortions seen with other diseases. Abortions can occur at any time but are more common during the second trimester, and cows can abort more than once during lactation. Clinical signs of the disease are limited to the reproductive tract and fetus.

Current evidence indicates that the disease is not transmitted directly from cow to cow but, rather, is spread by ingestion of the organism. Calves infected at birth remain infected. It follows, then, that control is best accomplished by preventing fecal contamination of feedstuffs by dogs. Positive animals, dog and cow, can be identified by blood tests. Where circumstances permit, negative cows can be kept in a separate herd and those that are positive can be culled as rapidly as is economically feasible. Ultimately, a negative herd will result, provided good sanitary practices are followed.

A promising vaccine is currently being evaluated.

Toxoplasmosis

The protozoan *Toxoplasma gondii* is capable of infecting all mammalian species, although among livestock it is most significant in swine and sheep. Sows may be infected without showing any signs of illness and may transmit the organism to their piglets *in utero* or via milk. Clinically affected piglets may show evidence of pneumonia, enteritis, hepatitis, and nephritis. The clinical infection is not common, but occasional serious outbreaks have been reported. Some individuals involved in an outbreak may show signs of encephalitis. Cats are the primary reservoir of the organism.

Toxoplasmosis is an important cause of abortion in sheep in some parts of the world. Ewes themselves rarely show signs of illness, but fetal tissue and the placenta are apparently quite susceptible. Although not a significant problem in the United States, that *T. gondii* is widely prevalent makes the infection a possibility in otherwise unexplained flock abortion problems. Correlation of characteristic microscopic lesions in the fetus with positive serologic tests on the ewe would confirm the diagnosis.

The mechanism by which toxoplasmosis spreads is not clearly defined. *In utero* transfer, ingestion of contaminated meat and milk, and inhalation of infective droplets are all possible routes. With so many routes of infection and others probably unknown, control recommendations other than the usual recommendation for good sanitation are difficult to make. The fact that the organism is widespread and the clinical disease uncommon leads one to believe that specific control procedures are probably unnecessary A word of caution is in order, however. Toxoplasmosis also infects humans and is particularly hazardous for the unborn infant. Although the family cat has been implicated in human infections far more often than livestock, people handling known infected animals should be cautious and, at the very least, scrub thoroughly with soap and water when through.

Trichomoniasis

Trichomonas foetus causes a true venereal disease in cattle, resulting in early embryonic death or abortion and pyometra. Irregular heat periods at long intervals are characteristic of the disease. Infection of the bull is inapparent and persists for the life of the animal. The disease is spread to the cow at the time of coitus, and if the cow is given complete sexual rest, the disease will generally disappear after several months. The principal effect is economic loss through delayed breeding. Occasionally, there will be some discharge of pus from the vagina, but other clinical signs of illness are rarely noted.

Trichomoniasis is a problem only in herds where natural service is used. Artificial insemination prevents infection because dilution of semen and, in most cases, freezing reduces the number of trichomonads to a very low or non-existent level. Artificial insemination is the single most important means of preventing the disease.

Diagnosis

Trichomoniasis is an insidious disease, and the entire herd may be infected before its presence is realized. Diagnosis is based on history and identification of the organism, either by direct microscopic examination of vaginal mucus or preputial washings or by fluorescent antibody test using the same fluids. The organism may also be found in fluids from the placenta and in stomach fluid of an aborted fetus. It is not easy to find, however, and a single negative sample can be misleading. Fluids from a number of cows in the herd should be checked, and where the history is compatible, finding a single trichomonad confirms the diagnosis.

Once the diagnosis is made, steps can be taken to eliminate the infection from the herd. It may take a year or more to accomplish. The first essential step is to stop all natural breeding and to exclusively use artificial insemination. The disease is self-limiting in the cow, provided the source of infection — the bull — is removed. A few cows develop sufficient resistance to carry a calf to term, despite infection, which only confuses the history and diagnosis. Infected bulls remain infected, and the best place for them is the slaughterhouse. Although infected bulls can be treated, treatment is laborious. It must be repeated several times, and samples must be checked over a period of several months to determine effectiveness of treatment. Even then, there is a chance that the last organism may not be killed and the infection will recur once the treatment and surveillance procedures are stopped. Nationwide, prevalence of the disease is low, and it isn't worth the risk of perpetuating it by trying to salvage infected bulls.

Prevention

Prevention of trichomoniasis is easily accomplished by exclusively using artificial insemination. If a bull must be used, select as herd sire a young virgin bull that has never bred cattle before. And for added insurance, mate him with a couple of virgin heifers first before putting the bull with the herd. If the heifers become pregnant, confirmed by rectal examination, you can be reasonably sure the bull is not carrying trichomoniasis. You will also have the added assurance that the bull is fertile. A vaccine is now available, to be used prior to the breeding season.

Parasitism

TECHNICALLY SPEAKING, any organism that lives at the expense of its host is a parasite. Under this definition, pathogenic bacteria, viruses, yeasts, molds, fungi, and protozoa are parasites. In common usage, however, when we speak of parasites in animals, we are referring to several types of worms (internal parasites) and insects (external parasites). There is also a third category, wherein the larval stage of an insect becomes an internal parasite. A good example of the latter is the stomach bot of the horse.

Internal Parasitism

All species of animals, including humans, are susceptible to a variety of internal parasites. Among livestock, sheep, horses, goats, and cattle are most susceptible to parasitism. Although there are exceptions, some general statements can be made about internal parasitism that will be helpful in designing a parasite-control program suitable for your circumstances.

First, most internal parasites are host specific, and those that thrive in one species — the swine ascarid, for example — will not infect other animal species, except perhaps for brief periods. Second, most internal parasites have direct life cycles — that is, they develop to maturity in the intestinal tract; lay eggs that are passed out in manure, contaminating pastures and drinking water; and infect other animals when they consume the contaminated feed or water. Last, it is virtually impossible under farm or range conditions to raise parasite-free animals. Generally, the best that can be hoped for is to keep parasitism at a sufficiently low level so that the effect on the animal is minimal.

There is a school of thought among many competent parasitologists that a low level of infection may actually be desirable because it stimulates some immunity (premunition), thereby protecting the animal from overwhelming exposure. This has been demonstrated with haemonchosis in sheep. The premunition concept is being actively pursued, and in the not too distant future, we may see vaccines cleared for use in the United States that will prevent major worm infestations. Such products are currently in limited use in Europe.

Physical Condition

Another important generality that can be applied, particularly to the stomach and intestinal worms, is that they are most prevalent in and detrimental to the animal that is in poor physical condition for some other reason, the major one being malnutrition. The biological interrelationship of living things, whether it be mutualistic, commensalistic, or parasitic, is complex, interesting, and sometimes even logical. In the case of parasitism, a delicate balance is maintained in nature between the welfare of the parasite and its host. All other things being equal, the parasite will persist in numbers sufficient to maintain its race but not in numbers lethal to the host. Because the parasite must have a host to survive, destruction of the host would be self-defeating. Among wild animals, internal parasitism is universal and rarely fatal. Among domestic animals, parasitism is also universal but is frequently fatal because people, either through lack of knowledge or lack of caring, upset the delicate host/parasite relationship. A well-nourished animal not under stress can withstand a parasite burden far in excess of what would kill one that is half-starved.

Susceptibility of Sheep

Of all livestock species, sheep are the most susceptible to infection with gastrointestinal worms, and the principal genera affecting sheep, goats, and cattle are *Haemonchus, Ostertagia, Trichostrongylus, Oesophagostomum, Bunostomum,* and *Cooperia.* Of these, *Haemonchus* is perhaps the most pathogenic for sheep. It and *Bunostomum* are bloodsucking worms, and the major signs of serious infection are anemia and edema, particularly of the submandibular region, giving rise to the term *bottle jaw.* Under certain conditions, haemonchosis in sheep can give the impression of a peracute infectious fatal disease. Sheep grazing a heavily contaminated pasture a few days after a warm rainfall can undergo massive infection, resulting in rapid death with no other clinical signs noted. The warm rain favors egg maturation, so large numbers of worm larvae are infective all at the same time.

General Symptoms

Watery diarrhea, rough hair coat, and general unthriftiness are typical signs of infestation with the other gastrointestinal parasites. If the worm burden is moderate and nutrition is adequate, external evidence of parasitism will usually be lacking. Diagnosis is generally confirmed by identification of worm eggs in manure samples using concentration techniques and the microscope. A tablespoonful of fresh manure is an adequate sample, and egg concentration is

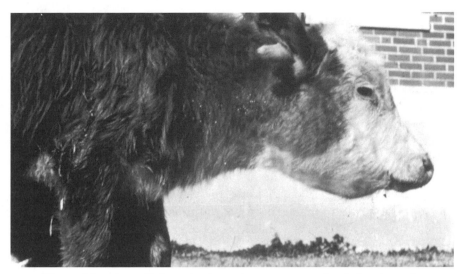

Edema of the submandibular region, hence the common name bottle jaw, *is a major sign of serious infection.*

usually expressed in terms of eggs per gram. The technique is simple and inexpensive. Your veterinarian can readily check samples for you, and a routine check of samples from several animals in the herd at least twice a year is a good precaution. If the count trend is upward, it indicates a break in control procedures somewhere that must be corrected to prevent trouble. Some people have the false impression that if they don't see worms in the manure, it's because the animal doesn't have worms. Similarly, if they don't see worms after giving the animal an anthelmintic, they think the drug didn't work. Both assumptions are false because the worms we have named thus far are extremely small and rarely can be seen without a magnifying glass. Ascarids common to swine and foals are an exception. These are large worms whose diameter approaches that of a pencil, and occasionally an adult worm will be passed in the manure. If you see one, you can be sure there are many more.

Control

It is possible to devise programs that will keep parasitism to a minimum. The approach favored by the drug companies is frequent therapeutic use of anthelmintics or continuous low-level feeding of anthelmintics. Most of the newer anthelmintics work by destroying the adult worms or rendering them sterile so that fertile eggs are not passed out in the manure. If other control measures are not adopted concurrently, this method has two obvious disadvantages. It involves a continuing expense for medication, and some species of worms become tolerant to the anthelmintic after prolonged exposure. Also, in food-producing animals, the range of drugs that can be used legally is limited.

Where the need for control of intestinal worms is not acute, management methods will in most cases prove more productive and economical. Remember that eggs are passed out in the manure and that reinfection is by ingestion. Anything that reduces the concentration of eggs will reduce the level of reinfection. The corollary to this is that high concentrations of infected animals will cause greater ground contamination and higher infection rates. Conversely, contamination can be reduced by weekly pasture rotation, periodic plowing and reseeding of pastures, paving holding areas and cleaning them daily, and protecting feed bunks and water supplies from fecal contamination. Pulling a drag over the pasture at weekly intervals helps distribute manure piles, thereby exposing worm eggs to the destructive effects of sunlight. Some species of intestinal worms go through a period of embryonation in the egg stage that lasts several days before they become infective. This process is facilitated by conditions of warmth and moisture. It is helpful, therefore, to keep pastures mowed short so tall grass doesn't trap moisture, favoring egg development.

These approaches are really methods of sanitation, which is the key to control of most internal parasites. Sanitation is especially important in controlling the swine roundworm, a major destructive parasite of baby pigs. A proven, effective method is to worm the sow prior to farrowing, keeping her in a paved yard or pen that can be hosed down periodically for the next few days. She is then scrubbed thoroughly with soap and water to remove all traces of dirt and manure *before* she is put in the farrowing crate or pen. If the piglets are destined for pasture at weaning, trucking them to a clean pasture rather than having them walk over contaminated ground helps to ensure that roundworms will not be a problem. This procedure, known as the *McLean County system,* was effective long before the advent and popularity of anthelmintics.

Simply put, control of common gastrointestinal worms depends on sanitation, management, and judicious, timely use of proper anthelmintics. A number of good medications for use orally, topically, or by injection are available, but these alone will not do an adequate job. Accurate diagnosis is important because worm life cycles and season of the year influence the effectiveness of the anthelmintic. Your veterinarian can help you devise a control program compatible with your circumstances that will reduce the detrimental effect of these parasites to a minimum.

Thus far we have been talking primarily about the gastrointestinal worms that affect sheep, goats, and cattle. It's convenient to group them together because their life cycles are similar and their response to anthelmintics is similar. There are, however, other internal parasites, equally or more important, that differ substantially and deserve special mention.

Ascarids (Roundworms)

The swine roundworms, *Ascaris suum,* and the horse ascarid, *Paracaris equorum,* are important species affecting livestock. The adult worms are large and easily recognized. Except where they are sufficiently numerous to mechanically block the intestine or bile duct, however, they do little harm to the animal. It's the migrating ascarid larvae that do the most damage. Adult female ascarids lay up to a quarter million eggs a day. These are passed out in the manure onto the ground, where they readily withstand freezing, drying, and chemicals, so ground contamination reaches high levels rapidly and persists. The eggs become infective in 2 to 3 weeks, and when ingested, the larvae emerge in the intestine. These penetrate the intestinal wall and are carried in the bloodstream, eventually reaching the liver, where they migrate and develop further. As development progresses, they are carried in the blood to the lungs, where they emerge into the alveolar spaces, eventually getting to the bronchi. From there they are coughed up and swallowed, ending up in the small intestine to become adults.

Symptoms

With this pattern of larval migration, it's not surprising that the symptoms of ascarid infection may bear little relationship to those we generally associate with worms. The migration to the liver may take a circuitous route, and larvae migrating in the sow or mare can cross the placenta and infect foals or piglets prior to birth. That's why it's important that pregnant animals be as free of ascarids as possible and be confined to areas that are relatively uncontaminated. Visceral larva migrans is a serious disease of children caused by migrating canine ascarids. It can cause blindness and brain lesions. In foals and piglets, larval migration causes damage to the liver, leaving lifetime scars. In pigs the white spots and streaks in the liver resulting from larval migration are cause for liver condemnation. Extensive infestation may cause enough liver inflammation to result in jaundice. Blockage of the bile duct by adults has the same outward effect. In heavily parasitized swine, verminous pneumonia is not unusual, causing labored breathing and all other signs associated with pneumonia.

In foals and young pigs, a potbelly, rough hair coat, unthriftiness, failure to gain weight, and frequent coughing should lead one to suspect roundworms as the cause. Roundworms respond well to administration of anthelmintics such as piperazine, but the life cycle illustrates why a single oral dose of the drug has no lasting value. It may kill all the adults, but many larvae will be inaccessible to the drug and will soon come back to the intestine to become adults. Many other drugs, diclorvos, levamisole, and pyrantel to name a few, are effective against ascarids. The drugs ivermectin and fenbendazole are used to eliminate migrating larvae. Treatment with oral anthelmintics must be continuous or repeated frequently, and reinfection must be prevented using the principles of the McLean County system mentioned earlier (see page 266). Debilitation due to parasitism increases susceptibility to other diseases.

Habronemiasis (Summer Sores)

Habronema species and *Draschia* species are relatively innocuous stomach worms of the horse. However, when their larvae are transferred by flies from manure to moist or abraded skin, they invade the skin to cause a chronic, red, weeping sore that becomes thickened and bleeds easily. The lesions itch and the horse keeps them raw from rubbing. Treatment with the usual antiseptics alone typically fails. Larvae carried by flies to the eye may migrate in the lacrimal discharge to the conjunctiva and establish a chronic infection there.

Fly control and protection of wounds with fly repellents help to prevent habronemiasis. Treatment with ivermectin is highly effective.

Horse Bots

These are not worms such as we have been discussing but instead are the larval stage of one of several species of flies belonging to the genus *Gasterophilus.* They are included here because the larvae are parasitic.

Life Cycle

The adult *Gasterophilus intestinalis* lays its eggs on the hair, particularly of the lower foreleg. These are cream-colored, slightly smaller than a pinhead, and attached so tightly that it is impossible to brush them off. They remain there until, under the stimulation of warmth and moisture from the animals licking, they hatch. The larvae then ride on the tongue to the mouth, where they embed themselves in the mucosal surface of the gums, cheeks, and tongue. *Gasterophilus haemorrhoidalis* deposits its eggs on the hairs around the mouth and they hatch without stimulation. *Gasterophilus nasalis* deposits its eggs in the throat region.

After a month or so in the mouth, the larvae travel to the stomach, where they attach themselves to the stomach wall and slowly enlarge over the next 8 to 9 months. When the larva is ready, it releases its hold on the stomach wall, passes out in manure, pupates, and finally emerges as a fly. The whole cycle takes about a year — yet the fly lives only 2 weeks or so.

The adult flies are annoying to horses, causing them to run or seek shelter in the brush or shade. But the most damaging aspect is when the bots are in the stomach. Digestive disturbances and colic are not infrequent with heavy infestations, although a few bots in a well-nourished horse usually do not cause any difficulty at all. Rarely, mature bot larvae in the pyloric end of the stomach may be sufficiently numerous to cause physical obstruction, leading to recurrent bouts of acute indigestion.

Control

Control of bots is by products such as ivermectin and related compounds that, when used as part of a regular internal parasite control program, will control bots as well. Wiping the attached eggs daily with a warm wet cloth or sponge during the fly season will stimulate hatching and reduce the number of bot larvae that find their way to the stomach.

Kidney Worm

Kidney worm, *Stephanurus dentatus,* is unique to swine and occasionally causes problems in some herds. The larvae, when ingested, migrate for several months, particularly in the liver, and eventually terminate their wanderings in cysts in the kidneys, ureters, and surrounding tissue. Eggs are passed out in the urine. Migrating larvae can infect piglets *in utero.*

The entire life cycle takes upwards of a year and a half, which lends itself to a control procedure by management alone. Because the life cycle is so long, slaughtered hogs go to the market before any eggs are laid. If breeding is confined to gilts using young boars and they are slaughtered when the litter is weaned, there is no opportunity for the kidney worm life cycle to be completed. Following this procedure for several years should render the premises free of kidney worm, provided no swine more than 2 years of age are retained. Fenbendazole and ivermectin are effective in controlling this disease.

Liver Flukes

Liver flukes, including *Fasciola hepatica* and *Dicrocoelium dendriticum,* are unique parasites in that part of their life cycles must be spent in snails. *F. hepatica* undergoes several developmental stages in an aquatic environment and in the snail, without which it cannot become infective. Ruminants, especially sheep, are their chief victims, and control is difficult at best.

Life Cycle

Eggs of the common fluke, *F. hepatica,* after about a week in water hatch into free-swimming miracidia, then enter snails, where they encyst in the tissue. Eventually, they emerge as cercariae and later become affixed to grass as encysted metacercariae, which are then eaten by sheep along with the blade of grass. In the intestine they emerge from the cyst, penetrate the gut wall, and wander through the peritoneal cavity until they find the liver. They penetrate the liver and migrate in it until they find the bile ducts, where they develop into adults. The duration of the life cycle is shorter in hot weather, longer in cold weather, and ceases in freezing weather. Most infections occur during the summer months. *D. dendriticum* is slightly different, in that it utilizes a terrestrial rather than an aquatic snail. Cercariae are in slime balls produced by the snail. Ants eat the slime balls, and sheep in turn eat the ants along with grass and become infected.

Effects

The effects of liver flukes on sheep and cattle may be acute or chronic. The acute disease occurs when there is massive invasion of the liver by the developing flukes. Symptoms include abdominal pain, lack of appetite, reluctance to move, and death. Chronic fluke disease is characterized by gradual weight loss, anemia, weakness, and edema. Liver damage caused by flukes predisposes to the rapidly fatal *black disease* caused by *Clostridium novyi.*

Control

Control of flukes is difficult. Reduction of the snail population through use of molluscicides such as copper sulfate is helpful, but usually runs afoul of environmental protection laws. Fencing sheep out of wet areas or draining the areas is helpful where practical. None of these methods is practical in areas where pastures must be irrigated.

Several drugs, such as albendazole and clorsulon, are available for removal of adult and immature flukes in sheep, but proper precautions must be observed in their use. With the limited control procedures available, it's not surprising that in some areas where the fluke population is high, it is simply not profitable to grow sheep.

Lungworms

Dictyocaulus viviparous in cattle and *Dictyocaulus filaria* in sheep and goats develop to maturity in the lungs. Other parasite larvae such as *Ascaris suum* may invade the lung and reside there temporarily. *Metastrongylus* species infect swine and play a role in the transmission of swine influenza.

Adult lungworms lay eggs in the lung, which are coughed up and swallowed with mucus. In ruminants, the embryonated eggs hatch and pass out in the manure as larvae, maturing on the ground, and then are ingested by animals. The earthworm is an intermediate host for *Metastrongylus,* and pigs get infected when they eat earthworms. The larvae thrive in moisture and warmth. Although most infections occur during the pasture season, serious outbreaks have occurred in winter when stabled calves lick walls wet with condensation, where infective larvae congregate. Ingested larvae penetrate the intestinal wall and are carried via the lymphatics to the lung, where they mature.

Except under unusual circumstances, lungworm infections do not reach serious proportions and may even be self-limiting. Young animals are more susceptible than are old. Clinical signs, when they occur in cattle, sheep, and goats, include chronic cough, unthriftiness, and abnormal lung sounds. Secondary bacterial pneumonia is not unusual.

Control by vaccination of young animals is widely practiced in Europe, but as yet a vaccine has not been licensed in the United States. Several drugs are available for treatment, when necessary, but because diagnosis is not easy, it would pay to consult your veterinarian. Infestation in pigs can be minimized by keeping them in paved feedlots, where they won't contact earthworms.

Pinworms

Pinworms have little significance as far as the health of the animal is concerned but are an annoyance. Adult female pinworms lay their eggs in masses at the anus, and their activity causes an intense itching. Affected horses swish their tails and rub their backsides against anything handy: fence posts, walls, or anything else that offers relief. In so doing, they may rub their tail head raw. Anthelmintic treatment is effective.

Strongyles (Bloodworms)

The large strongyles, *Strongylus vulgaris, Strongylus edentatus,* and *Strongylus equinus,* are perhaps the most important equine internal parasites, and of these, *S. vulgaris* heads the list.

Life Cycle

Adult strongyles inhabit the large intestine, where they lay eggs that are passed out in the manure. The eggs undergo several development stages in manure or soil until they become infective third-stage larvae, which migrate upward in water films on grass, stable walls, and so on. When ingested, these larvae pass through the stomach to the large intestine. There they penetrate the intestinal wall, become a fourth-stage larvae in about a week, and enter the walls of nearby small arterioles. Their migration continues in the walls of progressively larger blood vessels until the majority end up in the wall of the anterior mesenteric artery, the principal artery supplying blood to the intestines. A few go beyond to the aorta. This migratory period, lasting a few months, results in arterial inflammation, thrombosis, and embolism.

Eventually, the larvae are carried in the arterial supply back to the small arterioles in the intestinal wall, from which they emerge and undergo final development in nodules about the size of a pea. When sexually mature, the adults leave these nodules to enter the large intestine, lay eggs, and repeat the cycle. The complete cycle requires 6 months or more.

Considerable physical damage is done to the arterial vessels through which the larvae migrate. Thrombi in the smaller vessels decrease blood supply to the intestine until collateral circulation can develop. Recurrent colic is a clinical sign associated with strongylosis. A more serious complication occurs when an aneurysm develops ahead of an anterior mesenteric thrombus. As the aneurysm increases in size, its wall gets thinner until it eventually bursts and the horse dies rapidly from internal hemorrhage.

Control

Unfortunately, during the most damaging phase of their life, strongyles are beyond the reach of some of the common oral anthelmintics. It is necessary, therefore, to adopt control programs coupling prevention of reinfection with regular routine anthelmintic treatment. Deworming all horses on the premises regularly every 6 to 8 weeks will help to keep the strongyle population down, but it will not eradicate it. A number of good drugs are available, among them tenbendazole, pyrantel, and ivermectin. To forestall development of future resistance, drugs should be alternated. In northern climates, deworming horses two or three times during the pasture season may be adequate, but in the warmer climates, worming every 6 to 8 weeks may be required. Periodic microscopic examination of fecal samples is necessary to monitor efficacy of the control program. Boarding horses or horses that have been elsewhere for an extended period should be wormed before being pastured with resident animals.

Strongyle control is an essential component of an equine health program.

Tapeworms

Tapeworms in livestock are, in most cases, relatively innocuous as far as the animal is concerned, and clinical disease due to tapeworm is uncommon in the United States.

The beef tapeworm and the pork tapeworm are really human tapeworms that spend their larval stages in cattle and hogs. Animals get these worms when they ingest feed or water contaminated by human feces. Prevention, therefore, is dependent on improved sanitary habits by humans. In societies where people are not sufficiently fastidious and live so close to their animals that human and animal fecal contamination occurs readily, these parasites cause significant health problems.

External Parasites

External parasites, as the name implies, are those that either reside on the skin or attack the animal via the skin. Some external parasites are primarily a nuisance for the animal, whereas others may cause significant disease.

Flies

Several different flies are important to livestock for the annoyance they cause, because they are vectors of other diseases, or because they are parasitic. Because the attack of a fly is quick and transitory, control is generally based on repellents incorporating insecticides rather than on insecticides alone.

Horseflies, deerflies, stable flies, and horn flies are all bloodsucking flies that cause great annoyance to livestock and consequently reduce productivity.

The bite of the first three is painful, and when these pests are about, animals will run trying to get away from them. Horseflies are important vectors of equine infectious anemia, and any of the biting flies can transmit anaplasmosis. Efforts to control these pests are worthwhile but not always successful. The tabanids — horseflies and deerflies — are particularly hard to control. Their feeding habit is to swoop in, get a quick suck of blood, and take off again, leaving little time for exposure to insecticides. Where it can be done practically, the best way to protect livestock from these pests may be to allow them to run inside, out of the sun. The tabanids don't care much for shade, and they usually stay outside when animals go inside.

Control

Stable flies (and houseflies) breed in manure and decaying vegetable matter. An essential part of their control is good housekeeping, particularly keeping manure from accumulating around the barn. Residual sprays inside and outside the barn are also helpful. What may become the most important manner of control is feeding insecticides to the animal that are carried through in the manure so that the manure is toxic to fly maggots. Horseflies, because they stay on the animal, are more susceptible to locally applied insecticides. Both back rubbers and dustbags give good control. These can be supplemented with insecticide-impregnated plastic ear tags or similar devices attached to the halter on horses.

Myiasis is the term given to invasion of animal tissues by fly larvae, and there are several flies capable of doing this. History tells us that at one time fly maggots were deliberately placed in wounds to clean up the cellular debris. The most dramatic myiasis is that caused by the screwworm in the Southwest. Adult screwworms deposit their eggs in open wounds — or anywhere there is a drop of fresh blood. These hatch, and the larvae burrow into living tissue, feeding as they go. Left untreated, a colony of screwworm larvae can literally eat an animal alive.

For years, prevention of wound infestation with repellents or bandages and frequent inspection and treatment of animals when necessary were all that could be done to prevent losses. A quirk in the screwworm fly's breeding habits has made it possible to almost eradicate this pest, however. The female mates only once and the males can easily be sterilized by irradiation. The U.S. Department of Agriculture (USDA) is raising flies by the millions, sterilizing and releasing them in the endemic area. When the female mates with a sterile male, no viable eggs are produced. This program has been spectacularly successful and is being extended to northern Mexico to create a buffer zone where no screwworms are present.

While the screwworm is the only fly maggot that regularly eats living flesh, the wool maggot occasionally gets just as voracious. These are blowfly larvae that hatch from eggs deposited in the wool next to the skin, particularly under the tail and between the hind legs, where the wool is most likely to be soiled and damp. The maggots start out feeding on the wool, but as they progress toward the head they begin to develop an appetite for skin and subcutaneous tissue. Such activity can be rapidly fatal to a sheep. Clipping the wool under the tail and between the rear legs (commonly called *tagging*), shearing, dipping, spraying, and use of repellents on wounds have all been used to prevent fly-strike.

Cattle Grub

Several flies spend part of their life cycle as parasites of animals. Of these, the most dramatic are the cattle grubs, *Hypoderma* species. Two species, *Hypoderma bovis* and *Hypoderma lineatum,* are recognized. The adult flies, which resemble small bumblebees, live only about a week, during which they lay eggs on the hair of the lower legs of cattle. These hatch, and the larvae, called *warbles*, penetrate the skin and begin a migration that takes almost a year. Larvae have been found in connective tissue throughout the body but particularly around the esophagus and spinal cord. After 6 months or more of apparently aimless migration, the larvae localize in the subcutaneous tissue along the topline. Then they encyst and bore a hole through the skin for a breathing pore. They gradually enlarge as spring wears on, and by May and June in the northern states have reached the size of about ½ inch in diameter and 1 inch long. At this time they emerge, fall to the ground, pupate, and become heel flies.

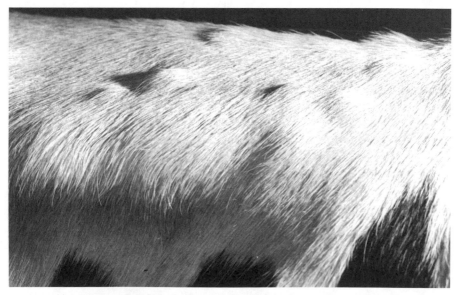

Larvae of the cattle grub, called warbles, *migrate to and encyst in the animal's topline, where they enlarge and emerge, eventually becoming heel flies.*

In yearlings there may be one hundred or more of these large lumps on the back, each containing a heel fly larva, but the numbers decrease in subsequent years as cattle get older. The principal economic effect of these grubs is through damage to the hide. The breathing pores leave scars, making that section of hide useless for fine leather.

Several systemic insecticides, in addition to the avermectins, are available for use on beef cattle. Timing of application, however, is important: It should be applied as soon as the active heel fly season ends. Once the grubs are in the back, the damage is done. Because of their size, attempting to destroy the encysted grubs with insecticides may lead to serious tissue reaction. Be sure to follow directions carefully when using systemic insecticides. Unfortunately, systemic insecticides may not be used on lactating dairy cattle. At present, only rotenone is approved for application to the animal's back, where presumably it comes in contact with the grubs through the breathing hole they have made. With only a few animals, it's about equally effective to manually express the mature grubs and then step on them.

Sheep Nose Bot

The sheep nose bot *Oestrus ovis* spends part of its life cycle residing in the nasal passages and sinuses of sheep and goats. The adult flies terrify sheep as they zoom in and deposit larvae at the nostrils. When the flies are active, it's not unusual to see sheep running or standing with their noses tucked tightly in each other's flanks. Sometimes, sheep will stand in a circle with their heads together for mutual protection, in a defense posture reminiscent of the wagon train.

Once deposited, the larvae migrate into the nasal passages and develop slowly over a period of months. As the larvae get larger and more active, the sheep sneeze and shake their heads in an attempt to dislodge them. Sufficient irritation may be produced to cause a blood-tinged mucopurulent discharge. At maturity, the larvae find their way out to the ground, pupate, and emerge as flies to repeat the cycle. Ivermectin is an effective treatment.

Lice

Of all the external parasites of animals, lice are ubiquitous and perhaps the most adaptable in terms of survival. They can afflict all livestock species and human beings anywhere in the world. They have been known for centuries as a pest of man and beast.

Lice are divided into two broad classes, those that suck and those that bite. The sucking lice actually suck blood from the host, whereas the biting lice feed on cellular debris and exudate on the skin. Many different louse species exist, but fortunately those that thrive on one species of animal generally will not colonize on another. If they did, most livestock owners would themselves have lice! Host specificity is helpful when considering control procedures.

Effects

As far as the effect on the animal is concerned, the one thing all lice, biting and sucking, have in common is that they make the animal itch. The itching is so intense at times that animals rub themselves raw. Sucking lice are occasionally sufficiently numerous on an animal to cause anemia and, in extreme cases, death.

Diagnosis

Diagnosis of *pediculosis,* or lice infestation, is not difficult, and a presumptive diagnosis can often be made from some distance away. For example, if you see bits of hair or wool stuck on posts, rails, wire, or trees in the barnyard, you can be sure the animals have lice or mange, and the odds favor lice. If on the animals themselves you see patches of hair pulled out or areas where the hair is broken off from rubbing, you are probably dealing with lice. If you part the hair at the periphery of these patches and look closely in good light, you will probably see lice on the skin or their eggs, called *nits,* stuck on the hairs. A magnifying glass makes observation easier and more certain. In cattle, horses, and goats, lice are more likely to be found along the topline, from the tail head to the withers. The head and feet are frequent sites of infestation in sheep. Nits, smaller than a pinhead and grayish white in color, will be found in great numbers attached to the hair near the skin. Finding these, even without seeing any adult lice, is adequate justification for a control program. Problems with lice are more likely to be encountered in winter than in summer and when animals are kept in close confinement.

Control

For the owner of an individual horse or two, lice are not likely to be a problem if the animals are groomed daily and if brushes are used on your animals only. The herd or flock problem is a different situation requiring mass treatment methods such as spraying and dipping. Dustbags and backrubbers laced with insecticide and placed where cattle have to use them are helpful.

Insecticide powders dusted on the topline of stabled cattle help to keep the louse population under control, and systemic insecticides or avermectins help control sucking lice. But when many animals are showing clinical signs of pediculosis, especially biting lice, dipping or high-pressure spraying or pour-on insecticide formulations are the only answers. There are many good insecticides on the market that will kill lice. Very few of these may legally be used on dairy cattle and dairy goats. In fact, the legal restrictions on the use of insecticides are so voluminous that they will not be listed here.

Suffice it to say, the livestock owner should follow the label warning on whatever insecticide he ultimately uses. Failure to do so could result in milk or tissue residues, which, if detected, could prompt condemnation of the product and legal proceedings against the producer.

Last, whatever product is used as a spray or dip should be repeated in about 2 weeks to allow time for the eggs to hatch. Insecticides do not affect the nits, but a second treatment will get those recently hatched. And because lice commonly spend time off the host, it's important to spray the stable area as well.

Mange

All classes of livestock are susceptible to mange, which is a dermatitis caused by one of the several species of microscopic mites. *Sarcoptes* is the mite found most often affecting horses and swine, but it can affect other species, including humans, as well. Intense itching, especially around the head and neck; papule and vesicle formation; acute dermatitis; and wrinkling of the skin characterize this form of mange. It spreads rapidly on the animal and to other animals. Left untreated, the disease can be sufficiently debilitating to be fatal.

Chorioptic mange is the type usually encountered in cattle. Like sarcoptic mange, it causes intense itching, but it starts most commonly around the tail head, escutcheon, and down the inside of the hind legs. Cattle mange is often called *barn itch.*

Psoroptes is the other major genus of mange mite generally associated with sheep. However, any of the three, *Sarcoptes, Chorioptes,* and *Psoroptes,* can infect any animal species. Distinction can be made among them on the basis of clinical signs and morphologic characteristics when examined under the

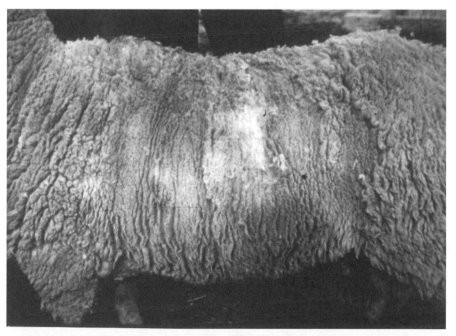

Psoroptic mange in sheep causes the wool to fall out in ragged patches, ruining the fleece.

microscope. *Psoroptic mange,* sometimes called *sheep scab,* is particularly serious in sheep because it causes the wool to fall out in ragged patches, ruining the fleece and causing great economic loss. Because of its seriousness, psoroptic mange is a legally reportable disease, which fortunately is rarely seen in the United States.

A fourth type of mange, *demodectic,* is of minor importance in livestock. The organism colonizes in the hair follicles and does not spread rapidly. It may occasionally cause small papules or nodules filled with cheesy material. Demodectic mange is frequently self-limiting, and treatment is of little avail.

Treatment

Treatment of the sarcoptic, chorioptic, and psoroptic mange is essential for the comfort and productivity of the animal. If you have reason to suspect mange in your herd or flock, have your veterinarian help you work out a treatment procedure that is practical. Drugs of the avermectin class are available in injectable, oral, and pour-on formulations. Some are approved for use in lactating cattle.

Sheep Keds

The ked, *Melophagus ovinus,* is an important bloodsucking parasite of sheep. It spends its entire life cycle on the sheep. The female, rather than laying eggs, gives birth to a larva that attaches to the wool and pupates. The life cycle spans a period of about 4 months.

Keds become quite numerous in winter and early spring, and the irritation of their feeding causes sheep to rub and bite, particularly around the shoulders, flanks, and rump.

Dipping is the most effective way to treat sheep, and the best time to do so is immediately after shearing. Unless a residual insecticide can be used, dipping will have to be repeated to get the keds that haven't yet emerged from the pupal case.

Ticks

Although ticks themselves are parasites depending on a blood meal for their survival, their primary importance may be as vectors of diseases such as tularemia, Rocky Mountain spotted fever, Q fever, and babesiasis.

Life Cycle

The typical tick life cycle involves mating on the host and engorgement of the female with blood. At that time, she drops to the ground and begins laying eggs that hatch in about 2 weeks into larvae, or *seed ticks.* These crawl up on vegetation and brush, and remain there as long as 8 months waiting for an animal to come by. When the animal brushes up against the plant, the larvae hop on for a ride and a blood meal. These then drop to the ground to become nymphs and the process is repeated. Ultimately, the nymphs develop into adults, which also wait in the vegetation for a blood meal to walk by. The animals attacked by larvae, nymphs, and adults may be all the same species or different, and humans may be one of them. A few ticks spend their life cycles on a single host. Adult ticks are most likely to be seen on animals in late summer and early fall.

A few ticks, although they suck blood, are usually tolerated by the animal. However, heavy infestations cause severe irritation and anemia, with affected animals being extremely uncomfortable as well as lethargic and unthrifty. The spinose ear tick prevalent in the Southwest crawls into the ear canal, causing pain and irritation.

Treatment

A few ticks on an animal can be removed manually, taking care not to break off the mouthparts, by which the tick is attached. Gentle traction is generally all that is required, but an old trick may accelerate the process. Light a match, blow it out, and apply the hot head to the body of the tick. This usually encourages it to let go in a hurry. This method is obviously impractical if many ticks are present, in which case dipping or spraying is the only resort. The same problems and precautions that apply to use of insecticides and avermectins for lice and mange apply to ticks. Because seed ticks tend to crawl to the highest point on grass and brush, clipping pastures reduces exposure to ticks. Grooming animals daily also helps prevent problems.

Metabolic Diseases

METABOLIC DISEASES ARE intrinsic in origin and represent a breakdown of normal body function. They are not contagious or infectious. However, the same external factors — nutrition, production, stress, and so on — that precipitate a disease such as ketosis in one cow may trigger it in others, giving the illusion of a contagious disease.

The metabolic diseases of livestock are not many in number, but collectively each year they cost the industry millions of dollars. Fortunately, if one understands the basis for them, most are preventable through management.

Azoturia (Black Water, Monday Morning Disease)

This once common disease of horses has declined in frequency, along with the decline in numbers of the draft horse. Nevertheless, it is still seen occasionally in horses that are worked hard, and may bear some relationship to the more frequently reported *tying-up syndrome.*

Typically, azoturia appears in a horse that has been routinely working hard and is maintained on full feed. Symptoms develop a few hours after work begins, following a few days or more of complete rest. The sobriquet "Monday morning disease" came about because it was seen most often on Monday following a weekend of rest.

Clinical Signs

Clinical signs begin soon after strenuous exercise starts. These include profuse sweating, stiff gait, and reluctance to move. If the horse is forced to continue working, signs get progressively more severe until the horse goes down in severe pain, unable to rise. If the horse is given complete rest as soon as signs begin, they may disappear in a few hours.

Theoretically, the disease comes about because excess glycogen is stored in muscle tissue at rest. When exercise begins, glycogen is rapidly metabolized, with one of the metabolic products being lactic acid. If this acid accumulates faster than it can be carried away by the bloodstream, coagulation necrosis of muscle tissue occurs. Whether or not the theory is correct, there is no doubt that muscle tissue necrosis occurs, involving especially the heavy muscles of the hip and loin. Breakdown of muscle cells releases myoglobin, which gives the urine a dark, coffee-colored appearance — hence the common name *black water*. The tying-up syndrome produces similar, although less severe, clinical signs under similar conditions.

The clinical signs of azoturia are sufficiently clear-cut that diagnosis is generally not difficult. If there is doubt, several chemical tests on the blood serum will clarify the issue and indicate the extent of the muscle damage. Your veterinarian should be called without delay, but what you do in the interim may determine whether the horse recovers, becomes permanently lame, or dies. The most important thing is to stop working the horse *immediately* and keep him at rest but on his feet. Even walking him to the barn should be avoided until the situation can be evaluated. Application of moist hot packs to the loin and rump may ease the pain and improve circulation, lessening lactic acid concentration.

Prevention

To prevent azoturia, feed your horse like your car. Just as the car uses more gas when pulling a load, so the horse needs more feed to produce energy. But when it's idling, the car doesn't use as much gas, and neither does the horse. When the horse isn't working, cut his grain ration in half. He won't love you for it but he will be much healthier.

Brisket Disease

This is of concern only to the owners of cattle pastured for long periods in high mountain areas, generally over 7,000 feet. The disease generally affects less than 2 percent of the herd and is the direct result of constant exposure to the low oxygen tension prevalent at that altitude and higher. In an attempt to meet the tissue demand for oxygenated blood, the heart works harder at those altitudes. In some animals this causes enlargement of the right side of the heart, a self-defeating attempt at compensation. Unless the valves increase in size proportionately to the body of the heart, leakage occurs, resulting in liver congestion and a call for even more oxygen.

The end result is brisket disease, leaving an animal with an enlarged heart, subcutaneous edema especially around the brisket, lack of stamina and appetite, loss of weight, rapid pulse, and labored breathing or collapse after exercise.

Treatment of these individuals is usually not practical, although obviously oxygen would help. The next best thing is to move them carefully and without excitement to a lower altitude, where spontaneous clinical recovery sometimes results. Pneumonia is a common sequel and may be prevented with antibiotics. Recovered animals should not be returned to high altitudes, nor should they be used for breeding on the chance that theirs may be a hereditary weakness.

Hypomagnesemia (Grass Tetany, Grass Staggers)

This disease, affecting lactating cattle, sheep, and occasionally goats, is the result of a decreased serum magnesium level. It occurs most often when animals are grazing lush pasture in early spring. Relatively low levels of magnesium in lush grass compared to potassium and nitrogen apparently are responsible for decreased magnesium absorption and the onset of clinical signs. Grass pastures top-dressed with either potassium or nitrogen or both have been shown to produce hypomagnesemia more often than those without such practices. Nitrogen and potassium apparently reduce the soil availability of magnesium, so grasses growing rapidly on such soils are themselves low in magnesium. The same circumstances prevail in some latitudes when fall rains again stimulate rapid pasture growth and on cereal crop pasture. In fact, in some areas the disease is called *wheat pasture poisoning.*

The precise mechanism by which hypomagnesemia comes about is not well known. Magnesium is excreted primarily in urine and to a lesser extent in milk. The ruminant lacks a good homeostasis mechanism for magnesium balance and is therefore more susceptible to rapid loss or lack of intake. In most cases of the tetanic form of the disease, there is hypocalcemia as well, and it is standard practice to treat grass tetany with intravenous solutions containing calcium and magnesium.

It appears that there may be two phases to hypomagnesemia, one being a chronic low level of serum magnesium that causes the second phase, the disease we know as *grass tetany,* only when triggered by some other factor: hypocalcemia, brief starvation, shipping, or weather stress.

Symptoms

Clinically, the symptoms range from chronic to acute. A few animals in a herd with low serum magnesium levels may show vague signs such as unthriftiness, poor appetite, and dullness. After a few days of this, they may develop more definitive signs, such as a wild attitude, throwing the head about, or unsteady gait with exaggerated leg movements. Loud noises or sudden movements may precipitate a convulsion lasting several minutes, with paddling motions of the legs. Similar signs are occasionally seen in calves on an exclusive milk diet as they approach 2 to 3 months of age.

The acute form of the disease in cattle and sheep may appear without warning, with the animal going from a normal grazing attitude to almost maniacal behavior. Tossing the head, bellowing, and galloping are common until the animal staggers and falls in a convulsion. During the convulsion, the eyes twitch and the legs paddle or are stiffly extended. Frothing and champing of the jaws are common. Pulse and respiration are rapid, and temperature is elevated due to exertion. When the convulsion subsides, the animal lies quietly, but a noise or touch may precipitate a recurrence.

Symptomatically, acute hypomagnesemia strongly resembles acute urea poisoning. Although response to treatment is good, mortality is high because it's generally only about an hour from onset of signs to death. Acute hypomagnesemia is one of the few diseases in livestock medicine that can be considered an emergency. Others become that way through neglect.

Control

Despite our lack of complete understanding of the pathogenesis of hypomagnesemia, control procedures have been worked out that are quite helpful. Feeding magnesium oxide as a feed additive during the period of greatest vulnerability, top-dressing pastures with dolomitic limestone or magnesium oxide, and placing one or more magnesium "bullets" in the animal's stomach with a balling gun have all given satisfactory results. A switch from all-grass to grass-legume pastures is helpful in climates where this is possible. Feeding some dry hay in addition to pasture will also help to prevent the disease. Protection from cold, inclement weather also helps, especially to prevent the winter tetany seen in cattle maintained on marginal diets.

Ketosis, Bovine (Acetonemia, Hypoglycemia)

This important problem of high-producing dairy cattle is not a discrete disease entity but, rather, a symptom of a sequence of events leading to an excess of ketones in the blood. *Primary ketosis* occurs when the cow metabolizes body fat for energy at a rate faster than ketones can be eliminated. This is most common during the peak of milk production when the cow is either not offered enough or cannot consume enough nutrients, particularly energy, to meet her needs for milk production as well as maintenance. *Secondary ketosis* may occur any time appetite is depressed as a result of diseases such as mastitis, metritis, and displaced abomasum, or as a result of malnutrition. It may be aggravated by feeding poor-quality grass silage that has a high butyric acid content.

The presence of a modest level of ketone bodies, acetoacetic acid, B-hydroxybutyric acid, and acetone in body tissues is normal. These are by-products of the breakdown of stored fat into fatty acids and, up to a point, can be used by the cow as an energy source. However, when energy requirements exceed energy intake, the rate of body fat catabolism accelerates, with production of these ketones in excess of the cow's ability to utilize them. When this happens, abnormal levels of ketones appear in blood, milk, and urine, where they are readily detectable by chemical means. Unfortunately, high ketone levels have a depressant effect on appetite, so the cow that needs more energy intake to counteract the ketosis usually has no interest in high-energy feeds.

While the foregoing is a simple rational explanation, it leaves some questions unanswered. For example, why is ketosis more prevalent in a given herd some years than it is in others, and why is it more common in some cow families than in others? Why do some cows of equal body weight, producing equal amounts of milk, have ketosis year after year while others never do? These are questions for which we don't have the answers, despite ongoing research.

Several factors have been suggested that may lead to primary ketosis:

■ **Glucose drain to meet lactation requirements.** Milk is high in lactose, which comes from glucose. It has been established that high-producing cows need as much as 1 kilogram of glucose daily from dietary carbohydrates to meet the need for lactose. If nutrient intake is inadequate, the cow will make up the deficit from body fat. This may be the most important factor, as ketosis almost invariably coincides with peak lactation.

■ **Endocrine disorders.** There is some evidence that exhaustion of the adrenal and pituitary glands during peak lactation accounts for gluconeogenesis failures. Substitution therapy, using adrenocorticotropic hormone (ACTH) or glucocorticoids, produces a favorable response in some ketotic cows, lending some credence to this hypothesis.

■ **Liver dysfunction.** The liver is an important organ in the conversion of free fatty acids to glucose and plays a role in the detoxification of ketones. A consistent finding in ketosis cases of long duration is a degenerative change — fatty infiltration of the liver. A similar change is seen in cows that are obese, lending support to the theory that fat cows are more prone to develop ketosis.

■ **Protein excess.** Ketosis has reportedly been produced experimentally by feeding excess protein. Protein may add extra ketogenic amino acids to the diet. In herds with a major ketosis problem, where protein was being fed in excess of requirements, reduction of protein intake has been beneficial.

■ **Vitamin or mineral deficiencies.** Over the years, ketosis has been ascribed to deficiency of a variety of minerals and vitamins. However, with the exception of cobalt, which is essential to the enzyme systems involved in gluconeogenesis, it is doubtful that deficiencies are a factor.

■ **High intake of ketogenic materials.** It is reasonably well established that intake of ketogenic materials such as butyric acid found in poor-quality silage will contribute to a herd ketosis problem.

Clinical Signs

Almost invariably, primary ketosis occurs in the range of 1 to 6 weeks after calving. Perhaps the earliest sign the alert herd manager will notice is a lack of eye luster. This is followed by a decline in milk production and a selective loss of appetite. Typically, the cow will refuse first grain, then silage, and finally hay. Concurrently, there will be rapid loss of body weight, and the manure will become dry and hard. Herd managers with a good sense of smell report that ketotic cows have a characteristic sweetish acetone odor in their milk and on their breath. Onset of the disease signs may be quite sudden or they may be insidious, spanning over several weeks.

A few cows with ketosis (about 1 percent) will exhibit signs of neurological disturbances such as pushing against walls, bellowing, and incoordination. Being a metabolic disorder rather than infectious in nature, ketosis rarely causes any elevation of body temperature.

A simple, rapid chemical test is available for the detection of acetoacetic acid and acetone in the milk or urine. The test is more sensitive when used with urine, as ketone levels are higher in urine than in milk.

Treatment

Because of the complexity of the disease and the poor response to treatment of some cases, hundreds of compounds and concoctions have been tried over the years. Most are worthless, but a few have real value.

Ketotic cows are always low in blood glucose. The standard therapy that produces good results is glucose solution given intravenously. Unfortunately, while it is very effective, its effect is transitory, lasting only about 2 hours, after which blood glucose levels begin to fall again. However, for many cows the brief respite it affords is often sufficient to allow their metabolic equilibrium to return to normal, and they proceed to recover. Glucose solution may be given as often as necessary to promote recovery. A more dilute solution given by slow intravenous drip over a period of 24 to 48 hours is more effective, but the apparatus and restraint required are cumbersome.

Orally, both propylene glycol and sodium propionate have been effective, and 6 to 8 ounces of either given three times daily to supplement intravenous glucose is helpful in refractory cases.

Use of steroid hormones such as dexamethasone provides good stimulus to gluconeogenesis, and it is often used in conjunction with glucose. However, overuse of corticosteroids has a depressant effect on antibody production that can lead to complications such as infection. For that reason, they should be used cautiously, keeping in mind that serious complications may result. The hormone ACTH to stimulate the adrenals is safer, but somewhat less effective.

The diagnosis in unresponsive cases should be carefully reevaluated for the presence of other concurrent disease problems. Displaced abomasum typically presents a clinical picture not unlike ketosis, even to the usual time of occurrence shortly after parturition.

Prevention

As with all diseases, prevention is far more valuable than treatment, and some recommendations can be made that will reduce the prevalence of ketosis.

■ Pay close attention to dry cows. Feed them to maintain the same body condition during the entire dry period.

■ Begin to feed some grain, 2 to 4 pounds daily, during the last 2 weeks of the dry period to condition rumen bacteria to utilization of grain.

■ Increase grain intake immediately after calving at the rate of 1½ to 2 pounds daily until milk production peaks. This will provide maximum energy intake when the cow needs it most. Increasing grain at a faster rate may induce indigestion with acidosis and precipitate ketosis.

■ Use good-quality hay and silage. Avoid using silage that has a spoiled or rancid odor.

Ketosis, Ovine (Pregnancy Disease, Ketosis, Pregnancy Toxemia)

Physiologically, this disease of sheep bears some resemblance to ketosis of cows in that the clinical signs are brought on by a metabolic failure resulting in an excess of ketones in the blood. The similarity ends there, although there are some common denominators.

Like bovine ketosis, ketosis in sheep is the result of a disparity in energy utilization compared with energy intake. In cows, the energy drain is from lactation; in sheep, the loss is brought about by the needs of a developing single large lamb or, more often, twin lambs. Characteristically, pregnancy disease occurs late in gestation, often during the last week or two, in ewes that have been on a gradually declining plane of nutrition. To the inexperienced observer, this may not appear to be the case when the body weight lost by the ewe is replaced by the bulk of the fetus. The disease can be precipitated in fat ewes by withholding feed 24 to 48 hours, abrupt change in diet, or the stress of inclement weather. Sometimes these factors combine to cause so many cases in a short period of time that it seems an infectious agent must be to blame.

Clinical Signs

Neurological signs characterize the disease in ewes. They will stand aloof from the flock, blunder into objects if they move, and sometimes stand with their heads pressing against a wall or fence for hours on end. Apparent blindness is common. As the disease progresses, muscle twitching, circling, and spasmodic jerking of the head may occur. Eventually, convulsions occur with intervals of rest between. This pattern continues for 3 to 4 days, followed by a period of prostration and death.

Treatment

While a dairy cow with ketosis will lose weight rapidly and milk production declines to a point where energy needs balance with energy intake, the cow recovers. Not so with sheep. Mortality from pregnancy toxemia, with or without treatment, is high. Once the clinical signs are fully developed, response to treatment is poor. Intravenous glucose repeated frequently will help, and an occasional ewe can be saved by a prompt cesarean or induced abortion if it can be done with minimal stress. Corticosteroids have not given consistently good results in sheep. Sodium propionate and propylene glycol given to other pregnant ewes in the flock may prevent additional cases from occurring if, at the same time, energy content of the ration is increased.

Management is the best prevention. Keep the ewe flock on a diet adequate for maintenance, and raise the energy content gradually during gestation. Be sure ewes get sufficient exercise, and protect them from the stress of inclement weather during late pregnancy.

Paresis, Postparturient (Milk Fever, Hypocalcemia)

Milk fever, sometimes called *parturient paresis,* is a metabolic disease seen primarily in dairy cattle manifested by onset at or near parturition, loss of appetite, stasis of the digestive tract, stilted gait, paresis, prostration, and death. This sequence of symptoms may occur over a period of 2 to 24 hours. There is usually some premonitory indication of the disease before the cow goes down. A similar condition is seen with less frequency in sheep and goats.

Calcium Loss

High-producing cows are most susceptible to milk fever, and it is seen more commonly in the Jersey breed. However, high milk production is not essential to the onset of the disease because it is occasionally seen in beef cows and mediocre dairy cattle. The precipitating factor is the sudden loss of calcium (up to 20 g/day) in colostrum, in excess of the rate of calcium replacement from the digestive tract and stored reserves in bone. The result is a hypocalcemia that, if uncorrected, leads to progressive development of the symptoms listed above.

Serum calcium levels are controlled by an interrelationship between calcium and phosphorus intake, serum phosphorus levels, vitamin D, calcium and phosphorus reserves, the parathyroid and thyroid glands, and the age of the animal. The normal serum calcium level ranges from 9 to 12 mg/100 mL.

Calcium Mobilization

Normally, the lost calcium is replaced within a few hours through mobilization of stored calcium reserves in bone, under the influence of parathyroid hormone and vitamin D. This happens only if the parathyroid is physiologically active. In cows that develop milk fever, the parathyroid is frequently inactive, resulting in failure of calcium mobilization. The rate of calcium intake has an important bearing on parathyroid activity. If the rate of intake is very high, as, for example, on a high legume diet, absorption from the gut alone will be adequate to maintain serum calcium levels during the dry period. There will be little exchange of calcium in bone and the gland becomes more or less dormant. Also, calcium and phosphorus in serum are normally in equilibrium. A deficiency of one will simulate an excess of the other as far as the parathyroid is concerned. Therefore, to maintain parathyroid activity, calcium and phosphorus intakes should be approximately in balance, and the total intake of each should be in line with established recommendations.

Vitamin D

Vitamin D has an important influence on calcium metabolism. It has some effect on the absorption of calcium from the intestine but has a profound influence on calcium in bone. Excessive doses will cause a rapid increase in serum calcium at the expense of bone reserve. The serum calcium level may increase beyond the animal's capacity to eliminate it, resulting in precipitation of calcium in soft tissues, especially heart muscle. At the same time, there will be a loss of bone strength due to depletion of mineral content. Therefore, although many researchers have established that the prevalence of milk fever can be reduced by administration of 20 million units of vitamin D daily for 5 days prior to calving, the procedure is not without risk.

The effect of vitamin D raises the question of deficiency. Under normal conditions in mature cattle, vitamin D deficiency probably does not occur. It is synthesized in the skin through the action of sunlight. However, in total-confinement housing where the cattle are rarely, if ever, outside, our thinking may have to be revised, and we may find it advantageous to supplement the diet with small amounts of vitamin D.

Age plays a part in calcium metabolism, too. As cows get older, the rate of absorption from the gut decreases. More important, calcium in bone tends to become more tightly bound with increasing age and, therefore, is not as readily mobilized on demand. This is a possible explanation of the observation that milk fever rarely occurs in first-calf heifers but increases in prevalence among older cows.

Treatment

It has been established that the thyroid gland has an indirect influence on calcium mobilization. Excessively high levels of serum calcium stimulate release of thyrocalcitonin from the thyroid, inhibiting the parathyroid. This mechanism can be triggered by intravenous administration of calcium. Standard treatment of milk fever is intravenous administration of 500 mL of 25 to 25 percent calcium gluconate. This will cause a transitory rise in serum calcium to about 20 mg/100 mL. The excess is dissipated rapidly, so within a few hours the serum calcium level is back down to normal or below normal again, if some mobilization has not occurred. It is postulated that this sudden high increase in calcium may precipitate the thyrocalcitonin response, leading to the relapses that sometimes occur.

Prevention

As with every disease, prevention is infinitely more valuable than treatment. Total intake of calcium and phosphorus must be adequate according to the body weight of the cow. The National Research Council recommendations — as found in *Nutrient Requirements of Dairy Cattle,* available from the U.S.

Government Printing Office, Washington, D.C. — are a good guide. Second, the intake of each should be balanced so that there is not a substantial excess of either. The calcium:phosphorus ratio in the diet should not exceed 2:1 and should be close to 1:1. In problem herds, this need will usually necessitate a forage analysis and alteration of the ration and/or addition of an additive such as dicalcium phosphate or other phosphorus supplement. Injection of large (10 million) units of vitamin D per week prior to calving seems to prevent some cases of milk fever, but if the cow doesn't calve within that time, milk fever is more likely to ensue. Oral administration of calcium gel the day before, the day of, and the day after calving may prevent many cases of milk fever.

The "Downer" Cow

One question that always arises in connection with milk fever is the problem of the alert "downer" cow. These cases usually begin as milk fever and respond to therapy to the extent that they are alert, eat reasonably well, and attempt to rise but cannot do so, hence the name "downer" cow. At one time it was thought that this condition might be a manifestation of potassium deficiency. However, results of potassium replacement therapy were disappointing.

It now seems apparent, from numerous necropsies, that many of these cases are the result of muscular, ligamentous, or skeletal injuries sustained during the initial hypocalcemic paresis. Cows down with milk fever in a cramped position for as little as an hour have been shown to develop degenerative muscle changes that make them physically unable to rise. Ruptured ligaments and tendons and, occasionally, fractures have been found. These lesions are probably due to the weight of the animal and the exertion of trying to get up during the hypocalcemic period when coordination is poor. The problem is compounded when the cow is confined in a stanchion or is lying on a hard slippery surface with no bedding. Good nursing care is essential for downer cows, and the longer they are down, the poorer the prognosis. Rotating them from one side to the other every hour helps prevent decubital sores, and if cows will tolerate it, use of a sling to help them to their feet frequently is worthwhile.

Most milk fever can be prevented by paying attention to calcium and phosphorus intake during the dry period. By forage analysis and arithmetical calculation you can keep intake of both within recommended limits and in proper ratio. For the few that don't respond to dietary management, don't delay treatment until the cow goes down. Milk fever almost always occurs within 24 hours of calving, and affected cows always have a glassy eye, absence of rumen activity, and a stilted gait before they go down. Treatment before they go down brings about uneventful recovery, although it may need repeating. Waiting until the cows are down carries with it a risk of injury from which they may never recover.

Deficiency 13 Diseases

STRANGE AS IT MAY SEEM, the most commonly reported deficiency disease is inadequate protein and energy intake, a polite way to describe starvation. Whether through ignorance or indifference on the part of their owners, thousands of animals are maintained in a state of malnutrition, particularly during winter months when feed must be brought to them.

The business of raising livestock is certainly governed by economics, and feed costs are generally the largest single item of expense. It's logical, then, that cutting back on feed costs by reducing consumption is the most likely place to save money. But is it? Cutting back on feed consumption will save money in the long run only if you are presently overfeeding and your animals are too fat. It's common practice to "rough" the young stock by giving them only enough to stay alive, on the premise that because they are only growing, not producing meat or milk, they don't need much to eat. That's a false assumption, resulting in retarded growth, delayed sexual maturity, and decreased disease resistance.

If breeding must be delayed several months because the animal didn't grow large enough fast enough on a marginal diet, it means that many more months must elapse before the animal starts producing income. Where is the economy in that? Similarly, if you can get a hog to market in 6 months, why hold back on feed and wait 8 months? Restricting feed intake below the needs of the animal is false economy.

When animals are fed adequate quantities of a variety of feedstuffs such as hay or pasture, grains, and silage, deficiency diseases are generally not a problem. Occasionally, however, specific mineral, trace element, or vitamin deficiencies will occur as a result of such things as deficiency in the soil where the crop was grown, feed spoilage or weather damage, oxidation in storage, and overabundance of one element tying up another to make it unavailable. The following deficiency diseases of livestock are of sufficient importance to warrant some discussion.

Anemia

Anemia has many causes — hemorrhage, parasitism, and diseases of red blood cells, to name a few. Nutritional deficiencies can also result in depressed hemoglobin formation. *Iron deficiency anemia* of baby pigs is perhaps the most common and universal. Piglets are born with virtually no iron reserve, and the iron content of sow's milk is usually inadequate to sustain them. Signs of iron deficiency anemia begin to appear at about 1 week of age, gradually increasing until the piglets are 1 month old. Affected piglets do not grow well, are prone to develop enteric infections, and usually show signs of respiratory distress.

Although piglets are most susceptible, iron deficiency anemia can occur in any species raised on an exclusive milk diet. It is not uncommon in veal calves raised in total confinement on milk or milk replacer. In some parts of the United States, there is a premium market for fancy veal that requires a very pale meat. To achieve this, some growers maintain calves on an iron-deficient diet. Such calves are anemic, and the stress of rough handling when they are being loaded may cause some to collapse.

Deficiency Correction

Iron deficiency anemia is most common in piglets raised in total confinement on impervious floors. If they are outside on the ground, it rarely occurs, and one of the early and still effective control procedures is to place a shovelful of sod in the pen for them to root around in. But this approach doesn't fit into modern management schemes and is contraindicated for parasite control; therefore, other means of supplementing iron have been devised. One is to add ferric citrate to the sow's diet for a couple of weeks prior to farrowing, in hopes of raising the iron content of her milk. This is not very effective, as the composition of milk remains quite stable regardless of diet. Swabbing the sow's udder daily with ferrous sulfate so the piglets get some when they nurse, or dosing the piglets daily with a 1 percent solution, is effective but laborious. The method adopted by most swine growers is to give each piglet oral iron or an injectable iron preparation such as iron dextran at 1 week of age. For early-weaned pigs, a single dose may be sufficient. If weaning is delayed to 5 or 6 weeks, a second dose may be necessary. The same preparation is suitable for the young of other species suffering from iron deficiency anemia.

Other Deficiencies

Deficiencies other than iron can also cause anemia in animals but are not as clear-cut or so easily diagnosed. *Deficiency of copper* is responsible for unthriftiness, depressed milk production, and anemia in many parts of the world. It may be *primary,* in which there simply isn't enough copper in the soil or forage, or *secondary,* in which case copper is there but made unavailable by an excess of molybdenum. The latter is most common on muck-type soils such as are found in many areas of the United States. *Cobalt deficiency* also causes anemia in ruminant animals and has been identified as one factor leading to reproductive inefficiency. Anemic animals do not come into heat regularly, nor do they readily conceive if they do.

Symptoms of copper or cobalt deficiency are often obscure, and diagnosis is not easy and is often retrospective. If the animal improves when the specific element is added to the diet, then the assumption is that deficiency is the cause. The best procedure is to prevent deficiency by adding trace mineralized salt to the ration or giving animals free-choice access to it.

Goiter

Goiter is enlargement of the thyroid gland due to deficiency of iodine. Soils in some areas, notably the upper Midwest and West Coast, are deficient in iodine, and animals as well as people raised in these areas may have goiter. The condition is most prevalent in the newborn, and pigs and lambs are most susceptible, although it can occur in any species. Severely deficient animals will be weak at birth or stillborn. Those that survive, if untreated, fail to grow and develop normally due to thyroid hormone deficiency. The disease is readily recognizable by the obvious enlargement of the gland located in the neck. Frequently, the skin is thick, edematous, and flabby.

Those that are born alive respond reasonably well to supplementation of the diet with iodine. The disease is readily preventable by feeding iodized salt, and this practice is now so general that the disease is rarely seen.

Osteomalacia

Sometimes called *adult rickets,* the underlying cause of osteomalacia is a deficiency of calcium in the diet, but the clinical signs are attributable to overactivity of the parathyroid gland. You may recall in our earlier discussion of milk fever that, as serum calcium levels drop, the parathyroid gland mobilizes stored calcium reserves in bone. Although with this disease the problem is with dietary calcium deficiency rather than calcium metabolism, the parathyroid activity is triggered the same way.

When calcium is deficient in the diet over a period of weeks or months, parathyroid hormone pulls compensating amounts out of the bones. Eventually, the

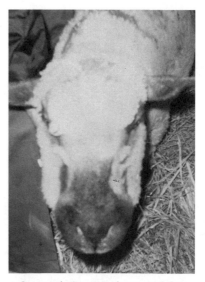

Osteomalacia causes bones to deform and fracture, here resulting in "big head."

bones become sufficiently demineralized that they become deformed or fracture. Clinical signs include reluctance to move, nonspecific lameness, and general unthriftiness. The disease is most common in pigs and horses, perhaps because calcium deficiency is more likely to occur in animals maintained on high-grain diets. Given a choice, most livestock will eat grain in preference to hay because it tastes good. Perhaps that is why adult rickets is seen more often in "pet" animals whose owners think feeding more grain is a kindness.

In the horse, the disease is occasionally referred to as *bran disease* or *big head,* the latter because of the characteristic changes that occur in the bones of the head.

Treatment

After diagnosis, treatment consists of rest and supplemental calcium to the diet in the form of calcium carbonate or limestone. Restoration of normal calcium levels will not correct bone deformities but will restore normal bone strength, reducing the possibility of future fractures.

This disease is readily and economically preventable by keeping calcium and phosphorus intake adequate and in balance. Refer to chapter 2 on nutrition for specific recommendations.

Parakeratosis

This skin disease occurs in pigs and occasionally calves raised in confinement and fed exclusively on commercial diets. It does not occur in animals with access to pasture. The cause is an actual zinc deficiency in the diet or a relative deficiency induced by an overabundance of calcium. It responds well to addition of zinc to the ration.

Symptoms

In pigs, the principal effect of the disease is reduced rate of gain due to depressed appetite and less efficient feed conversion. The skin lesions appear first as reddened areas. These areas become papules, which develop crusts that may coalesce. There is symmetrical involvement of limbs, ears, and head. The crusts become quite thick and crack easily. Secondary bacterial infection of the affected skin is not unusual.

The skin lesions in cattle may be more extensive with alopecia and wrinkling of the skin over the joints, scrotum, and neck. The disease has been diagnosed in sheep grazed on zinc-deficient soils. Loss of wool, wrinkling of the skin, and ram infertility are the prominent signs in sheep.

Prevention

Zinc in the form of carbonate or sulfate added to the diet relieves the symptoms rather rapidly. The disease can be prevented by being certain, through analysis, that the diet contains adequate amounts of zinc, and by supplementation if necessary. If the calcium level is excessive, adjusting the ration composition to bring it down to normal will have a sparing effect on zinc, so a marginal level will be adequate.

Rickets

This is a disease of young animals caused by dietary deficiency of calcium or phosphorus or a wide ratio between the two, and/or inadequate vitamin D, resulting in a failure of mineralization of long bone. Lesions are most pronounced as enlargements at the ends of the long bones *(epiphyses)*, where the longitudinal growth of bone occurs. Lameness and fractures are common, but by themselves they are not sufficient basis for an accurate diagnosis. Other diseases such as hyperparathyroidism can cause similar signs. Rickets is not common but is most likely to be found in young animals raised in total confinement in an area of the barn where there is little or no sunlight. Specialized cells in the skin produce vitamin D under stimulation of ultraviolet

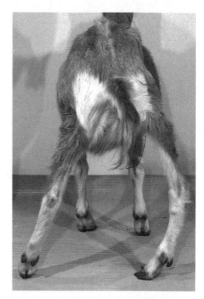

Crooked legs such as these are due to improper bone development resulting from rickets.

rays from the sun. Although vitamin D can be added to feedstuffs such as milk replacer and grain, it does not occur naturally in sufficient quantity to prevent deficiency signs from developing if an animal is deprived of sunlight.

Prevention of rickets is contingent on adequate phosphorus and calcium intake and regular exposure to sunshine or vitamin D supplementation. Before embarking on treatment of suspected rickets with vitamin D, be sure of the diagnosis. If the condition is actually due to calcium deficiency, injection of vitamin D would only make matters worse. In advanced cases, physical examination of the animal coupled with consideration of the diet, including adequacy of calcium and phosphorus intake, usually lead to the diagnosis of rickets. When clinical signs are less apparent early in the disease, x-rays and histopathologic examination of bone sections may be necessary for an accurate diagnosis.

Vitamin A Deficiency (Avitaminosis A)

Vitamin A is one of the most important vitamins for livestock and is required in comparatively large amounts. Green feeds, pasture grasses, hay, and corn contain ample amounts of carotene and carotenoids, which animals readily convert to vitamin A, and deficiency is unlikely to occur in animals with access to these feed-stuffs. Very young animals depend on colostrum and milk for their vitamin A needs. If the dam's reserves are low, deficiency may occur in the offspring.

Carotene is absorbed as vitamin A in the intestine and converted back to carotene for storage in the liver. A high proportion of carotene may be destroyed in the intestine, and the rate of absorption and conversion is influenced by availability, presence of phosphorus, calcium:phosphorus ratio, vitamin E, and levels of serum vitamin A. Required intake is higher during any disease due to lowered efficiency of conversion. If carotene intake is marginal, the liver reserve will be depleted in 2 to 3 months and deficiency signs will begin to appear.

Carotene (vitamin A) is rather unstable, tending to oxidize quite rapidly. Hay that has been weather damaged or in storage more than 6 months will have a low carotene content, and supplementation is recommended for animals maintained on this type of diet. Grains, especially corn, have a high carotene content, but most commercial grain rations have vitamin A added as a precautionary measure. Vitamin A deficiency is most likely to occur in animals maintained on diets that do not include forage crops and during the late-winter months when the carotene stored in the liver is depleted.

Symptoms

Vitamin A exerts its principal effect on epithelial tissue. Epithelial tissues include the skin and the lining of the gastrointestinal, respiratory, and reproductive tracts. Signs of deficiency relate to problems of these areas, particularly lowered resistance to such things as ringworm, respiratory disease, and reproductive disorders — infertility and retained placenta, for example. Classic descriptions of vitamin A deficiency include reference to such things as night blindness, swollen joints, convulsions, and diarrhea. These are extremes, and long before these severe signs are seen, less definitive aberrations occur. The cumulative losses from lowered resistance, stillbirths, weak offspring, and so on are much more significant and difficult to diagnose.

Prevention

Vitamin A deficiency can be prevented by including good-quality hay in the diet or by addition of vitamin A to the grain ration. Where this is not feasible, intramuscular injection of vitamin A will provide a reserve lasting several months.

Water Deprivation

It seems so obvious that most texts don't even mention it, but water is the single most important dietary component for all species. Adult animals can go a week or two without feed but 1 day without water and they are pretty uncomfortable, 2 days and they are obviously sick, and in 3 days many will be dead. Hot weather hastens the onset of clinical signs. These include restlessness, bellowing, depression of milk flow and appetite, dehydration, and constipation. Convulsions and coma may occur prior to death. Similar signs occur when there is overconsumption of salt with restricted water intake (i.e., salt poisoning).

It's important that animals have adequate fresh water available at all times. Check your watering equipment daily, because equipment failures account for the vast majority of water-deprivation problems.

White Muscle Disease (Nutritional Myopathy, Stiff Lamb Disease)

White muscle disease is a nutritional disease seen occasionally in young calves and lambs. In some areas it reaches serious proportions, causing losses of 50 percent or more of the calf or lamb crop. It is caused by a deficiency of the element selenium. The effect of selenium deficiency is more pronounced when levels of vitamin E are also low.

Selenium is a part of the enzyme glutathione peroxidase, which plays a part in detoxification of naturally occurring peroxide at the cellular level. Peroxides are toxic to cell membranes and, unless detoxified, cause muscle cell necrosis. This hyaline degeneration of muscle tissue gives the affected areas a white, cooked appearance, hence the name *white muscle disease.*

Vitamin E, also an antioxidant, has a sparing effect on selenium, so that if selenium intake is low but vitamin E is adequate, clinical signs of white muscle disease will not appear. However, if selenium is absent, vitamin E alone will not prevent symptoms from occurring.

Selenium is an essential trace element with a rather narrow margin of safety. A daily intake of as little as 0.1 ppm is adequate for health. Higher levels may be toxic, and the element in high doses has been shown to be carcinogenic for laboratory rodents.

Selenium content of soils varies widely. It is deficient in many parts of the Northeast but overabundant in some of the western range areas in the United States. Some seleniferous plants growing in such areas may contain in excess of 10 ppm, a level toxic to animals that eat those plants.

Although seen more commonly in the young, the effect of selenium deficiency is not limited to that age group. Adult animals can be affected as well. There is increasing evidence that retained placenta as a herd problem in dairy cattle may be due in part to inadequate selenium in the diet. Also, careful necropsy of so-called downer cows will sometimes reveal the lesions typical of white muscle disease in the heavy muscles and particularly the heart.

Symptoms

The condition may be seen any time but it is most common in the age range of 3 weeks to 3 months. Clinical signs vary from stiffness of the hind limbs and reluctance to move, to sudden death with no premonitory signs.

Exercise aggravates the condition, and a typical history is that the calves seemed healthy, but when they were turned out on pasture the first time and started to run and play, several dropped dead.

Occasionally, the condition may be manifested by a pneumonia-like syndrome, with fever and labored breathing that is unresponsive to antibiotics.

Diagnosis

The disease can usually be readily diagnosed on the basis of clinical signs, but the stiffness and stilted gait must be differentiated from injury, blackleg, and conditions such as foot rot.

At necropsy, characteristic white areas of degenerated muscle tissue will be seen in the heavy muscles of the hind leg, the loin area, the intercostal muscles, and occasionally in the diaphragm and heart. In advanced cases, some calcification of the necrotic tissue occurs, and it may have a gritty feel when cut with a knife. However, most cases terminate fatally before this occurs.

Treatment

If detected early, many cases respond well to injection of sodium selenite, vitamin E, or a proprietary combination of the two. However, sodium selenite is quite toxic, and treatment should be administered only under direction of your veterinarian. Unfortunately, many cases are not detected until it is too late. The muscle damage that occurs is not reversible. The animal that survives may compensate to some degree, but it is frequently unthrifty and therefore uneconomical. Prevention is easier and more effective than treatment.

Prevention

The disease is most prevalent in calves that are basically on a milk diet. The easiest and most logical preventive, therefore, is to be sure there is adequate selenium and vitamin E in the dam's milk

One method is to buy hay and grain from a variety of sources on the assumption that at least some of it will be grown on soils adequate in selenium. A more practical method for most people is to inject the dam with a vitamin E–selenium preparation during the last month or two of gestation. A single injection usually is sufficient.

Alternatively, a smaller dose of the same material can be given to each calf when it is born. However, this won't help the occasional calf that is born with white muscle disease or the few that are stillborn for the same reason. Creep feeding grain will help to prevent the disease in older calves.

Perhaps the most convenient way to ensure adequate selenium intake is to incorporate small amounts of it in the grain. Because the amount required and legally permitted is so small, this should not be attempted with home-mixing equipment. It can be done on a prescription basis by your feed dealer.

Miscellaneous Diseases

THERE ARE A NUMBER of commonly encountered disease conditions of livestock that cannot be readily grouped by cause. Nevertheless, they occur with sufficient frequency that the owner should have some knowledge of them. A few are uncontrollable, but the majority, if you know what to look for and plan ahead, can be prevented. These conditions are described briefly in this chapter.

Abomasum, Displaced

This is a problem of the dairy cow close to the time of parturition, seen almost exclusively in cows on high-concentrate, high-silage, or complete-feed diets. The condition is one of torsion of the *abomasum,* or fourth stomach, to either the left or the right, resulting in depressed appetite and reduced milk production. The majority of displacements are to the left, with the abomasum sliding under the anterior part of the rumen and upward, where it becomes distended with gas. The clinical signs are almost identical to ketosis, with the cow showing preference for hay and silage over grain, intermittent constipation, and occasionally diarrhea and gradual weight loss. The test for ketones in urine and milk is positive.

Many theories have been advanced as to the cause, including abomasal and rumen atony due to hypocalcemia, vitamin E or selenium deficiency, and lifting of the rumen by the gravid uterus to allow the abomasum to slip underneath. Diet, however, appears most important, because the condition can be prevented almost entirely by feeding 4 to 5 pounds or more of long hay daily.

Treatment

Conservative treatment consists of rolling the cow on her back and rocking her back and forth to get the abomasum back in position. This sometimes produces dramatic recovery, but relapses are frequent. A heavy suture placed through the abomasum from the outside will hold it in place, but this approach carries a risk of infection. Many veterinarians have found the rate of relapse declines if the animal is given calcium gluconate and a laxative. When these methods fail, surgery is the only resort and is quite successful.

Abscesses

These are accumulations of dead and living bacteria, cellular debris, and body fluids, otherwise known as *pus,* walled off in a connective tissue capsule. They can occur anywhere and vary in size from microscopic to the size of a basketball. Microabscesses occur in the liver, kidney, and occasionally the brain, secondary to generalized bacterial infection. The larger abscesses are generally located subcutaneously or intramuscularly and are the result of wound infection. Subcutaneous abscesses due to *Arcanobacter (Corynebacterium) pyogenes* are common in goats, and the same organism commonly causes abscesses on the lateral side of the hocks and on the knees of cattle confined to stalls with inadequate bedding. The constant bruising they undergo each time the cow lies down injures and devitalizes tissue, and infection results. This is a serious problem in some herds that can best be controlled by steam-cleaning the stall beds to reduce the bacterial population and then using more bedding and/or rubber mats. Poor sanitation aggravates the problem. Lung abscesses may be secondary to pneumonia. Umbilical abscess is not uncommon in animals about 1 week old, due to infection occurring at or soon after birth. Dipping the navel in tincture of iodine usually prevents the problem.

When first detected, abscesses are usually hot and painful to the touch. They may or may not cause fever and lack of appetite. Without treatment, they commonly terminate in one of two ways: (1) the abscess may continue to enlarge, with the capsule thinning out at the surface until it ruptures to discharge pus; or (2) active infection may subside, with inflammation disappearing and pus remaining inside the capsule. These so-called sterile abscesses may persist for months, with the pus gradually being replaced by scar tissue.

Treatment

Treatment of abscesses is determined by the location. Long-term antibiotic therapy is the only way to handle abscesses in the internal organs such as the lung, and it isn't always successful. Fair success has been obtained in controlling liver abscesses of cattle and hogs by constant low-level antibiotic feeding.

Surgical drainage of abscesses that are accessible is the treatment of choice, followed by daily irrigation with antiseptics and concurrent systemic administration of antibiotics. If you decide to open an abscess yourself, be sure you know what you are doing. Abscesses can easily be confused with hematomas, joint capsule distention such as bog spavin, and umbilical hernia.

On more than one occasion, I have been called on to rescue a calf that supposedly had an umbilical abscess that the herdsman incised, only to find himself holding a handful of intestines. When in doubt, call your veterinarian!

Allergy

Like people, some animals suffer from allergies, most notably horses and cattle and occasionally goats. The mechanism of allergy is complex and beyond the scope of this text. Suffice to say it is a generalized adverse reaction to prior sensitization by an allergen. In animals the allergenic substance is usually certain weeds or grasses, mold spores, or drugs. The reaction may take the form of urticaria or hives, characterized by edema of the eyelids and hairless skin areas such as the vulva, and by wheals on the neck and back. *Pulmonary edema* is a complication of hives in which the lungs fill with fluid, causing respiratory distress. It can be rapidly fatal if untreated. *Allergic dermatitis* occurs as a result of insect bites and contact with chemicals or harness.

Photosensitization is a form of allergy that occurs when animals ingest certain plants such as Saint-John's-wort, rape, white clover, and sometimes alfalfa. Substances in the plant render the animal more susceptible to sunlight, and the lesions resemble sunburn. The lower leg and muscle are the main areas affected.

Although allergy is usually an individual problem, it occasionally affects a high proportion of the herd. A good example is the acute respiratory disease seen in cattle grazing on aftermath or improved pastures. This disease is more common in climates noted for wet weather and frequent fogs, hence the name *fog fever*. It is rarely reported in the United States as a herd problem, although we do see a similar condition in individuals, sometimes called *summer snuffles*.

An unusual type of allergy occurs in a small percentage of dairy cattle allergic to their own milk. Signs of urticaria develop when the udder is distended and subside when the cow is milked out.

Generally speaking, allergy is a self-limiting individual problem that disappears spontaneously in most cases. An exception is the complication of pulmonary edema, which can be very rapidly fatal. It requires prompt treatment with epinephrine, antihistamines, or corticosteroids and sometimes all three. In such cases, until your veterinarian arrives, the best you can do is keep the animal as quiet as possible to reduce the demand for oxygen. Urticaria that doesn't disappear promptly when the diet is changed can be successfully treated with antihistamines.

Anaphylaxis

This can best be described as a peracute, rapidly fatal allergic response to a foreign protein. In livestock, the triggering factor is usually injection of a vaccine, bacterin, or antiserum. The reaction can occur following the initial dose, but is more likely following a second or subsequent dose, with the first acting as a sensitizing dose. Products containing serum from another animal species (heterologous serum) cause anaphylactic shock more than any other. The older leptospirosis bacterins containing small amounts of rabbit serum frequently caused anaphylactic reactions.

Symptoms

Signs of anaphylaxis occur usually within an hour of the time of injection and often within minutes. These may include hypersalivation; rapid, labored breathing; shivering; and rapid temperature rise. Pulmonary edema or emphysema in the less acute case is common. Bloat in ruminants and diarrhea are occasionally seen. Release of large amounts of histamine from muscle tissue occurs, which in turn contributes to rumen atony (failure of normal rumen contractions) and vasodilation, with a fall in blood pressure and the eventual collapse of the animal.

The biological products in use today are highly purified to reduce the risk of anaphylaxis, but it still occurs occasionally. It's a good idea, therefore, to keep animals under close observation for an hour after vaccination. Immediate treatment is important if the affected animal is to survive, using drugs such as ephinephrine and antihistamines. Laminitis is a common sequel in the horse.

Anemia, Isoimmune Hemolytic

Isoimmune hemolytic anemia is unique in that it is rarely reported in species other than the horse and is most common in Standardbreds, Thoroughbreds, and mules. It occurs when, through placental injury, some of the foal's blood enters the mare's circulation. This acts as an antigen, and the mare produces antibody in response. When the newborn foal then nurses colostrum, he also gets a dose of antibody against his own red blood cells. This results in hemolysis and agglutination of red cells, causing the foal to show signs of anemia in 12 to 96 hours. The severity of signs is governed by concentration of antibody in the colostrum and how much colostrum the foal consumed.

Affected foals are lethargic and weak and have accelerated heart and respiratory rates without fever. Jaundice and hemoglobinuria appear as the disease progresses. These signs, coupled with age at onset and the breed, are presumptive evidence of isoimmune hemolytic anemia. Diagnosis can be confirmed by hemagglutination of the foal's red cells with serum or colostrum from the dam. The disease is more likely to occur in second or subsequent foals born of the same mating.

Treatment

Treatment depends on severity of clinical signs, but in any case the foal should not receive additional colostrum from the mare. Mild cases recover with good nursing care. Blood transfusion is indicated for those more severely affected, and in extreme cases a complete blood exchange may be necessary.

Prevalence of the disease can be reduced by blood-typing and test-matching serum from the mare with red cells from the stallion prior to breeding. If agglutination occurs, use another stallion. Alternatively, follow the same procedure with red cells from the foal before it nurses. If agglutination occurs, don't let the foal nurse. Instead, use colostrum from a different mare, if available, or a milk substitute. Milk out the mare by hand for 48 hours and then let the foal nurse. By that time, most of the antibody will be gone, but bear in mind that foals deprived of colostrum will be more susceptible to infection and will require special care.

Bloat

Bloat is a condition unique to ruminant animals and is generally more of a problem in cattle than in sheep or goats. Bloat is distention of the rumen with trapped gas that can become severe enough to cause death in an hour or less. That bloat is more than a simple mechanical problem of accumulated gas has been demonstrated by experimental inflation of the rumen with air with no adverse effect on the animal. It just belches the air out as fast as it is pumped in. With bloat, however, rumen contractions are sluggish or totally absent and eructation does not occur, so the distention continues as long as gas evolves from the rumen contents.

Bloat is more likely to occur when animals are grazed for the first time on lush legume pasture, which is especially dangerous when it is wet with early-morning dew or rain. Bloat is also a problem in the feedlots when cattle or lambs are placed on full feed. Some of them become chronic bloaters and fail to gain as they should. Early marketing is the best answer for them. Chronic bloat is occasionally seen in cattle whose rumen function is impaired by irritation of the vagus nerve, either from traumatic gastritis *(hardware disease)* or from tumors.

Legume bloat is not a simple matter of free gas trapped in the rumen but is often called *frothy bloat* because the gas is trapped in bubbles. This greatly complicates resolution of the problem.

Diagnosis

Diagnosis of bloat is a simple matter. Affected animals usually stop eating and stand apart from the herd. When viewed from the rear, the animal shows a pronounced swelling on the upper left side, behind the last rib and below the lateral processes of the lumbar vertebrae. When palpated, this area feels as tight as a drumhead. Depending on severity, the animal may breathe in rapid, short breaths with the mouth open. The least exertion aggravates the shortness of breath, and the animal may fall to the ground and expire from anoxia. Death due to bloat may be acute, with animals found dead in the pasture. For that reason, it's a good idea to check them periodically for the first few days they are put into a legume pasture. If no clinical signs are seen prior to death and a dead bloated animal is all you see, a distinction must be made between death due to bloat and other diseases such as anthrax, blackleg, and urea poisoning.

Treatment

Severe bloat requires prompt emergency treatment. Call your veterinarian, but while you wait there are some things you can do to help. Get all the animals out of the pasture immediately. A few tablespoons of household detergent given orally helps reduce surface tension of bubbles in the rumen, releasing trapped gas. A pint of vegetable or mineral oil will do the same thing, but the volume of fluid makes it more risky to give orally. Tying a 1-inch-diameter piece of wood in the mouth, as you would place a bit in a horse's mouth, will stimulate salivation and eructation. This procedure has saved many animals.

If veterinary help is not available, a makeshift cow stomach tube can be made using a 10-foot length of smooth garden hose. Lubricate it with mineral oil and pass it gently down the throat into the rumen to relieve the pressure. This procedure takes practice, but if you can't get professional help in a hurry, it's worth a try.

As a last resort, use a trocar, if available. This instrument, available from most livestock supply houses, is especially made to relieve bloat when inserted directly into the rumen. If the diameter of the cannula is inadequate to relieve the bloat, enlarge the hole in the rumen with a sharp knife and insert a piece of larger pipe. This is not a time to be squeamish. If the animal is so badly bloated that a cannula is necessary, the pain of cannula insertion will be inconsequential. Complications may ensue, but these will be manageable, whereas unrelieved severe bloat is fatal. Medication such as poloxalene, detergent, or oil can be put directly into the rumen via stomach tube or through the cannula. Use of the cannula is quick in an emergency to save the animal's life, but because infection frequently follows, routine use is not recommended.

Prevention

Bloat can be largely prevented through management. Feeding some dry hay to cattle or sheep prior to putting them in legume pasture and waiting until the grass is dry before turning them out are very helpful procedures. Leaving them in the pasture for only half an hour or so until they are accustomed to it also helps. Feedlot bloat is not so easy to manage, but various techniques have been used with fair success. Addition of surface tension–reducing agents such as poloxalene and vegetable oils to the feed are helpful.

Calculi

Urinary calculi are sometimes a problem in feedlot steers or wethers and less often in intact males. *Calculi* are hard aggregations of mineral salts and epithelial cells that form either in the renal pelvis or the bladder, where they may produce a mechanical irritation and a chronic cystitis. A more serious complication results when they become lodged in the urethra to block the flow of urine, partially or completely.

Symptoms

Affected animals evidence colicky pain such as kicking at the belly, treading with the hind feet, and switching the tail. Attempts to urinate are frequent, with straining and grating of the teeth. Urine passage is scanty, often blood-tinged, and sometimes totally absent. When the obstruction is complete, the urethra or bladder ruptures. Rupture of the urethra results in diffusion of urine into the subcutaneous tissues of the belly extending toward the chest, causing obvious fluid swelling. This is often accompanied by infection and occasionally by sloughing of a section of skin, which permits urine to escape. Rupture of the bladder brings immediate relief from pain, but urine accumulating in the abdomen causes a toxemia and death in about 48 hours. The characteristic appearance of animals with abdomen distended by urine gives the disease the common name *water belly.*

Treatment

Surgical intervention is the only effective treatment once the clinical signs appear, but dietary management helps to reduce prevalence of the condition. Adequate and balanced amounts of calcium and phosphorus are important, as is adequate vitamin A. Addition of sodium chloride to the diet, up to 5 percent of daily dry matter intake, will prevent the problem almost entirely, provided adequate amounts of fresh water are available. Feeding ammonium chloride to alter urine pH has also been found to reduce the formation of calculi.

Colic

This is really not a disease but, rather, a group of symptoms in response to abdominal pain. The underlying cause is almost always a gastrointestinal disturbance, and it occurs in the horse far more often than in any other species. It may range from simple indigestion with gas formation to mechanical blockage such as volvulus or intussusception. A not-infrequent occurrence in the horse is thrombus formation in the mesenteric arteries due to strongyle larvae. When a thrombus forms in an artery, the blood supply to tissue served by it is cut off and that section of the bowel dies. Large masses of bots may cause sufficient inflammation of the stomach wall in the horse, and even partially obstruct the pyloric end, to cause gastric distress. Engorgement and impaction often occur when a horse gets accidental access to the feed bin or is fed finely chopped indigestible hay. Some horses get chronic indigestion because their teeth are bad and they can't chew properly.

Symptoms

Regardless of the cause, clinical signs of colic in the horse are essentially the same, varying only in severity. Restlessness, kicking at the belly, getting up and down frequently, and rolling are common. Standing in a stretched-out, "sawhorse" attitude is characteristic. More severe pain causes sweating, rapid pulse, and onset of a shocklike syndrome. Movements may be quite violent, with self-inflicted injury common. With volvulus or cecal torsion, onset is sudden; with impaction, engorgement, or simple indigestion, onset is more gradual.

Early accurate diagnosis is important in the management of colic. Volvulus, torsion, and sometimes impaction require surgery to save an animal's life, and the longer it is delayed, the poorer the prognosis. Aside from calling a veterinarian immediately, the most useful thing an owner can do is to keep the horse from injuring himself. The best way to do this is to keep the horse on his feet and walking. Walking also helps to stimulate peristalsis and passage of gas and manure.

Prevention

As with everything else, prevention of colic is far better than treatment, and several things should be done as a matter of routine good husbandry. Control internal parasites, and have the horse's teeth checked and floated at least once a year. Make any feed change gradually, and, most important, be sure the horse doesn't have an opportunity to overeat grain. Feed coarsely ground rather than finely ground grain, and avoid hay composed primarily of young, tender legumes. Some horses develop a habit of bolting their grain as soon as it is put out and regularly get indigestion as a result. Putting a couple of clean stones the size of softballs in their feed buckets will slow down consumption because they have to work around the stones to get at the grain. Some horses regularly get indigestion from eating straw used as bedding. The logical thing to do in this case is switch to shavings or sawdust for bedding.

Founder (Laminitis)

This painful condition of the foot occurs in all hooved animals but is most commonly thought of in connection with horses and ponies. The predisposing factors in the horse are well defined, but the mechanism by which they cause founder is less well understood. These factors include overeating grain, consumption of large amounts of cold water when the animal is hot, serious illness such as pneumonia or metritis, and concussion during fast road work, especially by an unconditioned horse. Overeating grain or pasture is the most common cause. Acute allergic reactions may also produce founder.

Normally, only a small portion of the animal's weight is borne on the sole of the foot. Most of the weight is borne on the walls through soft laminae that attach the coffin bone to the wall. With acute founder, swelling of the laminae occurs, and because the walls of the hoof can't expand to accommodate the swelling, excruciating pain results. The swelling is probably the result of excess histamine combined with impairment of circulation in the foot. In more advanced cases, separation of the laminae occurs with rotation of the coffin bone downward at the tip — even to the point, in extreme cases, where it protrudes through the sole. This rotation results in deformity of the foot and chronic lameness.

Symptoms

Acute laminitis in the horse has a sudden onset, with acute pain, sweating, fever, and extreme reluctance to move. The horse will stand with the feet tucked up or stretched out to relieve pain, and after considerable effort may lie down and refuse to get up. Prompt treatment is required if the animal is to recover without permanent lameness. Antihistamines, analgesics, a laxative, and alternating hot and cold packs on the feet to stimulate the circulation are the usual therapy.

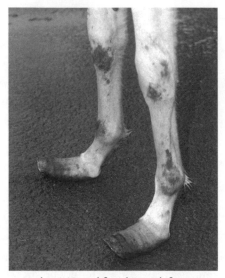

Laminitis and founder result from inexcusable neglect.

The horse may recover in a few days, or the disease may become chronic, with the coffin bone rotating downward, the forward part of the hoof wall becoming concave, and the entire wall assuming a corrugated appearance. The effects of chronic laminitis can be relieved somewhat by corrective shoeing, but the foundered horse is usually unable to do hard work without again becoming lame.

Laminitis in the other livestock

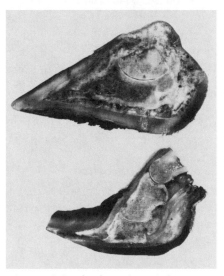

A normal claw (top) emphasizes the severe deformity typical of laminitis (bottom).

species is more insidious and occurs over a period of time. It is rarely acute, as in the horse. Almost invariably it is the result of high grain feeding and is a particular problem for exhibitors of beef cattle who want their animals fat at show time. The high-concentrate feeding necessary to get adequate fat covering contributes to laminitis. Because their feet hurt, cattle with laminitis don't gain weight or produce milk as they should, and in some herds the resulting economic loss is substantial.

Alleviation of the problem is difficult. Frequent trimming of the feet to be sure they bear weight evenly is about the best that can be done. Prevention through dietary management is most important.

Fractures

Fortunately, fractures don't occur very often in livestock, although the frequency increases in the presence of other conditions, such as rickets and phosphorus deficiency. From a theoretical medical standpoint, fractures in livestock should heal as well as they do in smaller animals and in people. And they do, depending on location. Broken ribs due to kicks, crowding through gates, or fighting are not unusual, and they heal uneventfully. But leg fractures are a different matter in mature animals, and the problem is mechanical rather than medical. It's extremely difficult to immobilize a long-bone fracture in an animal weighing 1000 pounds or more, particularly when the animal doesn't understand what you are trying to do and does its best to take off the splint or cast. With calves, foals, sheep, and goats the problem is not as great, but even then it taxes the ingenuity of the orthopedic surgeon. Fractures of the small tarsal and carpal bones, occurring most frequently in the horse, are amenable to surgical repair using internal fixation such as screws, nails, and/or external casts.

But given the guarded prognosis for long-bone fractures and the finite value of commercial livestock, most owners elect euthanasia. The expense and tribulations of fracture repair generally can be justified only for valuable purebred animals.

Prevention

Fractures are accidents, and most accidents are preventable if one uses a little forethought. In this case, the owner has to do the thinking for his animals. Try to foresee the hazards and take steps to remove them. Simple things — such as putting sand on slippery floors to prevent falls and keeping animals confined when it's icy outside — will help. Keeping machinery and junk out of the pastures will reduce accidents of all kinds. Cattle frequently fracture the end of the tuber coxae (hip) when crowding through narrow doors, especially when some impatient soul is chasing them from behind. Padding the sides of the door frame and moving cattle slowly will keep this type of injury from occurring. All it takes is a little forethought, a little more intelligence than the animals possess, and the realization that whatever can go wrong will.

Gastritis, Traumatic (Hardware Disease, Traumatic Reticulitis)

This is a disease almost exclusively of cattle and occurs because of the eating habits of the cow coupled with the anatomical arrangement of the stomach compartments. Cattle swallow forage with minimal chewing and regurgitate it later for more complete mastication. Because they don't chew initially and only wad the forage sufficiently to swallow it, they occasionally swallow nails and pieces of wire that are mixed in with it. Being heavier than grass or silage, these objects gravitate to the lowest part of the stomach, the reticulum. Because the outlet from the reticulum to the omasum is not located at the bottom of the reticulum, accumulated hardware remains there, sometimes until it rusts out.

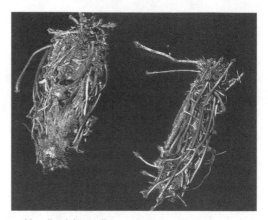

Metallic debris adheres to rumen magnets, which are given prophylactically to protect against hardware disease.

When field choppers and pickup balers first came into use as a method of harvesting the hay crop, *hardware disease* was almost an epidemic on some farms because all the stray wire lying in the fields was chopped into pieces about 2 inches long and harvested along with the hay. Now that most of this debris has been gleaned from the fields, the condition is much less common.

Symptoms

The vast majority of cows have some metal lying loose in the reticulum, and it normally does no harm. Occasionally, though, a piece will become lodged in such a way that during the normal reticulum contractions it perforates through the wall. This causes immediate pain, cessation of stomach contractions, loss of appetite, and typically a low-grade fever of 103°F to 104°F. Affected cows are reluctant to move, and may stand with a "humped-up" appearance. When forced to move, they do so very gingerly because every movement causes pain. Local abscessation or peritonitis or even sudden death due to penetration of the heart by the foreign object may occur.

Treatment

In an attempt to prevent damage to the heart, it is standard practice in cases of traumatic gastritis to confine the cow in a stall with her front legs raised on a platform about 4 inches high. The objective of this procedure is to direct the center of gravity back away from the forward wall of the reticulum. In early cases, if the metal has not passed all the way through the wall, this technique alone may bring about recovery. Special cylindrical magnets given to the cow orally with a balling gun are a further aid to retrieval of the metal from the rumen or reticulum wall. These magnets last as long as the cow, and, given prophylactically to every cow in the herd, they will prevent hardware disease almost entirely.

If these conservative methods fail, the only recourse for the affected cow is a surgical operation known as a *rumenotomy*. Through an opening in the rumen, the surgeon, preferably one with long arms, reaches in and removes the offending object. If undertaken before too much damage is done, the surgery is highly successful. Vigorous antibiotic therapy is necessary, of course, to combat the peritonitis that invariably accompanies the condition.

Keeping nails, wire, and other hazards separated from the feed and putting a magnet in each cow will almost completely prevent hardware disease. Not surprisingly, it's unclear whether a cow has had a magnet put in her or not. To find out, hold a magnetic compass near her left elbow. If she has a magnet, north will always be toward the cow no matter which way she is headed.

Heatstroke

This is a seasonal problem encountered primarily in swine, but any animal can be affected. High temperatures, high humidity, and inadequate ventilation are the predisposing factors, and fat animals are more susceptible. Panting, collapse, and very high body temperature are the principal signs.

The condition requires prompt treatment, and the cost-effective procedure is to reduce body temperature with cold showers. As soon as the animal can stand, move it to a shady or cooler area.

Prevention measures are obvious. In hot weather, provide shade for pastured animals and cool the barn with fans and/or evaporative coolers. Avoid the stress of trucking animals during the hot period of the day, and don't overcrowd them in the pens. In feedlots, the use of overhead foggers during the heat of day is advantageous, not only for cooling but also to keep dust down.

Hematoma

This is an accumulation of blood, generally subcutaneously, resulting from rupture of a blood vessel. Injury is the usual cause and the location can be anywhere. Swelling is the obvious clinical sign, and bleeding may continue for several hours, with the hematoma becoming quite large. Hematomas must be distinguished from abscesses and, depending on location, hernias. Compared with an abscess, hematomas develop rapidly, are not hot to the touch, and generally are not acutely painful.

In most cases, no special treatment is necessary and the blood will eventually be reabsorbed, although some scar tissue may remain. Surgical drainage may be necessary if the hematoma is located in a position to cause interference with breathing or eating. Occasionally, secondary infection will occur, and what started as hematoma becomes an abscess. In dairy cattle, hematomas of the teat due to injury are difficult to handle. The teat becomes swollen, hard, and difficult to milk. Soaking the teat frequently in a warm water and Epsom salts solution (1 tablespoon Epsom salts per pint of warm water) will help reduce the swelling, but a cannula may have to be used for several days to remove the milk without further injury. When using a teat cannula, follow careful aseptic procedures to avoid causing mastitis.

Hernia

Hernias occur in all species and are usually umbilical, scrotal, or inguinal in location. Hernias at other sites are ruptures — the result of injury. A hernia is an interruption of the continuity of the abdominal wall, with an outpouching of the peritoneum. The condition is serious if a loop of intestine passes through the opening. It may become strangulated, causing severe pain, with necrosis of that part of the bowel due to interruption of the circulation, and ultimately death of the animal. If the intestine has been there long enough for adhesions to form, surgery is the only solution.

Umbilical hernias are obvious at or soon after birth, but must be distinguished from an umbilical abscess or hematoma. They are most common in calves, and there is good evidence that the condition is hereditary; therefore, calves with umbilical hernia should not be used for breeding purposes. Small hernias of an inch or so in diameter will usually close spontaneously. Closure can be hastened by maintaining reduction of the hernia with a band of wide adhesive tape around the abdomen. Larger hernias require surgical repair.

Scrotal hernias are found most commonly in baby pigs, usually at the time of castration. Anyone who castrates very many pigs soon learns to keep suture and needle handy to make on-the-spot repairs. This lesson is brought home rather forcefully the first time one sees a just castrated piglet run to the far side

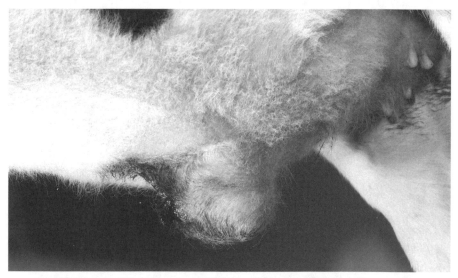

A calf with an umbilical hernia such as this should not be used for breeding purposes, as the condition is hereditary.

of the pen dragging a loop of intestine behind him. Closure of the external inguinal ring with a few sutures is a simple matter if you have the materials at hand. Scrotal hernia is really an extended inguinal hernia.

Strangulated inguinal hernias occur in stallions and occasionally bulls, and are extensions of bowel through the internal inguinal ring. Such a hernia is often manifested as colicky pain immediately after breeding, and the diagnosis can be made by rectal examination. If the hernia cannot be reduced by way of the rectum, surgery is necessary.

Hernias result from omission of nature or accident, and, except in the case of hereditary umbilical hernia of calves, little can be done to prevent them. Although a definite hereditary link has not been established, it would be prudent not to use littermates of pigs with scrotal hernia as breeding stock.

Lameness, Equine

Lameness in horses has many causes, but perhaps the single most important factor is the stress of training to race as 2-year-olds. This has nothing to do with the horse but, rather, is a reflection of human greed, to get horses on the track and earning money as soon as possible. The skeletal development of many horses until they are about 3 years old is not sufficiently progressed to withstand the concussion and the stresses of hard work. An analogous situation is the disproportionately high prevalence of injuries sustained by high school athletes on the football field.

Terms for Equine Lameness

Because sound feet and legs are so important to the horse, diagnosis and management of lameness should be left to an experienced veterinarian. Over the years a bewildering array of terms, many of which make no sense at all, have evolved to name the various lamenesses. The following definitions may help you understand the various types of lameness, making it possible for you to converse intelligently with the veterinarian when the diagnosis is made.

Bog spavin. Accumulation of fluid causing distention of the joint capsules of the hock.

Bowed tendon. Severe strain on the flexor tendons of the foreleg. Swelling gives a "bowed" appearance from the knee to the ankle.

Bucked shin. Seen in overworked young horses. Swelling and heat appear on the front of the foreleg from the knee to the ankle.

Canker. Inflammation or infection of the frog, resulting in an overgrowth of imperfect frog tissue.

Capped elbow (shoe boils). Swelling at the point of the elbow. Caused by bruising due to inadequate bedding, or self-inflicted in high-stepping horses.

Capped hock. More or less chronic swelling at the point of the hock as a result of injury.

Coffin joint. The joint formed by the second and third phalanges and the navicular bone. It lies within the wall of the hoof.

Contracted tendon. Shortening of the flexor tendons of the leg. Seen primarily in young horses.

Corn. A bruise resulting from pressure from the heel of the shoe. Occurs at the angle of the sole, between the bar and the wall.

Curb. A swelling starting about 4 inches below the point of the hock. Results from ligament rupture due to strain from jumping, running, or slipping.

Founder (laminitis). An inflammation of the sensitive laminae inside the wall of the hoof. It is seen most commonly in overweight horses and ponies, and in mares as a complication of foaling. Congestion within the hoof weakens the attachment of the sensitive laminae, and the sole drops so that it appears convex rather than concave. The condition is acutely painful in the early stages.

Knee spavin. Injury to the inside of the knee produced when turning at high speeds. May result in a chronic arthritis.

Navicular disease. A chronic inflammation of the navicular bone, which with the coffin bone and the second phalanx forms the coffin joint. Usually starts as a bursitis and continues with erosion and exostosis. Most common in Quarter Horses.

Osselet. Hot, painful, and relatively soft swelling at onset along the front margin of the fetlock. Due to bone disease in the area of the joint capsule attachment. The affected area later becomes calcified.

Quittor. A draining sinus at the coronet, usually from infection or necrosis of the lateral cartilage.

Ringbone. A term generally applied to erosion of bone at the joint surfaces, from the fetlock down. May be called high or low depending on which joint is affected. With *false ringbone* there is excess bone (exostosis) formed at the edges of the joint surface, but the joint surface is unaffected. In true ringbone, the joint surface is affected.

Sandcrack. A crack starting at the wearing surface and extending partway up the wall of the hoof. Quarter cracks may start at the hairline and extend downward.

Seedy toe. A separation of the toe between the wall and the sensitive laminae of the foot. The space is filled with a crumbly type of horn tissue, hence the name *seedy toe.* May be evidence of past foundering.

Sidebone. Bone formed as a result of ossification of the lateral cartilage of the foot.

Spavin. *True spavin,* or "jack" spavin, is an inflammation of the periosteum of the bones on the inside of the hock, resulting in bone enlargement at this point. *Blind spavin* is an inflammation of the joint surfaces of the bones at the hock, with no visible bony enlargement.

Splints. Exostoses occurring usually on the inside of the foreleg, just below the knee. They may also occur on the outside of the foreleg below the knee and rarely appear on the rear leg. They are found principally in young horses, and though they may be present in older horses, they usually are not a cause of lameness in this group.

Stringhalt. A condition in which the hock is overflexed and forcefully extended when the horse moves, resulting in a jerky motion. The true cause is unknown.

Thoroughpin. Soft swelling due to distention of the tendon sheath of the hollow area forward of the point of the hock.

Lightning Stroke

In pastured animals, death due to lightning stroke can be confused with other diseases causing sudden death such as anthrax, blackleg, and bloat. Lightning stroke is usually fatal, so one might wonder what difference a diagnosis makes. There are two good reasons that diagnosis is important. First, if death was due to lightning, insurance may cover the loss. Second, if it was due to an infectious disease or bloat, steps can be taken to protect the balance of the herd.

Symptoms

Obviously, lightning stroke occurs only in conjunction with electrical storms. On several occasions, I have had farmers try to convince me that a cow found dead on a bright day was killed by lightning. These were blatant attempts at insurance fraud. Death due to lightning stroke is sudden, with no evidence of struggle such as trampled ground. Sometimes the animals even have the last bite of grass in their mouths. Occasionally, singed hair will be found around the muzzle or lower leg where sparks have jumped. Necropsies are frequently entirely negative, so circumstantial evidence is all there is to go on. Often the animals are found lying near a fence or gathered around an isolated tree that shows evidence of having been hit by lightning.

Surprisingly, lightning stroke is not always fatal. It may render the animal unconscious for a time, with no other injury. It may also cause partial or complete paralysis, from which the animal may or may not recover. The most unusual case I ever saw was a cow with a clean cut all the way through the skin and subcutaneous tissue extending from the backbone in a straight line to a point below the hock, a distance of almost 3 feet! A sharp knife couldn't have done better, and after the wound was sutured she made an uneventful recovery. Three others in the pasture with her were killed instantly.

Little can be done to protect against lightning stroke. The safest place for animals during an electrical storm is in a barn equipped with lightning rods. But if these are nonexistent or not functioning properly, cattle confined in steel stanchions may all be electrocuted if lightning hits the barn or they may suffocate if the barn burns. Most people philosophically accept lightning stroke as one of the risks of raising livestock.

Myoclonia Congenita

This is a disease of piglets, the cause of which is obscure. It begins as fine tremors at or shortly after birth. The trembling increases to a point where the piglets have difficulty nursing and then die of starvation. Those less severely affected gradually improve over a period of several days.

At one time, vaccination of pregnant sows for hog cholera was thought to be a factor, but since vaccination is no longer permitted and the disease has been eradicated, this is not a factor. However, other viruses infecting the sow and thus the piglets during gestation may be a factor. Nutritional deficiencies have been suggested but not proved. Heredity may be a factor in some breeds, and it is suggested that boars that have sired litters in which the disease appeared not be used for further breeding. For the same reason, recovered pigs should not be used for breeding stock. Assuming a virus is responsible for some cases, it may be useful in herds where the disease has appeared to expose open sows and gilts to affected piglets so they become infected and develop immunity prior to breeding.

Obturator Paralysis

This partial paralysis of the rear legs is the result of trauma to the dam's obturator nerves during a difficult birth. It is seen in cattle more than any other species. For part of their length the right and left obturator nerves run along the inside forward edge of the pelvic inlet against the bone, where there is no protective fat covering. Prolonged pressure from an oversized or malpresented calf injures the nerve, causing paralysis of the adductor muscles that the cow uses to hold her hind legs together. The cow with obturator paralysis is either unable to stand or, if she does, may lose control of the legs so they spread outward. When this happens, dislocation of the hip or splitting of the pubic symphysis frequently occurs.

Treatment

Affected animals may or may not recover, depending on the extent of the nerve injury and the quality of the nursing care. Use of lots of bedding to prevent decubital sores and turning the paralyzed cow from one side to the other every hour or so are important parts of the nursing care. Tying the hocks together with soft rope will help prevent "splitting" of the hind legs. If the cow will tolerate it, supporting her for a few minutes several times a day with a hip sling is very helpful. When using a sling, raise the animal just high enough that the feet touch the floor in the normal extended position. The idea is to encourage her to support her own weight with the sling in place to keep her from falling. The longer the paralysis persists, the poorer the prognosis. Those that don't recover within a week usually don't recover at all.

The moral of the story is to be sure the fetus is in a normal position for delivery and then to use gentle traction rather than brute force. See chapter 4 for more information on normal and abnormal delivery.

Poisoning, Silo Gas

This is not a common problem, fortunately, but it occurs often enough to deserve mention, particularly because it is also a hazard to people. Early in the fermentation of ensiled corn, oxides of nitrogen form that are extremely irritating to lung tissue and may even involve an allergic response. Most texts describe the first 3 weeks after the silo is filled as being the most dangerous period, but I have seen acute respiratory distress in cattle caused by silo gas toxicity as long as 3 months after the silo was filled. This is probably the exception rather than the rule, however.

The condition is more likely to occur when cattle are fed corn silage in a tightly closed barn. The first signs noted are coughing when the silage is placed in front of them. Continued exposure leads to copious salivation, labored breathing, elevated temperature, and depressed milk flow. In severe cases, abnormal lung sounds can be heard even without the aid of a stethoscope. Continued exposure without treatment may cause death due to anoxia.

In most cases, removal of the offending silage from the diet brings about spontaneous recovery, although the cough may persist for several months. More severely affected animals require treatment with atropine, antihistamines, and corticosteroids, as well as antibiotics to prevent secondary bacterial pneumonia.

It is best to wait several weeks before feeding out of a newly filled silo and to observe cattle carefully the first day or two when feeding begins. If they seem to cough excessively, stop feeding the silage or aerate it outside for a few hours prior to feeding, and keep the barn well ventilated during the feeding period. If these measures don't control the problem, it may be necessary to wait several months before the silage can be safely fed.

Poisoning, Urea

The economic advantage of adding urea to cattle feeds as a substitute for part of the protein has made this one of the more common poisonings of dairy and beef cattle.

Urea is highly toxic to livestock not conditioned to it. However, through repeated daily exposure to small amounts, rumen microorganisms adapt to it and convert the nitrogen in urea to amino acids, which are absorbed and utilized by the animal. Without this bacterial intervention, urea hydrolyzes to ammonia, which is rapidly absorbed from the rumen and highly fatal. It takes about 6 weeks to build a rumen flora that can safely handle sizable amounts of urea. However, if urea feeding is interrupted for as few as 48 hours, this urea-adapted population dies off. If urea feeding is then resumed at the previous level, toxicity may result. Most cases of urea poisoning occur following interruption of urea feeding, following inadequate mixing of urea in the grain or silage, following accidental addition of too much, or when cattle accidentally get access to a bag of urea.

Symptoms

Regardless of the cause, acute urea poisoning is a dramatic disease. Onset usually occurs within half an hour of consumption. The first sign is hyperesthesia, with the animals appearing unusually alert and responsive to external stimuli. They move quickly in the pen or pasture, finally breaking into a full run, bawling as they go. This progresses to more aggressive, mindless behavior, and they run into walls or fences and occasionally charge other animals or people in the pasture. This progresses to staggering, and they crawl before finally collapsing. Hypersalivation, bloat, panting, and fever are consistent findings. The symptoms closely parallel those of acute grass tetany and the furious form of rabies. The entire episode, from onset of signs to death, usually takes less than an hour.

Treatment

Treatment of animals that have consumed a fatal dose is, in my experience, of little value. Theoretically, neutralization of the ammonia with weak acids, such as vinegar, given orally or pumped directly into the rumen should help. But it takes a couple of gallons to do any good, and it's a rare occasion when that much vinegar is available in time.

Most commercial dairy rations contain some urea, and it is a perfectly safe protein substitute when properly used. The important things are to be sure that cattle are conditioned to it and that it is thoroughly mixed. It's also important that cattle being fed urea get sufficient high-energy feed to maintain a rumen flora adequate to handle it.

Prolapse

This can be simply defined as an eversion, or a turning inside out, through a normal body opening of the rectum, vagina, uterus, or prepuce.

Prolapse of the Prepuce

This occurs in some bulls, particularly those with Brahma breeding. The preputial tissue protrudes from the sheath, where it is subject to injury, infection, and scarring that may be sufficiently severe to prevent coitus. Surgical removal of the excess tissue is the only alternative to salvage by slaughter.

Prolapse of the Rectum

This is the result of prolonged straining due to enteritis or constipation. It is most common in young animals, particularly pigs. The rectum everts through the anus and appears as a red, inflamed, cylindrical mass. This soon becomes black and necrotic due to interruption of circulation. The condition is fatal if not promptly corrected. If detected early, the mass can be replaced and retained with a purse-string suture in the anus. Longstanding cases require amputation and resection. Regardless, it's a job for the veterinarian. The condition is most likely to occur when the straining is induced by chronic diarrhea or constipation. Prevention, therefore, depends on either control of diarrhea or modification of the diet to produce a normal soft stool. High-fiber diets for young pigs should be avoided.

Prolapse of the Uterus

Uterine prolapse is a complete eversion of the uterus following parturition. It can occur in any species but is most frequent in cattle. In most cases, muscular atony induced by hypocalcemia is a contributing factor. To the uninitiated, a prolapsed uterus is a terrifying sight. The only thing good to be said about it is that it makes it easy to remove the placenta because you can see what you are doing. The sooner it can be replaced, the better for the life of the animal and her future productivity, but replacement is a job for a veterinarian. It is physically difficult due to the bulk and weight of the organ, if nothing else, so be prepared to help the veterinarian do the work. Until then, the best you can do is to protect the uterus from injury. Confine the animal so she can't bang the pendulous uterus around when walking. Wrap it in a clean cloth (a bedsheet is ideal) to protect it from dirt and manure, and keep it moist with warm water. Cows that continue to strain after the calf is born are more likely to prolapse their uterus (cast their withers). If you have a cow in that category, have the veterinarian give her an epidural anesthetic to block the straining reflex.

Prolapse of the Vagina

This condition occurs during advanced pregnancy and is first noticeable when the animal is lying down, especially if her hindquarters are lower than the front. It is most common in fat cows that have unusually relaxed pelvic ligaments. The increased intra-abdominal pressure when the cow lies down causes the vagina to balloon outward though the vulva. In most cases, it slides back into place when the animal gets up. However, exposure of the vaginal mucosa to the elements causes irritation and swelling, and the swelling may become so great that the vagina does not go back into place. The protruding vagina stimulates a straining reflex that further aggravates the problem. There are several ways to alleviate prolapse of the vagina. It is helpful to confine the animal in a straight stall with the floor built up higher under the rear legs to throw the abdominal weight forward.

For cattle, a truss is commercially available that has been used with some success. It is simply a heavy aluminum rod shaped in the form of a

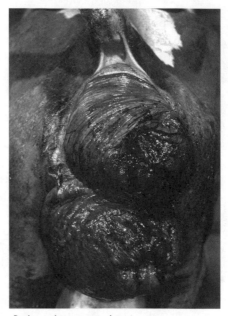

Prolapsed rectum and vagina appears as two red, inflamed, cylindrical masses.

Y. Placed so that the arms of the Y pass on each side of the vulva and tied tightly to the neck with rope, it provides enough external pressure to keep the vagina in place.

If these methods fail, surgical repair is the only recourse. Once parturition takes place, the problem is solved. Vaginal prolapse is much less common in animals that have ample exercise and are not too fat.

Pulmonary Emphysema (Heaves)

This is a chronic, irreversible, noninfectious disease seen primarily in the horse. Pathologically, the condition is one of rupture of the walls of the lung alveoli, with some escape of air into the surrounding tissue. The result is loss of lung elasticity such that they fail to collapse during expiration. Because they don't collapse completely, neither do they fill completely during inspiration, and the seriously affected animal has difficulty inhaling air sufficient to meet its oxygen needs.

Pulmonary emphysema may occur secondary to pneumonia in all species, but in the horse the condition appears to be more of an allergic response, with dusty surroundings and mold spores from spoiled hay being triggering factors. A few horses develop signs of heaves in the spring when put out to pasture, but most cases originate when animals are stabled. The symptoms may be more pronounced in hot weather.

Symptoms

The disease is progressive, with dry hacking cough especially after exercise, gradual weight loss, flaring of the nostrils during inspiration, and contraction of the abdominal muscles during expiration. The latter is noticeable at the heave line (margin of the ribs) and by a pumping action of the anus as the horse tries to expel the residual air. It occurs more often in older horses. There is no specific treatment for heaves, although antihistamines, corticosteroids, clenbuterol, and aminophylline may relieve the symptoms in some cases. Keeping the barn free of dust and well ventilated, using shavings instead of hay or straw for bedding, and substitution of feeds such as beet pulp for hay in the ration are all helpful. When hay must be fed, wetting it with water prior to feeding may be worthwhile.

Prevention by keeping horses in dust-free surroundings and avoiding the use of moldy hay is most important

Quittor

Quittor is a nondescript term that means different things to different people. To the horse owner, it means chronic inflammation of the lateral cartilage in the foot, with pus formation, necrosis, and sinus tracts extending from the cartilage to the outside at the coronary band. It is the result of penetrating wounds, either down from the coronet or up through the sole. Surgery to remove the diseased tissue is the only recourse.

To the cattle owner, *quittor* means protrusion of a pad of fat and connective tissue down into the interdigital space, which in time may extend halfway to the tip of the toe. This pad, or quittor, keeps the toes splayed apart when the animal walks and chafes to cause chronic lameness. It is most common in fat cattle, and surgical removal is the only lasting cure.

Note the splayed appearance of the toes due to the quittor between them.

Spastic Syndrome (Stretches)

This hereditary disease of dairy cattle, unfortunately, doesn't make its appearance until they reach maturity. Signs are most evident when the cow gets to her feet. Crampiness is apparent, and the animal treads from one hind leg to the other, intermittently extending one leg rapidly backward and then the other. Concurrent muscular tremors of the leg and back may occur. The condition gets progressively worse, and eventually, affected animals stand in an abnormal posture with the rear legs extended backward. They are in constant discomfort and have difficulty walking. As a result, milk flow drops to a point where they are uneconomical to keep.

Treatment is of no value. Prevention through selective breeding is the only recourse. Unfortunately, because of the long delay in onset, this is easier said than done, but certainly offspring of cattle known to have the disease should not be used for breeding purposes.

A similar condition called *spastic paresis* or *Elso heel* occurs in calves. It, too, is an apparently inherited incurable condition. Neither condition is likely to appear in herds where artificial insemination with semen from responsible suppliers is used exclusively. Before placing a bull in service, responsible suppliers will carefully screen his ancestors and siblings for any indication of inherited defects.

Tumors (Neoplasms, Cancer)

With the exception of bovine lymphosarcoma and papillomatosis, the cause of cancer in animals as well as in humans is obscure. Although many substances have proved carcinogenic in massive doses, it is doubtful that normal limited exposure to any of these is responsible for cancer in animals. The cause, therefore, remains unknown.

Tumors can occur in any tissue or organ, and where there is organ involvement, the symptoms are usually those of malfunction of that organ. For example, tumors in the brain result in abnormal behavior or problems with locomotion. Tumors may be benign or malignant, in which case they metastasize to other parts of the body. Surgical removal of accessible benign tumors is the only practical cure in livestock. While some tumors are responsive to radiation therapy or chemotherapy, the cost — except, perhaps, for valuable racehorses — cannot be justified.

One of the most frequently encountered and therefore costly tumors of livestock is adenocarcinoma of the third eyelid *(cancer eye),* seen almost exclusively in Hereford cattle. Other breeds are rarely affected. In some herds, a rather high percentage of cattle develop this tumor each year, leading to the possibilty that a transmissible agent maybe involved, although none has yet been demonstrated. Lack of pigment in the eye and constant exposure to bright sunlight seem to increase the frequency of these tumors. Treatment is surgical removal. When the tumor is small, with no evidence of spread to adjacent structures, removal of the tumor alone is adequate. With more extensive involvement, the entire eyeball and adjacent structures must be removed.

Wounds

These come in a variety of shapes, sizes, and locations and have about the same variation in severity. Wound management is determined by all these factors. If there is hemorrhage, the most urgent thing is to stop the bleeding, either with a tourniquet or by pressure applied to the wound. Once the bleeding is arrested, then a decision can be made as to whether sutures are required or the wound should merely be treated with antiseptics and left to heal as an open wound. As a general rule, lacerations extending through the skin will heal faster if they are sutured. However, a ragged, heavily contaminated gash may be better if left open and allowed to heal from the bottom. Alternatively, the damaged tissue should be thoroughly debrided and the wound sutured. When scars are a consideration, the latter technique is preferable. In either case, antibiotic therapy generally hastens healing.

Dairy Cattle

A fairly common accident in dairy cattle is a puncture wound through the mammary vein, usually acquired going through a barbed-wire fence. These wounds bleed profusely, and the hemorrhage can be fatal. The area does not lend itself well to application of a pressure pack or tourniquet. As an emergency measure, apply a spring-type clothespin directly on the puncture wound, which will suffice until a veterinarian arrives to suture it.

Horses

The horse is perhaps more susceptible to lacerations than other species because of a comparatively thin skin and less protective hair covering. By nature, horses are also more prone to accidents because of their normally quick movements and excitability. Cuts on the lower legs, where there is only a little connective tissue between skin and bone, and over the joints, where there is constant movement, frequently develop a complication known as *granulation tissue* or *proud flesh*. Granulation is a normal part of the healing process for open wounds, and granulation tissue is basically unorganized, highly vascular connective tissue. In the horse, it tends to grow exuberantly, filling the entire wound cavity and bulging, cauliflower-like, beyond the margins of the skin. At that point it actually impedes healing, because the skin won't cover it and it bleeds and becomes infected easily. Proud flesh can be retarded by keeping a pressure bandage over wounds on the lower leg. If proud flesh does overgrow, it must be cut back surgically or with chemicals until the skin heals.

Management of wounds is largely a matter of good judgment and nursing care. Sheep and horses with lacerations should routinely be given a prophylactic dose of tetanus antitoxin, and during the fly season wounds in all species should be covered with a bandage, ointment, or repellents to protect against myiasis. This is particularly important in screwworm-infested areas.

Foreign Animal Diseases

THE CASUAL READER, seeing the title of this chapter, may wonder why a discussion of foreign animal diseases is included. If we don't have a disease in the United States, why worry about it? It's precisely because we don't have some of these catastrophic foreign animal diseases that we should worry about them. Our livestock have no prior experience with these diseases and therefore no immunity, making them highly susceptible. A rapidly spreading disease such as foot-and-mouth could decimate our cattle, sheep, and swine industries in a matter of weeks, causing an economic disaster the magnitude of which cannot be appreciated until it happens. It is not a question of *if* one of these major diseases enters this country; it's only a question of *when.*

The foot-and-mouth virus can readily be transported via animals, meat and dairy products, and frozen semen, and even on shoes and on clothing of people who have recently visited infected farms. The magnitude of traffic in people and goods from foreign countries makes it inevitable that disease will be imported in the United States someday.

Although a major outbreak of a foreign animal disease is sure to be costly, the speed with which it can be contained will determine how costly. Early diagnosis is most essential, and the first person to see a cow with foot-and-mouth disease or a pig with African swine fever in all probability will be the owner. If that owner or herd manager recognizes that the animal may have a foreign animal disease and calls a veterinarian immediately, emergency state and federal disease-control procedures will be set in motion that may contain the disease before it spreads very far.

That's the reason for the brief descriptions of the major foreign animal diseases that follow. If you learn the clinical signs, you may someday be instrumental in preventing a catastrophic disease outbreak.

There is another aspect of foreign animal diseases that should be mentioned. Every country is concerned about the health of its livestock, and some are free of a few diseases that we have in the United States, such as rabies and bluetongue. Naturally, they impose restrictions on importation of animals and animal products just as we do. Although sometimes these requirements may seem silly, it is their prerogative and our obligation to comply honestly and accurately if we value the market. Exportation of animals and animal products is an important part of our foreign exchange, and we mustn't jeopardize it by being less than honest with foreign buyers.

African Horse Sickness

This equine disease is transmitted by biting flies and mosquitoes. It is endemic in most of Africa, and since the late 1950s, outbreaks have occurred in Turkey and the nearby island of Cyprus. Several outbreaks have been reported in Spain, the latest in 1989. Clinically, the disease can be confused with equine piroplasmosis, equine infectious anemia, and viral arteritis. However, the mortality is much higher, ranging up to 90 percent.

Symptoms

High fever lasting 4 to 5 days and obvious discomfort are consistent findings. Edema of the eyelids, conjunctiva, and along the jugular veins, extending to the brisket, are the most obvious external signs. In the later stages, there may be copious frothy exudate from the nostrils. Oddly, most horses continue to eat until they die, leading to speculation that there may be some central nervous system involvement as well.

At least seven types of African horse sickness virus have been identified, and a polyvalent vaccine that apparently protects against all types has been used effectively to control outbreaks. Should the disease appear in the United States, whether via imported horses or via accidentally imported insect vectors, it is virtually certain that many thousands of horses would die before adequate numbers could be vaccinated.

African Swine Fever

As the name implies, this swine disease was first found in Africa and is endemic there. In Africa, warthogs appear to be the natural reservoir of the virus, and most outbreaks in African domestic swine have occurred when warthogs were seen in the vicinity. Aside from Africa, the disease was endemic in Spain and Portugal but has now been eradicated. Outbreaks have occurred in France, Italy, Haiti, and Cuba, but the disease has apparently been eradicated from those countries. In Haiti and Cuba, the disease was eradicated by slaughtering the entire swine population.

Symptoms

The African strain of swine fever virus is particularly lethal for domestic swine. Persistent high fever ranging up to 105°F is the earliest clinical sign noted, but characteristically pigs continue to eat and act normally during the early febrile period. After about 4 days, more definite signs develop, including lack of appetite, huddling together, reluctance to move, and rear leg weakness. Very rapid pulse, cough, labored breathing, discharge from eyes and nose, and occasionally vomiting and diarrhea follow the high fever. Reddish blotches on the ears and legs are common. Death due to the African strain usually occurs about 7 days from the onset of fever. Serial passage of virus through domestic swine, such as occurred in Spain and Portugal, renders it less virulent, and in those countries more swine survived.

African swine fever closely resembles hog cholera, a serious swine disease present in the United States until the mid-1970s. While vaccination played an important role in hog cholera control and eradication, as yet there is no vaccine for African swine fever. Preventing its introduction, therefore, is of utmost importance.

Bovine Spongiform Encephalopathy

This apparently new disease of cattle, sometimes referred to as *mad cow disease,* was first reported in Great Britain in 1986 and has since been reported in several other European countries. It has not yet been reported in the United States. The disease closely resembles scrapie in sheep and goats, in that it is primarily neurological, has a long incubation period, is seen only in adult animals, and is slowly progressive, terminating in death.

Clinical signs that appear over a period of several weeks or months include apprehension, reduced milk yield, loss of weight, hyperesthesia, aggression, frenzy, incoordination, ataxia, and paresis. The intense itching characteristic of scrapie is not seen with bovine spongiform encephalopathy (BSE). The clinical signs could be confused with rabies, urea poisoning, or hypomagnesemia, but these are of much shorter duration. Generally, only about 1 percent of a herd has been infected.

The assumption in Great Britain is that the source of the infective agent was scrapie-contaminated processed protein and bonemeal in cattle feed. Feeding ruminant-origin animal protein in ruminant rations is now prohibited.

The disease is thought to be caused by a proteinaceous infective agent called a *prion.* There is no present evidence of animal-to-animal or insect-to-insect vector transmission. However, historically, a few cases of a very similar disease in humans, called Creutzfeldt-Jakob disease, are thought to have been due to contaminated neurosurgical instruments. The similarity of symptoms and lesions of this disease to BSE, and the evidence that a number of young people have apparently contracted a new variant of the disease by eating meat from infected cattle, has devastated the beef industry in Great Britain and Europe. Although the risk of human infection is slight, one cannot argue with people's decision to stop eating beef raised in the endemic areas.

If BSE appears in the United States, which is unlikely because of our heightened surveillance techniques and import restrictions, a cattleman somewhere will be the first to see it. If you see a mature cow showing any of the clinical signs previously listed, don't allow any animals to leave the herd, and if the animal was not home raised, locate records relating to its point of origin.

Contagious Bovine Pleuropneumonia

This disease, caused by *Mycoplasma mycoides* var. *mycoides,* was formerly one of the major cattle epizootics in the world. It has been eradicated from Europe, North America, South Africa, and Australia but still persists in other areas of southern Africa and parts of Asia, including China and Mongolia. A related organism, *M. mycoides* var. *capri,* has been isolated from goats in the United States but does not cause disease in cattle.

The disease has an incubation period lasting at least 3 months. It is spread primarily through inhalation of aerosol droplets exhaled or coughed by infected cattle. High concentrations of cattle, therefore, encourage spread of the disease.

Symptoms

The principal clinical sign is pneumonia, which may be very severe prior to death. Fever, lack of appetite, depression, and evidence of acute chest pain are characteristic. Respiration is shallow and rapid with frequent coughing. Mortality is about 50 percent, and many of those that recover become chronic carriers. Carrier animals are the source of greatest risk for new infections.

In terms of that with which we are familiar, contagious bovine pleuro-pneumonia perhaps resembles severe shipping fever pneumonia more closely than anything else. Areas of necrosis occur in the lungs, and adhesions occur between the lungs and chest wall. Large amounts of fluid accumulate in the chest cavity, further increasing respiratory difficulty. In calves, the organism invades the joints to cause arthritis more often than pneumonia. Serological testing to detect carrier animals and vaccination have been useful to controlling spread of the disease.

Exanthema, Vesicular

Vesicular exanthema, a disease of swine and identical in appearance to foot-and-mouth disease and swine vesicular disease, is no longer important. It was first reported in California, and during the 1950s became widespread in the United States. Restrictions on the movement of swine and the feeding of garbage, coupled with slaughter of infected herds, resulted in eradication of the disease. It has not been reported elsewhere in the world.

A virus isolated from sea lions off the coast of California and designated *San Miguel sea lion virus,* however, has been shown to be physically and chemically identical to vesicular exanthema virus. Moreover, when injected into swine, it produces disease very similar to vesicular exanthema. Serologically, there is some difference, but at the moment there is debate about whether the sea lion virus is a new virus or a different antigenic strain of vesicular exanthema. The major concern is that it will come ashore one way or another and start a new wave of infection in swine.

As an illustration of how foreign animal disease can occur when least expected, 2 months after graduation from veterinary college, I had the dubious distinction of diagnosing the first case of vesicular exanthema to appear in Maine.

Foot-and-Mouth Disease

This viral disease is prevalent in most parts of the world except North and Central America, Australia, and New Zealand. Foot-and-mouth disease (FMD) is widespread in Europe, Africa, the Middle East, and South America. It is one of the most contagious of all animal diseases and affects all cloven-hoofed animals such as cattle, sheep, goats, swine, and deer.

Symptoms

Symptoms include fever, and vesicles in the mouth, on the tongue, at the bulb of the heel, between the toes, and on the teats. Copious salivation accompanies the mouth lesions. The vesicles rupture and slough, leaving raw, denuded areas. Lameness is common with the foot lesions; affected animals are reluctant to move and they stand with their feet tucked up under them to relieve pain. Lacrimation and nasal discharge are common. Affected animals refuse feed during the acute phase and lose weight rapidly. Milk production may stop entirely. The disease is usually not fatal but lasts about a month in the individual animal. It takes several months longer for weight to be regained and milk production to resume. The economic loss is severe.

In some countries where the decision has been made to live with the disease rather than attempt eradication, vaccination is the only control program. It is a major continuing expense, and occasional outbreaks still occur. In the United States, for example, with about two hundred million susceptible animals, the cost of a vaccination program would approach a billion dollars annually. Furthermore, there are seven distinct serotypes of foot-and-mouth virus and sixty-two subtypes. No single vaccine will protect against all of these different strains of virus.

The clinical signs of FMD can be confused with malignant catarrhal fever and mucosal disease in cattle as well as with vesicular stomatitis in cattle, sheep, and goats. Vesicular exanthema produces similar signs in pigs but is no longer present in the United States.

An outbreak of FMD in Great Britain late in 2000 has virtually destroyed a livestock industry already decimated by the outbreak of bovine spongiform encephalopathy. The cost to its economy in lost production and loss of export markets is incalculable. Reports as of June 2001 indicate that more than three million animals have been slaughtered thus far in an attempt to control the spread of FMD.

The most important thing is to keep FMD out of the United States. The second most important is to identify it immediately when it does get here.

Rinderpest

This viral disease of cloven-hoofed animals is one of the oldest recognized animal diseases. Since the fourth century, it has occurred in many parts of the world. Its distribution at present is limited to parts of Africa, India, and Southeast Asia. Although cattle are the only species to be seriously affected, the virus is capable of infecting sheep, goats, and swine, some of which may become unaffected carriers.

Symptoms

The clinical signs in cattle vary with the pathogenicity of the particular virus strain and with the natural resistance of the animal. Infection occurs via the respiratory or digestive tract, resulting in fever, depression, lack of appetite, and decreased milk production. The mucous membranes of the mouth, eye, and vulva become reddened and congested, and the muzzle is dry. This is followed by lacrimation and a clear nasal discharge that becomes mucopurulent.

After 4 to 5 days of fever, small necrotic areas form on the lips, gums, tongue, and the inside of the cheek. These coalesce to form larger areas of ulceration. Excessive salivation coincides with the appearance of mouth lesions. Weight loss is quite rapid, with dehydration due to diarrhea prior to coma and death. In highly susceptible herds, mortality may be as great as 90 percent. On the basis of clinical signs alone, rinderpest is virtually indistinguishable from bovine virus diarrhea and malignant catarrhal fever, making laboratory confirmation essential. In some areas where the disease is endemic, it is kept under control by vaccination.

Sheep Pox

At present, this pox disease is limited to southeastern Europe, North Africa, and Asia. It is the most severe of the pox diseases of domestic animals. Pox eruptions occur on the cheeks, nostrils, lips, and wool-free skin. Unlike most pox diseases, systemic reactions occur frequently, with lesions occurring in the trachea, lungs, and digestive tract. The pox vesicles frequently become hemorrhagic, with development of pustules.

Goat pox virus is closely related to sheep pox, but the lesions in the goat are less extensive. Mortality from sheep pox may be as high as 50 percent. Sheep or goat pox can easily be confused with sore mouth.

In areas where these diseases occur, vaccines are used to control the outbreaks.

Swine Vesicular Disease

The lesions of swine vesicular disease (SVD) closely resemble those of foot-and-mouth disease, vesicular exanthema, and vesicular stomatitis. In swine, these four vesicular diseases are indistinguishable, except by serological means. It has been reported in Europe and the Far East. The virus is an enterovirus of the picornavirus group and is closely related to coxsackievirus B-5 in humans. In fact, there is some speculation that it is coxsackievirus that has become adapted to pigs. Infection with it has occurred among laboratory workers, so it must be considered a public health hazard.

Symptoms

Swine vesicular disease starts with high fever, quickly followed by numerous vesicles on the snout, in the mouth, and on the feet. Affected pigs refuse feed and are very lame. The vesicles rupture in a day or two, leaving raw denuded areas that, in the mouth, heal rather quickly. Although the lesions are similar, the disease is not generally as severe as foot-and-mouth disease; fewer pigs are affected and recovery is more rapid. Encephalitis is an occasional complication, with shivering and an unsteady gait. Experimentally, the virus has been shown to be lethal for baby pigs, but the principal economic effect is due to weight loss and a protracted recovery period. Additional loss occurs due to the embargo placed on pork products from countries where the disease exists by those countries that are free of the disease.

Swine vesicular disease, like foot-and-mouth disease, is very hardy and has been shown, for example, to survive in salami for more than 200 days. Feeding contaminated garbage to swine is the route by which most outbreaks have occurred.

Summary

We must constantly be on guard against introduction of any of these diseases because our livestock, having no immunity through prior exposure or vaccination, are completely susceptible. Inspectors of the Animal and Plant Health Inspection Service (APHIS) do an excellent job at our ports of entry, but the task they face in our mobile society is awesome. Despite the tons of potentially disease-bearing animal products confiscated at our ports of entry each year, not all such products are detected. Our livestock population is always at risk.

Scientists working under tight security precautions at the Plum Island Animal Disease Center, USDA/APHIS, are constantly seeking additional knowledge about foreign animal diseases and working on development of vaccines to prevent them. Much of what they have learned is being applied in those areas of the world where these diseases are rampant. Veterinary epidemiologists employed by the U.S. Department of Agriculture and the U.S. Public Health Service travel worldwide to assist nations with animal health problems. They not only assist the nations to which they are invited, but in so doing, they also develop a body of knowledge that will be invaluable if similar problems occur here.

But they can't do it all. The ultimate responsibility lies with you and with me and with everyone else who either works with livestock or is tempted to bring back from abroad animals or animal products that could harbor disease agents.

Recommended Reading

There are many excellent references in the field of veterinary medicine; following is a partial list.

Aiello, Susan E. (ed.). *Merck Veterinary Manual,* 8th ed. Whitehouse Station, N.J.: Merck & Co., 1998.

Bowman, Dwight D., Randy Carl Lynn, and Jay R. Georgi. *Georgi's Parasitology for Veterinarians.* San Diego: Harcourt, Brace & Co., 1998.

Jensen, Rue, and Donald Mackey. *Diseases of Feedlot Cattle.* Philadelphia: Lea & Febiger, 1979.

Kahrs, Robert F. *Viral Diseases of Cattle,* 2nd ed. Ames: Iowa State University Press, 2001.

Kimberling, Cleon V., Rue Jensen, and Brinton L. Swift. *Jensen and Swift's Diseases of Sheep.* Philadelphia: Lippincott Williams & Wilkins, 1988.

Lewis, Lon D. *Feeding and Care of the Horse.* Philadelphia: Lippincott Williams & Wilkins, 1995.

Osweiler, Gary D. *Toxicology.* Philadelphia: Lippincott Williams & Wilkins, 1995.

Radostits, Otto M., et al. *Veterinary Medicine*, 9th ed. Philadelphia: W. B. Saunders, 2000.

Rebhun, William C., Chuck Guard, and Carolyn M. Richards. *Diseases of Cattle.* Philadelphia: Lippincott Williams & Wilkins, 1994.

Robinson, N. Edward, and Lisette Bralow (eds.). *Current Therapy in Equine Medicine.* Philadelphia: W. B. Saunders, 1997.

Smith, Mary C., and David M. Sherman. *Goat Medicine.* Baltimore: Lippincott Williams & Wilkins, 1994.

UC Davis, Faculty and Staff. *UC Davis Book of Horses.* New York: HarperCollins, 1996.

Other Resources

The Nutrient Requirements series prepared by the National Research Council offers valuable, up-to-date guidelines on feeding and nutrition. The publications are available for purchase by calling 800-624-6242 or by writing the Printing and Publishing Office, National Academy of Sciences, 2101 Constitution Avenue, N.W., Lockbox 285, Washington, DC 20055, or by calling 1-800-624-6242. Many publications are available free on-line at the National Academy Press Web site: http://www.nap.edu/

The *Sheepman's Production Handbook* is available from Sheep Industry Development, Inc., American Sheep Industry Association, 6911 South Yosemite Street, Suite 200, Englewood, CO 80112-1414; 303-771-3500; http://www.sheepusa.org/

Metric Conversions Chart

Unit	Metric Equivalent	Round Equivalent
Distance		
1 inch	2.54 cm	2.5 cm
1 foot	30.5 cm (0.305 m)	0.3 m
Temperature*		
0°F	−18°C	
32°F	0°C	
70°F	21°C	
Volume		
1 teaspoon	4.92892 mL	5 mL
1 tablespoon	14.7868 mL	15 mL
1 cup	236.588 mL (0.236588 L)	230 mL
1 quart	946.353 mL (0.946353 L)	0.95 mL
1 gallon	3.78541 L	3.8 L
Weight		
1 ounce	28.35 g	28 g
1 pound	453.6 g (0.45 kg)	454 g

*To convert Fahrenheit to Celsius, subtract 32 from the Fahrenheit number. Divide that answer by 9. Multiply that answer by 5.

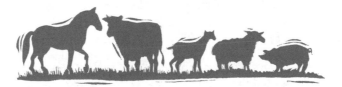

Glossary

Abomasum. The fourth, or true, digestive stomach of a ruminant.

Acidosis. A disturbance in the acid-base balance of the body, in which there is an accumulation of acids.

Adjuvant. Chemical added to a prescription to enhance therapeutic action.

Ad libitum. At pleasure, or as much as is wanted.

Aerosol dispersion. Spraying through the air.

Agalactia. Absence of milk secretion.

Alopecia. Lack or loss of hair from skin areas where hair is normally present.

Aneurysm. Localized abnormal enlargement of a blood vessel.

Anoxia. Deficiency of oxygen.

Anthelmintic. An agent used to control internal parasites.

Arthritis. Inflammation of a joint.

Ataxia. Muscular incoordination, usually of neurological origin.

Atony. Lack of normal tone.

Attenuation. Lessening of pathogenicity of an organism.

Avermectins. A class of broad-spectrum parasiticide of which ivermectin is one example.

Bacterin. Suspension of killed bacteria used to immunize against a specific disease.

Ballottement. A technique of feeling for a floating object in the body, such as an organ or fetus.

Biuret. A crystalline substance formed from urea.

Carcinogenicity. The property of being able to induce cancer.

Carotene. A precursor of vitamin A found in various plant and animal tissues. It is stored in the liver, where it is converted to vitamin A.

Caseous. Resembling cheese or curd.

Cerebellar hypoplasia. Incomplete development of the cerebellum.

Circling disease. Common name for listeriosis.

Collagen. A fibrous protein found in the connective tissue.

Comatose. In condition of a coma; a deep, abnormal sleep.

Conjunctivitis. Inflammation of the inner surface of the eyelid and adjacent tissue.

Coronary band. Junction of skin and hoof wall.

Corticosteroid. Adrenal gland hormone, natural or synthetic.

Crepitus. Crackling feeling due to gas accumulation in tissue.

Cyanosis. Slightly bluish or grayish discoloration of skin because of reduced oxyhemoglobin in blood.

Cyclopean. Malformed; having one eye.

Demyelination. Process of removing the myelin sheath of nerve tissue.

Downer. A cow that can't return to its feet due to any cause.

Dystocia. Difficult labor.

Edematous. Swollen; filled with fluid.

Electrolyte. A chemical salt that ionizes in solution. Ions increase the electrical conductivity of solutions, hence the name.

Encephalomyelitis. Acute inflammation of the brain and spinal cord.

Endocarditis. Inflammation of the endocardium, or heart lining.

Endometrium. The mucous membrane lining the inner surface of the uterus.

Endometritis. Inflammation of the endometrium.

Enteric. Pertaining to the intestinal tract.

Enterotoxemia. Disease caused by toxins in the intestinal tract.

Epididymis. Small oblong body resting on and beside the posterior surface of the testes. A part of the vas deferens or spermatic duct.

Epileptiform. Having the form of epilepsy.

Epiphyses. Enlargements at the ends of long bones from which bones elongate during growth.

Epithelium. Layer of cells forming the outer layer of skin and the surface layer of mucous membranes.

Eructation. Belching.

Estrum. The phase of the heat cycle during which the female is receptive to the male.

Etiology. Cause of disease.

Exostosis. A benign bony growth projecting outward from the surface of a bone.

Exudate. Accumulation of fluid containing tissue cells, bacteria, and other debris of infection.

FA test. Fluorescent antibody test.

Febrile. Feverish.

Fistulous tracts. A group of abnormal tubelike passages from one part of the body to another or to the outside, usually resulting from infection.

Founder. Lameness caused by separation of the sensitive laminae from the wall of the hoof.

Gilt. A young pig that has yet to produce a litter.

Goitrogenic. Tending to cause goiter.

Granulomatous mastitis. Inflammation of the udder due to chronic infection and scar tissue formation.

Hemoglobinuria. The presence of hemoglobin in the urine.

Hemolytic. Pertaining to breaking down of red blood cells.

Hernia. Bulging of an organ through a defect in the wall of the cavity that normally holds it.

Herpes. A class of virus.

Host-specific. An organism that matures in only one species of host.

Humoral. Pertaining to circulating body fluids such as blood.

Hypocalcemia. Abnormally low blood calcium.

Ingesta. Food and drink received into the body through the mouth.

Inguinal. Pertaining to the region of the groin.

Intradermal. Within the substance of the skin.

Intranasal instillation. Dropping or spraying a liquid into the nasal cavity.

Intussusception. Telescoping of the bowel; prolapse of one part of the intestine into the lumen of an adjoining part.

Ketone. Fatty acid that is the end product of fat metabolism.

Ketosis. Incomplete metabolism of fatty acids, usually from carbohydrate deficiency or inadequate utilization. Commonly seen in starvation, high-fat diet, following anesthesia, and in diabetes. A metabolic disease of cattle and sheep.

Lacrimation. Secretion and discharge of tears.

Lactate. To form or secrete milk.

Laminitis. Inflammation of the sensitive laminae of the hoof. Commonly called *founder.*

Leukocyte. White blood cell.

Leukopenia. Abnormal decrease of white blood cells.

Lymphangitis. Disease of the lymph glands and lymphatic ducts.

Lymphosarcoma. A malignant disease of lymphatic tissue.

Mastectomized. Having had the udder removed.

Metritis. Inflammation of the uterus.

Mucopurulent. Consisting of mucus and pus.

Multiparous. Having borne more than one offspring.

Mycotoxin. Toxic substance produced by molds.

Myiasis. Condition arising from infestation with larvae of flies or maggots.

Myositis. Inflammation of muscle tissue.

Necropsy. Examination of dead body to determine cause of death.

Neurotoxin. A toxin or poison that attacks the nervous system.

"Obligate" parasite. Parasite completely dependent on its host.

Oocyst. Infectious stage of protozoan life cycle.

Opisthotonos. An arched-back position of the head, caused by spasm induced by such things as strychnine poisoning or by brain disease.

Osmotic. Having to do with the passage of solvents, such as water, through semipermeable membranes.

Osteomyelitis. Inflammation of bone caused by infection.

Papule. Circumscribed raised area.

Parasite. Organism that lives within or on another one, which is known as the host.

Parenteral. Pertains to route of administration of drugs. Intravenous, subcutaneous, and intradermal are parenteral routes.

Paresis. Partial paralysis.

Parturition. Act of giving birth.

Pathogens. Organisms capable of producing disease.

Peracute. Excessively acute or sharp.

Perineal. Relating to the perineum, the area at the outlet of the pelvic region.

Peripheral. Pertaining to the outer part or surface of the body.

Peristalsis. Involuntary wavelike movement in the alimentary canal.

Peritonitis. Inflammation of the lining of the abdominal cavity.

Petechiae. Small, hemorrhagic spots.

Placenta. The structure in the uterus through which the fetus derives its nourishment. It is an organ of the fetus and is expelled from the uterus at or soon after birth.

ppb. Parts per billion.

ppm. Parts per million.

Propionate. A salt or ester or propionic acid.

Protozoan. A one-celled organism; the lowest division of the animal kingdom.

Pustule. Papule containing pus.

Pyometra. Pus accumulation in the uterine cavity.

Pyruvate. A salt or ester of pyruvic acid that plays an important role in the metabolism of carbohydrates, fats, and amino acids.

Rarefaction. Making bone more porous because of loss of mineral substances, or osteolysis.

Rumen. Large first stomach compartment of a cud-chewing animal.

Rumen atony. Lack of normal rumen contractions.

Rumenitis. Inflammation of the rumen.

Ruminant. Cud-chewing animal, including cattle, sheep, and goats.

Salmonella. A genus of bacteria causing intestinal disorders, which are sometimes fatal.

Saprophyte. Organism living on decaying or dead organic matter; nonpathogenic.

Schizont. A stage appearing in the life cycle of coccidia.

Scours. Severe diarrhea in farm animals.

Septicemia. Blood poisoning; bacteria and their products in the blood.

Septicemic. Relating to infection, when an animal's bloodstream has been invaded by disease-producing organisms.

Serologic testing. Laboratory examination of blood or blood serum.

Serovar. Type of bacterial species, as in serovar of *E. coli.*

Slough. Dead matter separating from living tissue.

Somatic. Pertaining to the body.

Sporulation. Production of spores, or one-celled reproductive organisms.

Staphylococcus. A genus of bacteria.

Stasis. Stagnation of normal flow of fluid, as of blood, urine, or intestinal products.

Subepithelial. Beneath the epithelium, the layer of cells forming the outer layer of the skin.

Symmetrical. Equally distributed throughout.

Systemic. Pertaining to a whole body.

Taxonomist. Specialist in the study of scientific classification.

Teratogenic. Contributing to the development of an abnormal embryo or fetus.

Theriogenologist: One who specializes in that branch of veterinary medicine dealing with reproduction, including the physiology and pathology of male and female reproductive systems and the clinical practice of veterinary obstetrics, gynecology, and semenology.

Titer. Standard of strength per volume.

Trocar. A sharp-pointed instrument equipped with a cannula, used to puncture the wall of a body cavity to withdraw fluid.

Turbinate. That portion of the upper respiratory tract between the nostrils and the pharynx through which air passes.

Uniparous. Producing or having produced a single offspring.

Urolithiasis. Formation of urinary stones and the illness associated with that condition.

Vasodilation. Dilation of blood vessels.

Vector. A carrier of disease from an infected animal to an uninfected one. Insects are common vectors.

Vegetative. Growing or having the ability to grow.

Viremia. Presence of viruses in the blood.

Viscosity. Density of fluid.

Volvulus. Intestinal obstruction due to a knotting and twisting of the bowel.

WBC. White blood cells or, commonly, white blood cell count.

Wheal. Smooth, slightly elevated area on the body surface that is redder or paler than the surrounding skin.

Withdrawal time. Interval between administration of a drug and the time of legal slaughter for meat or sale of milk. Also, the length of time it takes for a drug to disappear from the meat or milk.

Index

Page numbers in *italics* indicate illustrations; those in **bold** indicate tables.

Other Storey Titles
You May Enjoy

Making Your Small Farm Profitable by Ron Macher. A practical guide to operating a small farm in the new millenium, examining alternative ways to target niche markets and sustain a farm's biological and economic health. 288 pages. ISBN 1-58017-161-3.

Small-Scale Livestock Farming by Carol Ekarius. A grass-based approach to small-scale livestock farming, promoting stock health, greater profit, and farm sustainability. 224 pages. ISBN 1-58017-162-1.

Storey's Guide to Raising Beef Cattle by Heather Smith Thomas. A comprehensive guide to facilities, breeding and genetics, calving, health care, and marketing strategies. 352 pages. ISBN 1-58017-327-6.

Storey's Guide to Raising Chickens by Gail Damerow. A comprehensive guide to breeds, care, facilities, flock health. 352 pages. ISBN 1-58017-325-X.

Storey's Guide to Raising Dairy Goats by Jerry Belanger. A comprehensive guide to breeds, facilities, dairying, and care. 288 pages. ISBN 1-58017-259-8.

Storey's Guide to Raising Ducks by Dave Holderread. A comprehensive guide to breeds, breeding, feeding and housing, health care, and disease prevention. 320 pages. ISBN 1-58017-258-X.

Storey's Guide to Raising Horses by Heather Smith Thomas. A comprehensive guide to facilities, feeding and nutrition, daily health care, disease prevention, foot care, dental care, selecting breeding stock, foaling, care of the young horse. 512 pages. ISBN 1-58017-127-3.

Storey's Guide to Raising Pigs by Kelly Klober. Practical advice for buying, feeding, and caring for hogs, plus modern breeding and herd management techniques. 320 pages. ISBN 1-58017-326-8.

Storey's Guide to Raising Poultry by Leonard S. Mercia. A comprehensive guide to selecting birds for meat and egg production, housing and equipment, home processing of eggs and poultry, flock health, and brooding and rearing. 352 pages. ISBN 1-58017-263-6.

Storey's Guide to Raising Sheep by Paula Simmons and Carol Ekarius. A comprehensive guide to breeds, feeding and housing, breeding and lambing, pasture management, diseases and health care, and herding dogs. 400 pages. ISBN 1-58017-262-8.

These books and other Storey Books are available at your bookstore, farm store, garden center, or directly from Storey Publishing, LLC, 210 MASS MoCA Way, North Adams, MA, 01247, or by calling 1-800-441-5700. Or visit our Web site at www.storey.com